The Struggle for Health

The Struggle for Health

Medicine and the Politics of Underdevelopment

Second Edition

DAVID SANDERS
WITH WIM DE CEUKELAIRE
AND BARBARA HUTTON

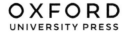

OXFORD
UNIVERSITY PRESS

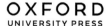

Great Clarendon Street, Oxford, OX2 6DP,
United Kingdom

Oxford University Press is a department of the University of Oxford.
It furthers the University's objective of excellence in research, scholarship,
and education by publishing worldwide. Oxford is a registered trade mark of
Oxford University Press in the UK and in certain other countries

Every effort has been made to contact copyright holders of material reproduced in this work.
We would be pleased to rectify any omissions in subsequent editions
of this work should they be drawn to our attention.

The moral rights of the authors have been asserted

First Edition published in 1985
Second Edition published in 2023

Published in the United States of America by Oxford University Press
198 Madison Avenue, New York, NY 10016, United States of America

British Library Cataloguing in Publication Data
Data available

Library of Congress Control Number: 2022946054

ISBN 978-0-19-285845-0

DOI: 10.1093/oso/9780192858450.001.0001

Printed and bound by
CPI Group (UK) Ltd, Croydon, CR0 4YY

Oxford University Press makes no representation, express or implied, that the drug dosages in this book are
correct. Readers must therefore always check the product information and clinical procedures with the most
up-to-date published product information and data sheets provided by the manufacturers and the most recent
codes of conduct and safety regulations. The authors and the publishers do not accept responsibility or legal
liability for any errors in the text or for the misuse or misapplication of material in this work. Except where
otherwise stated, drug dosages and recommendations are for the non-pregnant adult who is not breast-feeding

Links to third party websites are provided by Oxford in good faith and
for information only. Oxford disclaims any responsibility for the materials
contained in any third party website referenced in this work.

Editors

Ms Barbara Hutton (Research Consultant and Educational Writer/Specialist)

Dr Wim De Ceukelaire (Director, Belgian NGO Viva Salud)

Reviewers

Dr Richard Carver (Co-author of the first edition of The Struggle for Health; Visiting Research Fellow, Oxford Brookes University; Co-editor, Journal of Human Rights Practice)

Emeritus Professor Sue Fawcus (Senior Research Scholar in the Department of Obstetrics and Gynaecology, University Cape Town, and the wife of the late Emeritus Professor Sanders)

Ms Nikki Schaay (Senior Researcher, School of Public Health, University of the Western Cape)

Consultants

Professor Fran Baum (Director, Stretton Health Equity, University of Adelaide, Australia; Extraordinary Professor at the School of Public Health, University of the Western Cape; and Member, People's Health Movement, Advisory Council)

Dr Chiara Bodini (Researcher, Centre for International and Intercultural Health, University of Bologna; People's Health Movement)

Emeritus Professor David Legge (Emeritus Scholar, School of Public Health and Human Biosciences, La Trobe University, Australia)

Contributors

Ms Jesse Breytenbach (Book cover designer, illustrator and artist)

Ms Colleen Crawford Cousins (Illustrator and artist)

Support from School of Public Health, University of the Western Cape

Professor Uta Lehmann (Director, School of Public Health, University of the Western Cape)

Ms Carnita Ernest (Project Manager, School of Public Health, University of the Western Cape)

This book is dedicated to the children and their mothers living in poverty in Zimbabwe, who made me learn something about the struggle for health.

The untimely demise of David Sanders on 31st August 2019 was an irreparable loss to all of us personally, David's family, and the broader health movement globally and in South Africa. This second edition of his iconic book, The Struggle for Health is part of his legacy and an inspiration to us all to carry forward his vision of strengthening the struggle for Health for All.

Foreword

Some books sit on shelves and gather dust. Few books start a movement. *The Struggle for Health* was an example of the latter.

It wasn't just a book. It became a slogan, the name of an international university on the politics of health for young activists, and the battle cry of the People's Health Movement.

It also became my life.

And I was not alone. You could sit in the breakfast room of a hotel with David Sanders anywhere in the world preparing for an international health meeting and someone would walk up to your table to introduce themselves. Invariably the person would explain how much *The Struggle for Health* had meant for their personal development and choices in life. Some of them had made a career in health ministries or in the World Health Organization (WHO). Others were rural doctors, staff of non-governmental organisations or health activists. All of them testified how important the book had been for them.

In his foreword to the book's first edition, Professor David Morley wrote: "*Perhaps books such as this will awaken those, particularly in the less developed countries of the world, to realize that improvement in the health of the vast majority of their patients in the shanty towns and rural areas will come largely through political change rather than through pills and injections.*" And indeed, that came through. But Morley, a pioneering paediatrician in colonial and post-colonial Africa, was a giant of another era. It was the era of 'tropical medicine', a specialty that was taught in institutions that reeked of colonialism. Alternative analyses were rare and hard to come by, in particular, those which located health and disease in relation to the dynamics of colonialism, racism, capitalism, patriarchy and imperialism.

Even harder to find were books like *The Struggle for Health*, which brought together such an analysis with a strong ethical position around injustice, and which offered accessible pathways into activism for health and social justice. *The Struggle for Health* avoids a simplistic dichotomy between health care versus political activism; rather it points toward ways of approaching health care which also challenge the structures which reproduce avoidable and inequitable burdens of disease and injury.

Today, almost every medical faculty has courses on 'global health' and even well-established medical journals are publishing articles on the decolonisation of health and health care. There is a vast amount of critical material available on the internet. Nonetheless there remains an urgent need for the analysis presented in *The Struggle for Health* to be updated to recognise the changing context. Many of the ideas in the first edition have found their way into the thinking and writing of others. But there are very few books that present an accessible, radical and comprehensive analysis of the political economy of health. *The Struggle for Health* is accessible for anyone who wants to know more about the causes of the inequities in global health and health care. It is an invitation, an inspiration, to an activist engagement in the struggle for health.

As we are now entering the era of climate chaos and pandemics, the book needed an update. Whereas the first edition recognised the double burden of infectious diseases and non-communicable diseases, these burdens have multiplied. Changing geopolitics, the fracturing of neoliberal globalisation, the urgency of climate change and the emerging threat of a new fascism are changing the context in which the struggle for health is embedded.

The politics, the ethics and the activist orientation remain central to this second edition of *The Struggle for Health* while adapting to changing circumstances.

We hope it will inspire even more people to join the struggle and the movement.

Wim De Ceukelaire
Director
Viva Salud

Preface to Edition 1 (David Sanders, 1985)

Some time ago, a British volunteer agency published a recruiting poster which carried a picture of the renowned German medical missionary Albert Schweitzer and the legend: "*You won't be the first long-haired idealist to go into the jungle and teach his skills.*" Unwittingly, perhaps, this expressed a sentiment that has always underlain the relationship between developed and underdeveloped countries—the notion of the West's civilising mission.

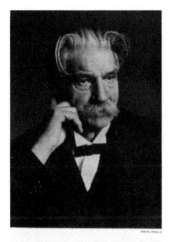

albert Schweitzer .

YOU WON'T BE THE FIRST LONG-HAIRED IDEALIST TO GO INTO THE JUNGLE AND TEACH HIS SKILLS.

Tradesmen and craftsmen, graduates and teachers, engineers and technicians, agriculturalists and foresters, medical auxiliaries, librarians and accountants, surveyors and architects, urgently needed for voluntary service overseas.

If you would like more information please contact: Voluntary Service Overseas, 14 Bishops Bridge Road, London W2. Tel. 01-262 2611

Hard work. Long hours. Low pay. The most memorable year of your life.

This book began life in the late 1970s as a manual for volunteer British health care workers going to work in the underdeveloped world. Over the years, it has grown into something rather broader, which I hope will be used by others as well—by health care workers anywhere, exploring the roots of ill-health in their societies and questioning their roles, indeed by anyone concerned with 'development'.

Many people can see that much ill-health is the result of widespread poverty, hunger or unsanitary conditions. And of course, common sense tells us that 'prevention is better than cure'—an idea that has been enthusiastically taken up by the international health bureaucracy. But there is still a firmly entrenched belief that the highly trained health professional is important to the well-being of those who live in the tropical climates of the underdeveloped world, with their 'reservoir of diseases'.

This book offers a far more radical approach than simply the need for more preventive medicine. It argues that medicine of any sort plays a very minor role in improving the health of peoples—that their health is inextricably linked to the context in which they live and work. Poverty and inequality impact on the patterns of ill-health *within* and *across* countries, whether they are rich or poor. Improvements in health can only be made by combining more appropriate health care with the struggle against inequality and underdevelopment. This struggle must involve health care workers, among others.

For an overall improvement in the health of populations we need more than a heavily doctor- and cure-oriented system of health care which only reaches a small and usually privileged minority. The failure to radically improve nutrition, water supplies, sanitation, living conditions and education, combined with the unequal distribution of resources and political power within and across nations, leave many millions of people suffering and dying from easily preventable conditions.

This book is no conventional health manual—though it has a similar starting point. It is dedicated to the proposition that problems of health, development and underdevelopment are intimately linked. It is for that reason that it might sometimes read like a lesson in history or politics, rather than a book on health care. There is no reason to apologise for this. For too long health has been widely looked upon as an issue apart from the real problems of society. The time has come to redress the balance.

A NOTE ABOUT THE TERMS DEVELOPED AND UNDERDEVELOPED

Some readers might object to the use of the word 'underdeveloped' to describe countries in the Global South. This book takes the same approach as John Berger:

> The term 'underdeveloped' has caused diplomatic embarrassment. The word 'developing' has been substituted. 'Developing' as distinct from 'developed'. The only serious contribution to this semantic discussion has been made by the Cubans, who have pointed out that there should be a transitive verb: **to underdevelop**. An economy is underdeveloped because of what is being done around it, within it and to it (Berger & Mohr, 1975).

Preface to Edition 2 (Sue Fawcus, 2022)

The first edition of *The Struggle for Health* was published in 1985 and has been widely read and endorsed by those who seek a broader and more political understanding of ill-health that went beyond the medical and commercial model. This revolutionary book charted new ways of understanding and tackling the causes of ill-health, and suggested strategies to enable *Health for All*. The book appealed to diverse audiences, including health care workers in both developed and underdeveloped countries, health care workers in training, academics in health science, sociology and health economics faculties, as well as activists for social change and community-based workers. Many said the book was for them a 'game changer', 'eye opener', 'career changer', to mention but a few of the comments received.

Since the book was written, the world has seen many changes in health and disease burdens, and their social, economic and political determinants. Developments and challenges related to *health* include, but are not limited to the HIV/AIDS epidemic; the COVID-19 pandemic; the increasing burden of non-communicable diseases; the dual burden of malnutrition (undernutrition and overnutrition); and the increasing burden of mental health disorders; whilst the plight of children which prompted the first edition has continued in many parts of the world.

In relation to *social determinants*, poverty remains a major driver of poor health, with the income gap between people who are rich and those who are poor increasing and lack of access to housing, land, water and sanitation persisting for many, despite some progress. Serious and urgent problems which have been more widely recognised in the twenty-first century include the climate change crisis and its influence on health outcomes, armed conflicts within and between countries that drive migration, and gender-based violence.

In the *broader political and global context*, we have seen globalisation with the consolidation of multinational corporations and the predominance of neoliberal politics, the fading of the welfare state and socially driven policies, and the emergence of new global power alliances. Developments in Information and Communication Technology (fourth and fifth industrial revolutions) have changed the nature of local, personal and global communications, with mixed implications, often reinforcing existing inequities.

To counter the adverse effects of the above developments, new forms of *social movements* have emerged to supplement that of organised labour, and include campaigns around social justice issues, homelessness, the right to health, equality in education, elimination of gender-based violence and combating climate change and its impacts.

In view of the major impacts on health from the 1980s due to the above factors, David Sanders was in the process of updating *The Struggle for Health* to incorporate these issues. He was assisted by Barbara Hutton and Wim De Ceukelaire. He was 75% through this task when his sudden death sadly prevented him from completing the process. This project was too important to be allowed to lapse, so a group of fellow travellers in health and politics from the University of the Western Cape, the People's Health Movement and others have collectively helped to finish the book. This was done out of respect for David's enduring legacy, but also because we all know how important the messages and analyses in the book are—continuing the urgent work of the struggle for health and equity.

When I first met David, I was a medical student considering giving up my studies due to disillusionment with the narrow focus of a London teaching hospital and having been exposed to the importance of the social determinants of health in a rural village in North India. David encouraged me to 'not give up', suggesting that as a doctor there would be the choice to be a kind, compassionate clinical doctor making individuals' lives better, *or* to go into public health and tackle the social determinants of ill-health, *or* to become a revolutionary and fight to change the political system that perpetuates inequality. For David it was not 'either/or'; remarkably he did all three in his life's work. All three archetypes can become activists for social justice in health; and all three archetypes require awareness of both the individual's needs and the broader context.

The second edition of *The Struggle for Health*, therefore, has not departed from the core message of the first edition: *Health for All* cannot be achieved without a change in the global economic order, community involvement and mobilisation, social justice and a Comprehensive Primary Health Care Approach—as enshrined in the 1978 Alma-Ata Declaration, but watered down considerably in the 2018 Astana Declaration. This second edition utilises the same approach as the first, with a narrative that starts with diseases, then describes historical trends and the limitation of the medical (and commercial) model of care, focuses on the social determinants of health, and examines the economic and political determinants which influence both health and health care systems. It asks the question 'WHY' at each juncture and has used a similar analysis as in the original book to understand and interpret all the changes since 1985. Most importantly, this second edition presents a strengthened call to action, building upon the original work and advocating for systemic changes to ensure justice and equity in *Health for All*.

Chapter 1 gives an overall impression of the conditions and diseases that most commonly affect people globally, especially those who live in poverty within and across countries.

Chapter 2 provides a deeper description of global disease patterns. It compares the disease pattern of European countries before they were industrialised, with diseases in underdeveloped countries today; and finds that many diseases we now regard as 'diseases of poverty or underdevelopment' were once prevalent in the northern hemisphere. However, instead of poorer countries following the same epidemiological transition as industrialised countries, another type of transition has evolved in which countries are struggling with more than one dominant disease pattern at the same time. Importantly, this is increasingly polarised across income groups, both across and within rich and poor countries.

Chapter 3 asks why this is so. How were the countries of the West able to eradicate those illnesses which were still prevalent in the early nineteenth century? Why are their former colonies—the underdeveloped countries—not able to? Why indeed are they still underdeveloped? Is there a connection between development in some countries and underdevelopment in others? In any given country, are health standards roughly equal for the whole population? Finally, this chapter discusses the question of population—so often seen as the crucial factor for explaining underdevelopment and poverty. Again, it compares the population structure of industrialised countries in the eighteenth and nineteenth centuries with that of underdeveloped countries today and asks: Is there a lesson to learn?

Chapter 4 looks at the history of medical services in those societies dominated by imperialism, which are the foundations of the present-day health care services in both developed and underdeveloped countries. It asks, what about the medical contribution? What about disease prevention, treatment and cure? Does the medical contribution significantly counteract the imbalance in the spread of health-promoting resources?

Chapter 5 examines what has happened within the context of neoliberal globalisation in the struggle for accessible and affordable health care for all. It explores some of the forces that have led to and shaped the privatisation and commercialisation of health care.

Chapter 6 isolates the various influences that have shaped the dominant medical model. It explores the role of doctors, of big business interests and of the State, looking at the areas where the three interact. Is it possible to make the necessary changes in this model, in either developed or underdeveloped countries, while the commercial determinants of health are still at work?

Chapter 7 asks, what are some alternatives to the medical model? To answer this challenge, the examples of China and Cuba in the twentieth century are given, where victorious popular struggles resulted in a change of economic and political systems, enabling underdevelopment to be successfully tackled and great improvements in peoples' health to be made. Significant changes and sometimes reversals in the last few decades for these two countries are discussed. State-led community health worker programmes in Ethiopia, Iran and India are examined as more recent examples of alternative approaches to health care and promotion. Finally, the chapter describes the global movement for the right to health, the People's Health Movement, which grew out of these alternative models.

Throughout his life David directed his energies to working with communities in struggle, whilst also challenging power and inequality in global forums, and performing rigorous academic research to provide evidence for the strategies he (and others) advocated for. These features are all central aims of the People's Health Movement which he helped to found and which he was a part of for many years. David never gave up on the struggle for health, against all the odds, and this second edition is part of his legacy.

Acknowledgements

The preface to the second edition would be incomplete without acknowledging all those who enabled its production.

Barbara Hutton and Wim De Ceukelaire worked with David on it. Wim's collaboration began in 2006 and together with David, he developed the concept of the second edition and updated the analysis and the data. Barbara joined the team in 2017 to help with writing and editing the actual chapters. She was also responsible for 'holding' the book after David's death and drawing the team and content together in preparation for publishing.

The University of the Western Cape permitted the funds from David's Author Fund to be used for completion of the book. Uta Lehmann, Nikki Schaay and Carnita Ernest were key in enabling this.

Fran Baum, Chiara Bodini and David Legge, all from the People's Health Movement, assisted Wim in writing sections and the last chapter.

Richard Carver, who co-authored the first edition and whom we tracked down, did the final edit of the second edition.

Jesse Breytenbach designed the front cover illustration, and was assisted by Colleen Crawford Cousins who also provided illustrations for the first edition.

Oxford University Press, who believed in the project and agreed to publish.

The plight of the world's children which inspired the first edition; and David's joy of having his own children, Ben, Lisa and Oscar whom he loved dearly.

And lastly, David Sanders, for his inspiration, clear analysis, compassion, courage and commitment, and of course his unique sense of humour.

Contents

1

Snapshots of (Ill)Health Around the World

The Child's Name Is Today
We are guilty of many errors and faults,
But our worst crime is abandoning the children,
Neglecting the fountain of life.

Many of the things we need can wait.
The child cannot.

Right now is the time his bones are being formed,
his blood is being made and his senses are being developed.
To him we cannot answer, 'Tomorrow'.
His name is 'Today'.

    Gabriela Mistral (Chilean Nobel Prize in Literature winner, 1945)

What are the world's main public health challenges? What are the most prevalent conditions and diseases that transcend national and international borders? Mainly through visual images and short scenarios, this chapter gives a broad impression of the health conditions and diseases that most commonly affect people around the world, especially those who are poor, both within and across countries (see Figure 1.1).

The scenarios include global hunger, which in 2019, impacted 8.9% of the global population; non-communicable diseases (NCDs), which in 2019 accounted for 74% of all deaths worldwide; communicable, maternal, neonatal and nutritional diseases (CMNN), which in 2019 accounted for 10.2 million deaths globally; and human-caused global warming, which has had a significant impact on the lives, health and livelihoods of the poorest and most vulnerable populations globally.

NOTE: Common health conditions and diseases mentioned in this chapter are explored in greater detail in the chapters that follow.

Scenario 1: global hunger

The child in the image in Figure 1.2 is receiving fluid replacement for dehydration caused by severe diarrhoea. Both an intravenous and a nasogastric route are being

The Struggle for Health. David Sanders with Wim De Ceukelaire and Barbara Hutton, Oxford University Press.
© Oxford University Press 2023. DOI: 10.1093/oso/9780192858450.003.0001

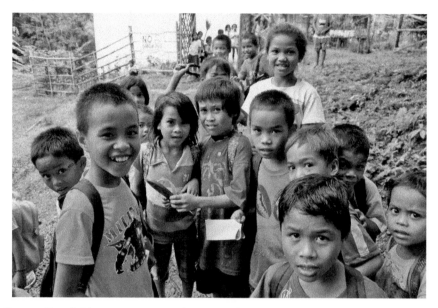

Fig. 1.1 To a child we cannot answer 'Tomorrow'. Their name is 'Today'.
Source: Wim De Ceukelaire—Viva Salud.

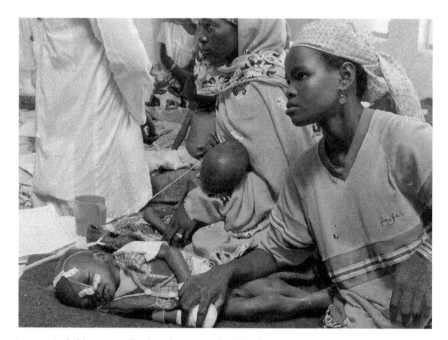

Fig. 1.2 A child receives fluid replacement for dehydration.
Source: UN Photo/Mark Garten.
http://www.unmultimedia.org/photo/detail.jsp?id=494/494704&key=0&query=494704&lang=en&sf=.

used as the child is critically ill and too weak to drink. The intravenous route entails inserting a needle into a vein in the forearm and requires sterile, accurately prepared solutions of glucose, salt and water. The nasogastric route requires the insertion of a polyvinyl tube into the nostril and down into the stomach. Both routes require trained personnel. The child is obviously extremely **undernourished** and has a form of **protein-energy malnutrition (PEM)** called **marasmus**.

Another form of PEM is **kwashiorkor** (see Figure 1.3). Marasmus and kwashiorkor are two forms of essentially the same disease, with the main difference being age distribution, although this varies somewhat from country to country. Marasmus typically occurs in children who are under the age of one year, whereas kwashiorkor generally occurs in children in the one- to five-year age group.

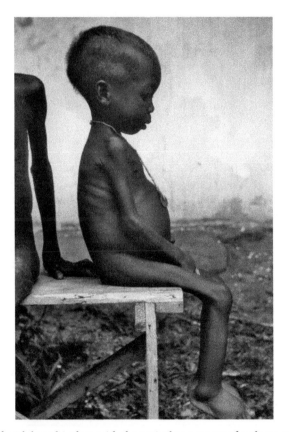

Fig. 1.3 A child with kwashiorkor, with the typical symptoms of oedema or swelling of the hands and feet, and bulging stomach.

Source: Dr Lyle Conrad (Public domain), via Wikimedia Commons.

https://commons.wikimedia.org/wiki/file%3astarved_girl.jpg.

GLOSSARY

Undernourished (hunger): a chronic condition that occurs when a person does not eat or absorb enough nutrients to grow (UNICEF, 2019).

Protein-energy malnutrition (PEM) or protein-energy undernutrition (PEU): a form of malnutrition that occurs due to a deficiency of protein and/or calories. It is likely to be due to malnutrition over a long period. It includes:

- **Wasting:** the child is too thin for their height. This is the result of sudden and quick weight loss or failure to gain weight. The child does not get enough calories from food and faces increased risk of death.
- **Stunting:** the child is too short for their age. This is the result of chronic or repeated undernutrition. The physical and cognitive effects can last a lifetime.
- **Underweight:** the child has low-weight-for-age. The child may be wasted, stunted or both.

Marasmus: a form of malnutrition that typically occurs in children who are under one year. It leads to dehydration and weight loss, and may include chronic diarrhoea and stomach shrinkage.

Kwashiorkor: a form of malnutrition that typically occurs in children in the one- to five-year age group.

From the early 1990s until 2014, global hunger gradually declined, despite a significant growth in world population (FAO et al., 2020). By 2019, more than 690 million people, or 8.9% of the global population, suffered from undernourishment, most of whom were in the underdeveloped regions of the world. This was 60 million more than in 2014. The COVID-19 pandemic has exacerbated global hunger, with undernutrition being experienced by a further estimated 132 million people in 2020 (FAO et al., 2020). It is expected that the pandemic will affect food systems, **food security** and hunger in multiple ways, so that by 2030, there will be approximately 909 million undernourished people globally (FAO et al., 2020).

GLOSSARY

Food security: relies on food being physically available; people having economic and physical access to the food; using the food in a way that satisfies energy and nutrient intake; and food stability over time (FAO et al., 2020).

Hunger and undernutrition are unevenly distributed throughout the world. There are marked differences across regions and sub-regions, as well as within individual countries. In almost every sub-region of Africa hunger is rising, with 19.1% of the African population (250 million people) being undernourished—more than double the world average of 8.9% (FAO et al., 2020). A detailed breakdown is presented in Table 1.1.

Figure 1.4 shows that by 2030, it is estimated that the African region will overtake the Asian region as having the highest number of undernourished people—433.2 million, i.e. 51.5% of the global undernourished (FAO et al., 2020).

In 2019, 2 billion people, a quarter of the world's population, experienced **food insecurity**—746 million faced **severe food insecurity** and an additional 1.25 billion experienced **moderate food insecurity** (FAO et al., 2020). Over half the population in Africa (51.6%), almost one-third in Latin America and the Caribbean (31.7%), and more than one-fifth in Asia (22.3%) were food insecure.

Table 1.1 Prevalence of undernourishment (PoU) in the world, 2005–2019 and projections up to 2030

	Prevalence of undernourishment (%)							
	2005	2010	2015	2016	2017	2018	2019[1]	2030[2]
WORLD	12.6	9.6	8.9	8.8	8.7	8.9	8.9	9.8
AFRICA	21.0	18.9	18.3	18.5	18.6	18.6	19.1	25.7
Northern Africa	9.8	8.8	6.2	6.3	6.6	6.3	6.5	7.4
Sub-Saharan Africa	23.9	21.3	21.2	21.4	21.4	21.4	22.0	29.4
Eastern Africa	32.2	28.9	26.9	27.1	26.8	26.7	27.2	33.6
Middle Africa	35.5	30.4	28.2	28.8	28.7	29.0	29.8	38.0
Southern Africa	4.9	5.4	7.0	8.0	7.0	7.9	8.4	14.6
Western Africa	13.8	12.1	14.3	14.2	14.6	14.3	15.2	23.0
ASIA	14.4	10.1	8.8	8.5	8.2	8.4	8.3	6.6
Central Asia	11.0	7.7	3.0	3.0	3.0	3.0	2.7	<2.5
Eastern Asia	7.6	3.8	<2.5	<2.5	<2.5	<2.5	<2.5	<2.5
South-Eastern Asia	17.3	11.7	10.5	10.0	9.8	9.8	9.8	8.7
Southern Asia	20.6	15.4	14.4	13.8	13.1	13.8	13.4	9.5
Western Asia	11.8	10.4	10.7	11.1	11.1	11.2	11.2	13.1
Western Asia and Northern Africa	10.9	9.7	8.6	8.9	9.0	8.9	9.0	10.4
LATIN AMERICA AND THE CARIBBEAN	8.7	6.7	6.2	6.7	6.8	7.3	7.4	9.5
Caribbean	21.3	17.5	17.3	17.0	16.6	17.0	16.6	14.4
Latin America	7.8	5.9	5.4	6.0	6.1	6.6	6.7	9.1
Central America	8.1	7.9	7.9	8.6	8.3	8.4	9.3	12.4
South America	7.6	5.1	4.4	4.9	5.2	5.8	5.6	7.7
OCEANIA	5.6	5.4	5.5	5.9	6.0	5.7	5.8	7.0
NORTH AMERICA AND EUROPE	<2.5	<2.5	<2.5	<2.5	<2.5	<2.5	<2.5	<2.5

[1] Projected values.

[2] Projections up to 2030 do not reflect the potential impact of the COVID-19 pandemic.

Source: FAO et al. (2020), p. 9.

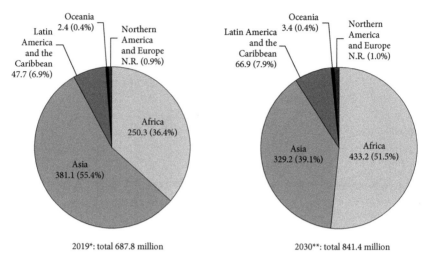

2019*: total 687.8 million   2030**: total 841.4 million

Notes: Number of undernourished people in millions. * Projected values. ** Projections to 2030 do not consider the potential impact of the covid-19 pandemic number = not reported, as the prevalence is less than 2.5%.

Fig. 1.4 Number of undernourished people in millions globally in 2019; and projections for 2030, without taking the COVID-19 pandemic into account.
Source: FAO et al. (2020), p. 16.

GLOSSARY

Food insecurity: people do not have access to sufficient, safe and nutritious food necessary to live a healthy and active life (FAO et al., 2020).

- **Severe food insecurity**: people have run out of food and have gone a day or a few days without eating (FAO et al., 2020).
- **Moderate food insecurity**: people are unsure about their ability to access food and are forced to compromise on the quality and/or quantity of food they consume (FAO et al., 2020).

Globally in 2019, of the children under five years old, an estimated:

- 144 million (21.3%) were stunted (see Figure 1.5).
- 47 million (6.9%) suffered from wasting.
- 38 million (5.6%) were overweight (UNICEF et al., 2020).

The global health community recognises that many countries are now facing a double or **triple burden of malnutrition**. This is defined as the coexistence of undernutrition, **hidden hunger** and **overweight** and **obesity** (UNICEF et al., 2020). Although in the 1990s, the triple burden was typically seen in middle-income countries, today it predominates in the poorest countries, particularly in south and east Asia and Sub-Saharan Africa (Popkin et al., 2019).

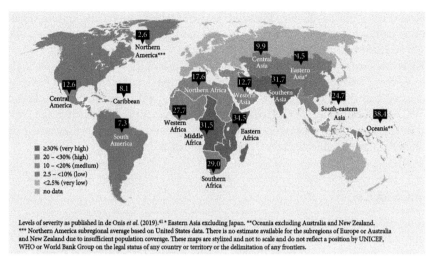

Levels of severity as published in de Onis *et al.* (2019).[41] * Eastern Asia excluding Japan. **Oceania excluding Australia and New Zealand. *** Northern America subregional average based on United States data. There is no estimate available for the subregions of Europe or Australia and New Zealand due to insufficient population coverage. These maps are stylized and not to scale and do not reflect a position by UNICEF, WHO or World Bank Group on the legal status of any country or territory or the delimitation of any frontiers.

Fig. 1.5 Percentage of stunted children under five years, by UN sub-regions, 2019. *Source*: UNICEF et al. (2020).

GLOSSARY

Triple burden of malnutrition (TBM): the simultaneous occurrence of under-nutrition, hidden hunger and overweight and obesity in the same country, community, household or individual.

Hidden hunger: not getting enough essential vitamins and minerals (UNICEF et al., 2020).

Overweight: a person's weight is too high for their height (UNICEF et al., 2020).

Obesity: a severe form of overweight (UNICEF et al., 2020).

Scenario 2: non-communicable diseases (NCDs)

I know that the food I buy from fast food outlets is unhealthy, but it's cheaper to feed a family of four at McDonald's than it is to cook a meal for them at home. But there is no such thing as cheap food because the real cost of this food is my health. I know I should get more physical exercise, but there are two factors which prevent this. Firstly, my weight and secondly, because I smoke tobacco, I suffer from shortness of breath. It is an effort to get out of bed in the morning, and generally, I just feel helpless, hopeless and very depressed (Paige Bagley [not her real name], Baltimore, USA).

The convergence of a sedentary lifestyle, the use of tobacco and a diet high in sugars, salt and fat has led to approximately 42% of American adults having obesity and the associated health issues (CDC, 2020).

Forty-two-year-old Paige Bagley represents just one of the 40 million people in the USA who in 2019 relied on the Supplemental Nutrition Assistance Program (SNAP—previously called the Food Stamp Program) for food aid. Against the backdrop of COVID-19, this number is expected to rise to more than 50 million (including 17 million children), with the most vulnerable being ethnic and racial minorities, and those with non-communicable diseases (Feeding America, 2020).

GLOSSARY

Non-communicable diseases (NCDs): non-infectious and non-transmissible conditions or diseases, such as heart attacks, stroke, cancer, chronic respiratory diseases, diabetes or a mental health condition (WHO, 2020b). NCDs may be chronic, i.e. of long duration and slow progression, or they may result in more rapid deaths.

NCDs affect people of all ages, in all regions and countries of the world. Globally, NCDs accounted for 74% of all deaths in 2019, with seven NCDs making up the ten leading causes of death: ischaemic heart disease; stroke; chronic obstructive pulmonary disease; tracheal, bronchus and lung cancers; Alzheimer's disease and other dementias; diabetes mellitus; and kidney disease (WHO, 2020a).

Approximately 36% (15 million) of all NCD deaths were in people under 70 years, and 85% occurred in low- and middle-income countries (WHO, 2014a; 2018a). People living in poverty are disproportionately affected by NCDs. For example, the probability of dying from one of these diseases before the age of 70 years varies across regions (see Figure 1.6), from 25% in South-East Asia to 15% in the Americas. This probability also varies between countries, from over 30% in low- and middle-income countries to less than 10% in high-income countries.

Mental health disorders and NCDs

Mental health disorders, including depression, anxiety disorders, bipolar disorder, eating disorders, schizophrenia, mental or substance use disorder and Alzheimer's disease (particularly dementia), can be experienced in isolation or co-morbid with other NCDs (NCD Alliance, 2017). Mental health disorders are experienced worldwide but are widely underreported, particularly in lower-income countries. In 2017, substance use and mental health disorders accounted for about 5% of the global **disease burden**, although this was as high as 10% in certain countries, with the highest contribution to the overall health burden being in Australia, Saudi Arabia and Iran (Ritchie & Roser, 2018).

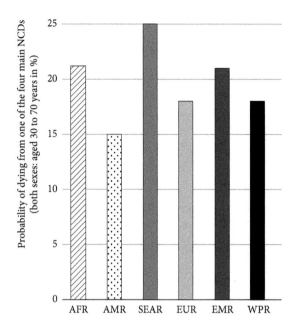

AFR=African Region, AMR=Region of the Americas,
SEAR=South-East Asia Region, EUR=European Region,
EMR=Eastern Mediterranean Region, WPR=Western
Pacific Region

Fig. 1.6 Probability of dying from one of the four main NCDs between the ages of 30 and 70 years, by WHO region, 2012.

Source: WHO. (2014a), p. 11.

GLOSSARY

Disease burden/burden of diseases: a comprehensive measure of the health status of a nation, attained by assessing the diseases, injuries and impairments, and death rate in a population in a certain period of time.

The COVID-19 pandemic has had major implications for mental health, and has highlighted how people living with NCDs and mental health disorders are at increased risk of becoming severely ill from the virus. This is due to, among other things, the disruption of critical health services, despite an increased demand for these services (WHO, 2020b).

Bereavement, isolation, loss of income and fear are triggering mental health conditions or exacerbating existing ones. Many people may be facing increased levels of alcohol and drug use, insomnia, and anxiety. Meanwhile, COVID-19 itself can lead to neurological and mental complications, such as delirium, agitation, and stroke. People with pre-existing mental, neurological or substance use disorders are also more vulnerable to SARS-CoV-2 infection—they may stand a higher risk of severe outcomes and even death (WHO, 2020c).

Following the outbreak of the COVID-19 pandemic, the pre-existing crisis of **gender-based violence (GBV)** intensified globally, as pressure and tension built up in the home, heightened by the cramped and confined living conditions of lockdown (UN Women, 2020). UN Women has declared GBV a 'shadow pandemic', which typically escalates in crisis contexts:

The Ebola pandemic demonstrated that multiple forms of violence are exacerbated within crisis contexts, including trafficking, child marriage, and sexual exploitation and abuse. COVID-19 is likely driving similar trends . . . (UN Women, 2020, p. 4).

GLOSSARY

Gender-based violence (GBV)/violence against women and girls: any form of violence—physical, sexual, psychological harm and controlling behaviour—that is perpetrated against an individual because of their gender. Prior to the outbreak of COVID-19, "*globally 243 million women and girls aged 15–49 [had] been subjected to sexual and/or physical violence perpetrated by an intimate partner in the previous 12 months*" (UN Women, 2020).

Scenario 3: communicable, maternal, neonatal and nutritional (CMNN) diseases

CMNN disorders include HIV/AIDS and sexually transmitted infections; respiratory infections and tuberculosis; diarrhoeal diseases; neglected tropical diseases and malaria; maternal and preterm birth complications; and nutritional deficiencies (*The Lancet*, 2020). In 2019, these diseases caused 10.2 million deaths globally—which represents a 36.3% decrease since 2010 (*The Lancet*, 2020). Despite this rather substantial decline, there are still important challenges around certain diseases, especially in certain regions of the world. In the African region, for example, the convergence of NCDs and communicable diseases like HIV/AIDS and malaria present ongoing health difficulties to the poorest and most marginalised populations.

Global HIV/AIDS statistics

According to UNAIDS (2020a), in 2019, 690 000 people died from AIDS-related illnesses, globally. However, in this same year:

- Approximately 38 million people were living with HIV—36.2 million adults and 1.8 million children under 15 years (see Figure 1.7). This number continues to rise for two main reasons:
  - With antiretroviral treatment (ART), more people are living longer (26 million on ART by mid-2020).
  - The number of new infections is still high—1.7 million (although there has been a 23% decline in new HIV infections since 2010).
- Outside Sub-Saharan Africa, women and girls accounted for about 48% of all new HIV infections worldwide. In Sub-Saharan Africa, women and girls accounted for 59% of all new HIV infections. Structural gender inequalities (perpetuated by patriarchal institutions and norms), discrimination and GBV undermine women's efforts to prevent HIV (UNAIDS, 2020b).
- Thirty-five percent of women worldwide experienced GBV and inequalities, making them 1.5 times more likely to become HIV-infected than those who have not experienced such violence. Female sex workers are 30 times more likely to acquire HIV than the general population.
- Tuberculosis remained the leading cause of death among people living with HIV. It accounted for about one in three AIDS-related deaths.

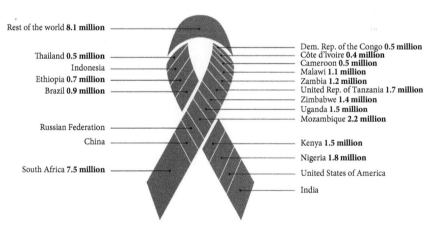

Fig. 1.7 People living with HIV globally, 2020: 38 million—36.2 million adults and 1.8 million children under 15 years.

Source: UNAIDS. (2020d). Estimates.

https://www.unaids.org/en/resources/infographics/people-living-with-hiv-around-the-world.

- It was speculated that the COVID-19 pandemic could disrupt the rate of increase in HIV treatment and services to prevent transmission. These disruptions could result in up to 293 000 new HIV infections and up to 148 000 additional AIDS-related deaths globally (UNAIDS, 2020c).

Scenario 4: climate change and related health hazards

Human-caused **global warming** has increased the likelihood of more frequent and extreme weather events, such as unprecedented heatwaves, droughts, heavy rainfall and floods (Diffenbaugh, 2020). The rising incidence of these events is having a significant impact on the lives, health and livelihoods of the poorest and most vulnerable populations globally. Hardest hit are low- and middle-income countries and populations, especially in Sub-Saharan Africa, South Asia and Small Island Developing States (SIDS) (see Figure 1.8).

GLOSSARY

Global warming: the effect of human activities, particularly the burning of fossil fuels (coal), that release heat-trapping greenhouse gases that profoundly affect our global climate system and cause the average temperature of the Earth to rise.

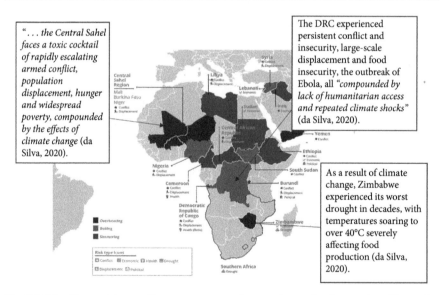

" . . . the Central Sahel faces a toxic cocktail of rapidly escalating armed conflict, population displacement, hunger and widespread poverty, compounded by the effects of climate change (da Silva, 2020).

The DRC experienced persistent conflict and insecurity, large-scale displacement and food insecurity, the outbreak of Ebola, all *"compounded by lack of humanitarian access and repeated climate shocks"* (da Silva, 2020).

As a result of climate change, Zimbabwe experienced its worst drought in decades, with temperatures soaring to over 40°C severely affecting food production (da Silva, 2020).

Fig. 1.8 The 18 countries needing emergency assistance due to the destructive effects of climate-induced disasters, conflict, economic crises and political instability.
Source: WFP. (2020).

Climate change impacts on crop yields and food production, water availability, land degradation, food security and rural livelihoods. Together with armed conflict, political instability and economic collapse, it forces people to flee their homes and places of work, and pushes a significant number of people worldwide into poverty and hunger (WFP, 2020). It affects population health, putting additional strain on already stressed health systems and social structures, and exacerbates social inequalities (WHO, 2015).

Climate change has an especially disproportionate effect on children's health and nutrition. After a flood or typhoon, for example, children are at the highest risk for waterborne diseases, such as diarrhoea, which also increases their risk of malnutrition and death (UNICEF, 2019). The impact falls most heavily on children from the poorest families who are the least able to cope. From 2030 onwards, climate change is expected to cause approximately 250 000 additional deaths per year, from malnutrition, malaria, diarrhoea and heat stress (WHO, 2018b).

Free riders and forced riders

Greenhouse gas emissions are felt beyond a country's own borders, and the effects of the resulting climate change in different countries are highly variable. Although some countries emit more greenhouse gas than others, they may be less vulnerable to the effects of the resulting climate change. Researchers have identified 'free rider' countries which contribute disproportionately to global greenhouse gas emissions but are the least vulnerable to the effects of the resulting climate change. The largest three contributors are China, the USA and India (Althor et al., 2016). 'Forced rider' countries are those that are most vulnerable to climate change but have contributed little to its actual emission, such as SIDS and some African countries (Althor et al., 2016). This inequity is increasing. In other words: those who will bear the burden of the climate chaos are not those who are responsible for it.

The two maps in Figure 1.9 show the global inequity in greenhouse gas emissions and those who bear the burden of its impacts for 2010 and predicted for 2030. Free riders, who are predominantly found in the industrialised world, are shown in black, while forced riders, who are mainly in less-industrialised and poorer countries, are in dark grey. Countries with intermediate levels of **equity** are shown in shades of grey, and countries that produce greenhouse gas emissions concomitant with their vulnerability are shown in the lightest grey.

GLOSSARY

Equity: different treatment and access to resources and opportunities, recognising that disadvantaged groups might need more support or resources in order to achieve equal outcomes; based on fairness.

(a) Climate change equity for 2010

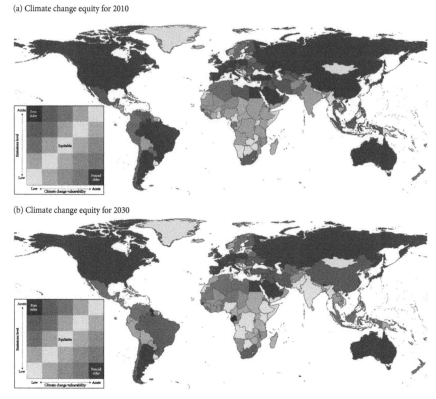

(b) Climate change equity for 2030

Fig. 1.9 Global inequity in the responsibility for climate change and the burden of its impacts.

Source: Althor et al. (2016).

In 2017/2018, 101 countries participated in a WHO Health and Climate Change Survey (WHO, 2018b), outlining climate hazards and their expected health impacts. Forty-eight of these countries had conducted vulnerability and adaptation assessments for health in relation to climate change. The following were some of the main climate-sensitive diseases identified:

- Vector-borne diseases, such as malaria and dengue, where the risk increases as a result of factors such as the rapid growth of parasites and pests, their spread into new areas, and the reduced effectiveness of control measures.
- Water- and food-borne diseases, such as diarrhoeal diseases in children, where the risk increases as a result of the rapid growth of pathogens and contaminated water sources due to flood damage to water and sanitation infrastructure.
- Heat-related illnesses, which may contribute directly to deaths from cardiovascular and respiratory diseases especially in older people.

A NOTE ABOUT OTHER HEALTH ISSUES

There are other significant health issues which have not been explored in depth in this chapter or this book, for example:

- The 2 billion people who live in conditions that are affected by warfare and conflict, which result in displacement, loss of livelihoods and food insecurity, all of which have ongoing physical and mental health implications for those affected, especially women and children (Garry & Checchi, 2019).
- The more than 5 million people who die each year due to injuries, violence against self or others, road traffic accidents, burns, drownings, falls and poisoning (WHO, 2014b). Road traffic accidents alone account for 1.35 million deaths globally, involving pedestrians, cyclists and motorcyclists. Ninety percent of these deaths occur in low- and middle-income countries, with the highest death rates being in the African region (WHO, 2020c).

Inequalities in health outcomes

There is no single indicator of health in a community. However, a number of statistics taken together can give us a broad view of the level of human development, **equality/inequality** (see Figure 1.10), well-being and the burden of disease.

GLOSSARY

Equality: equal treatment and access to resources and opportunities, regardless of need or outcomes; based on sameness.

Inequality: unequal treatment or access to resources and opportunities.

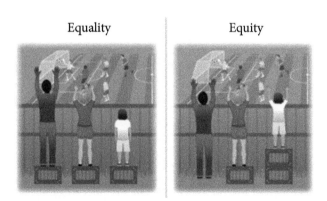

Equality   Equity

Fig. 1.10 Equality and equity.
Source: Figure reproduced with permission from the Interaction Institute for Social Change. Artist: Angus Maguire.

Pregnant women, children and adolescents account for more than one-third of the global burden of premature mortality (death), with most of their deaths being preventable or their conditions being treatable. In most cases these deaths reflect the huge disparities in access to health care between those who are rich and people who are poor, and between urban and rural dwellers within and between countries (WHO, 2015).

An important indicator of the most at-risk populations is the mortality rate of children under five years. Despite substantial progress being made over the past few decades to reduce under-five-year-old mortality from 12.6 million in 1990 to 5.4 million in 2017, the global burden of child deaths remains extremely high (Roser et al., 2019).

Of course, the death of every child is an enormous tragedy, and in many countries far too many children die because of causes we know how to prevent and treat ... today the highest child mortality rates are in Sub-Saharan Africa, where we still have countries with child mortality rates greater than 10%—this means that one out of 10 children born never reach their 5th birthday (Roser et al., 2019).

The gap between child mortality in underdeveloped and developed countries is particularly significant. In developed countries, the majority of people who die are old, while in underdeveloped countries the reverse is true—almost one in three deaths is in children under five years (WHO, 2019).

The problems of health, development and poverty or underdevelopment are intimately linked. In 2019, two regions alone accounted for 80% of the 5.2 million deaths of children under five years globally, despite these regions only accounting for 52% of the global under-five population—53% in Sub-Saharan Africa and 26% in Central and Southern Asia (UNICEF, 2020). Nutrition-related factors contributed to about 45% of these deaths (UNICEF, 2020).

Inequalities in health outcomes are not only between underdeveloped and developed countries, but also exist *within* communities of both underdeveloped and developed countries. In other words, the poorest areas within the poorest underdeveloped regions and countries have the highest levels of child mortality (UNICEF, 2019). Even among developed countries the mortality rate for children under five years differs. For example, in 2013, in the UK this rate was double that of Iceland (2.4 per 1000)—the country with the lowest rate globally (WHO, 2015). The reasons for these inequalities will be explored in more detail in Chapter 2.

Conclusion

This chapter has provided a broad overview of a few major public health challenges that transcend national and international borders—global hunger, non-communicable diseases, communicable diseases and some health risks associated with climate change. These illnesses and diseases interact within specific populations according to patterns of inequality deeply entrenched in our societies. In future chapters, this will be analysed historically for social and political determinants and solutions.

NOTE: The word 'underdeveloped' in this book is used to describe how economies in the Global South have been, and continue to be, underdeveloped by what is done around them, within them and to them (see the Note in the Preface to Edition 1).

References

Althor, G., Watson, J. & Fuller, R. (2016). Global mismatch between greenhouse gas emissions and the burden of climate change. *Scientific Reports*, 6(20281).

Berger, J. & Mohr, J. (1975). *A Seventh Man*. Penguin: Harmondsworth, p. 21.

CDC. (2020). Overweight and obesity, adult obesity facts. Centers for Disease Control and Prevention. https://www.cdc.gov/obesity/data/adult.html.

de Onis, M., Borghi, E., Arimond, M., et al. (2019). Prevalence thresholds for wasting, overweight and stunting in children under 5 years. *Public Health Nutrition*, 22(1):175–179.

da Silva, I.S. (2020). Climate change and conflict could fuel hunger in 2020. *SciDevNet*. https://www.scidev.net/global/news/climate-change-and-conflict-could-fuel-hunger-in-2020-1x/.

Diffenbaugh, N.S. (2020). Verification of extreme event attribution: using out-of-sample observations to assess changes in probabilities of unprecedented events. *Science Advances*, 6(12):eaay2368.

Feeding America. (2020). The impact of the coronavirus on food insecurity in 2020. https://www.feedingamerica.org/sites/default/files/2020-10/brief_local%20impact_10.2020_0.pdf.

FAO, IFAD & WFP. (2020). *The State of Food Security and Nutrition in the World 2020. Transforming Food Systems for Affordable Healthy Diets*. FAO: Rome.

Garry, S. & Checchi, F. (2019). Armed conflict and public health: into the 21st century. *Journal of Public Health*, 42(3):e287–e298.

NCD Alliance. (2017). Mental health and neurological disorders. https://ncdalliance.org/why-ncds/ncd-management/mental-health-and-neurological-disorders.

Popkin, B.M., Corvalan, C. & Grummer-Strawn, L.M. (2019). Dynamics of the double burden of malnutrition and the changing nutrition reality. *The Lancet*, 395(10217):65–74.

Ritchie, H. & Roser, M. (2018). Mental health. https://ourworldindata.org/mental-health#disease-burden-of-mental-health-and-substance-use-disorders.

Roser, M., Ritchie, H. & Dadonaite, B. (2019). Child and infant mortality. https://ourworldindata.org/child-mortality.

The Lancet. (2020). The Global Burden of Disease Study, 2019. *The Lancet*, 396(10258):1129–1306.

UNAIDS. (2020a). Global HIV and AIDS statistics—2020 fact sheet. https://www.unaids.org/en/resources/fact-sheet.

UNAIDS. (2020b). In South Africa, young women leading HIV and violence prevention say men's involvement is key. https://www.unaids.org/en/resources/presscentre/featurestories/2020/december/20201201_south-africa-young-women-lead-hiv-and-violence-prevention.

UNAIDS. (2020c). New modelling shows COVID-19 should not be a reason for delaying the 2030 deadline for ending AIDS as a public health threat. https://www.unaids.org/en/keywords/hiv-treatment.

UNAIDS. (2020d). 2020 estimates. https://www.unaids.org/en/resources/infographics/people-living-with-hiv-around-the-world.

UNICEF. (2019). *The State of the World's Children 2019. Children, Food and Nutrition: Growing Well in a Changing World*. UNICEF: New York.

UNICEF, WHO & the International Bank for Reconstruction and Development/World Bank. (2020). *Levels and Trends in Child Mortality. Key Findings of the 2020 Edition of the Joint Child Malnutrition Estimates.* WHO: Geneva.

UN Women. (2020). COVID-19 and ending violence against women and girls. https://www.unwomen.org/-/media/headquarters/attachments/sections/library/publications/2020/issue-brief-covid-19-and-ending-violence-against-women-and-girls-en.pdf?la=en&vs=5006.

WFP. (2020). WFP global hotspots 2020: potential flashpoints to look out for in New Year. https://docs.wfp.org/api/documents/wfp-0000111565/download/.

WHO. (2014a). *Global Status Report on Non-Communicable Diseases 2014.* WHO: Geneva.

WHO. (2014b). *Injuries and Violence: The Facts 2014.* WHO: Geneva.

WHO. (2015). *Climate and Health Country Profiles—2015, A Global Overview.* WHO: Geneva.

WHO. (2018a). Noncommunicable diseases fact sheet. https://www.who.int/en/news-room/fact-sheets/detail/noncommunicable-diseases.

WHO. (2018b). Climate change. https://www.who.int/health-topics/climate-change#tab=tab_1.

WHO. (2019). *World Health Statistics 2019: Monitoring Health for the Sustainable Development Goals.* WHO: Geneva.

WHO. (2020a). The top 10 causes of death. https://www.who.int/news-room/fact-sheets/detail/the-top-10-causes-of-death.

WHO. (2020b). *Noncommunicable Diseases Progress Monitor 2020.* WHO: Geneva.

WHO. (2020c). COVID-19 disrupting mental health services in most countries, WHO survey. https://www.who.int/news/item/05-10-2020-covid-19-disrupting-mental-health-services-in-most-countries-who-survey.

WHO. (2020d). Road traffic injuries. https://www.who.int/news-room/fact-sheets/detail/road-traffic-injuries.

2

Global Disease Patterns

In all probability it is the local conditions of society that determine the form
of the disease, and we can so far state as a fairly general rule that the simple
form is the more common, the poorer and one-sided the food and the worse
the housing (Virchow & Reinhardt, 1848, p. 248).

Why do more children die in underdeveloped countries than in developed countries? Why is this excess mortality especially seen in communities that are poor, in both rich and poor countries?

This chapter focuses on the changing pattern of health and disease worldwide. It first presents the 10 leading causes of death globally, before narrowing the focus to the leading causes of death among children under five years old as an indicator of the most at-risk populations. Disease patterns in underdeveloped countries are compared with those of European countries in the nineteenth century and we see that many diseases we now regard as 'diseases of poverty' were once prevalent in the northern hemisphere. Why is this so? Different theories have been put forward to explain the change in disease patterns that countries follow as they urbanise and modernise. Instead of poorer countries following the same epidemiological transition as rich countries, another type of transition is evolving. In this new transition, countries are struggling with more than one dominant disease pattern *at the same time*—there is often a double, triple and sometimes even a quadruple burden of disease. Importantly, this is increasingly polarised across income groups, occurring not only *between* rich and poor countries, but also across social class *within* poor and rich countries.

Facts and figures

Of the world's 7.5 billion people:

- More than 820 million are suffering from chronic undernourishment. Almost all live in underdeveloped countries, with most being in Africa (representing, for example, 20% of the population of Africa) (FAO et al., 2019).
- 2.2 billion people around the world do not have safely managed drinking water services (UNICEF & WHO, 2019).
- 2.4 billion people do not have access to any type of improved sanitation facility (UNICEF & WHO, 2019).

The Struggle for Health. David Sanders with Wim De Ceukelaire and Barbara Hutton, Oxford University Press.
© Oxford University Press 2023. DOI: 10.1093/oso/9780192858450.003.0002

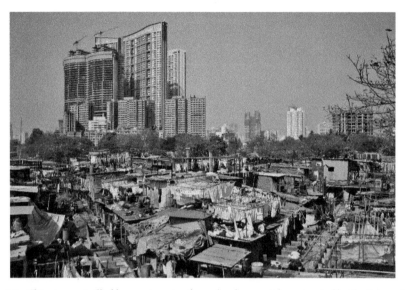

Fig. 2.1 Climate-controlled luxury towers of people who are rich contrasted by the improvised shacks of people who are poor, who are exposed to varying climatic conditions in Mumbai. *Source*: Nicolas Vigier, Flickr.

- Approximately 100 million people are homeless worldwide and one in four people live in inadequate housing or overcrowded conditions which are harmful to their health and safety (see Figure 2.1). It is estimated that by 2030, 3 billion people (about 40%) globally will lack affordable and accessible housing (UN-Habitat, 2021).

The global burden of disease

Everyone, all over the world, deserves to live a long life in full health. In order to achieve this goal, we need a comprehensive picture of what disables and kills people across countries, time, age, and sex. The Global Burden of Disease (GBD) provides a tool to quantify health loss from hundreds of diseases, injuries, and risk factors, so that health systems can be improved and disparities can be eliminated (Institute for Health Metrics and Evaluation [IHME], 2019).

In the early 1990s, the World Bank, World Health Organization (WHO) and Harvard School of Public Health commissioned the first Global Burden of Disease (GBD) study to systematically measure the world's health problems and disease patterns. The aim was to assist health policy-makers to determine the focus of their public health policies and actions. Since this first GBD study, researchers from various international organisations, led by the WHO, have continued to update the findings. The latest GBD report, *GBD 2017*, was published in November 2018. From such reports, GBD can

Table 2.1 The GBD study's classification of health conditions

Group	Type	Examples
1	Communicable diseases, maternal, perinatal, nutritional	Malaria, tuberculosis (TB), lower respiratory diseases, severe malnutrition, diarrhoeal diseases, conditions arising during pregnancy and childbirth, HIV/AIDS, COVID-19
2	NCDs	Heart attack, stroke, diabetes, dementia/Alzheimer's disease, chronic obstructive pulmonary disease (COPD) (e.g. chronic bronchitis, refractory [non-reversible] asthma and some forms of bronchiectasis), lung cancer (including trachea and bronchus cancers)
3	Violence and injuries	Injuries from road accidents

be measured for different countries and social classes and the disease patterns can be compared. In addition, the magnitude of emerging problems can be monitored, for example the increasing burden of mental health conditions in the NCD group; and most notably the occurrence of new epidemics (HIV/AIDS) and pandemics (COVID-19), both communicable diseases that have had profound impacts on **morbidity** and **mortality**.

GLOSSARY

Morbidity: illness, a diseased state, disability or poor health.

Mortality: death.

The GBD study combines health conditions into three broad categories (see Table 2.1). Drawing on these categories, countries are described as suffering from a double, triple or quadruple burden of disease, depending on which category or categories are dominant. Trends in each category can be monitored over time for different settings.

The global picture

In 2019 (pre COVID-19), 55% of the 55.4 million global deaths—in terms of total number of lives lost globally—were due to 10 main causes, as shown in Figure 2.2 (WHO, 2020a).

NOTE: By 3 May 2021, COVID-19 had claimed over 3.1 million lives globally, making it one of the leading causes of death worldwide (WHO, 2021).

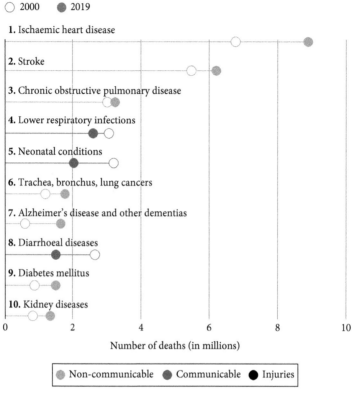

Fig. 2.2 Global health estimates: Leading causes of death. Cause-specific mortality, 2000–2019.

Source: WHO. (2020a). The Global Health Observatory. Global health estimates: Leading causes of death, Cause-specific mortality, 2000–2019.

In 2019, 7 of the top 10 causes of death globally (80%) were NCDs, which are all on the rise (WHO, 2020a):

- Ischaemic heart disease was responsible for 16% of all deaths—rising from 2 million deaths in 2000 to 8.9 million in 2019. This was followed by stroke (11% of all deaths) and obstructive pulmonary disease (6% of all deaths).
- Trachea, bronchus and lung cancers claimed 1.8 million lives (up from 1.2 million in 2000).
- Alzheimer's disease and other forms of dementia ranked seventh, with 65% of these deaths occurring in women.
- Deaths caused by diabetes have increased by 70% since 2000, with the largest increase being in male deaths.
- Kidney disease caused 1.3 million deaths (up from 813 000 in 2000).

In 2019, in the communicable disease category (WHO, 2020a):

- Lower respiratory infections ranked fourth in the top 10, claiming 2.6 million lives (down from 3 million in 2000).
- Neonatal conditions claimed 2 million lives (down from 3.2 million in 2000).
- Less than 295 000 women died in pregnancy or childbirth in 2017 (down from 451 000 in 2000) (WHO, 2019).
- Diarrhoeal diseases claimed 1.5 million lives (down from 2.6 million in 2000).

By the fourth quarter of 2020 there was an increase in deaths directly related to COVID-19, as well as **excess deaths** from other categories due indirectly to the effect of the pandemic on the health system and on underlying factors, such as increasing poverty and hunger. As an example, from the end of January 2020 to early October 2020, the USA had 299 000 more deaths than the normal number during the same period in previous years. Two-thirds were attributed to COVID-19, and the largest percentage increases were among Hispanic and Latino people and among adults aged 25–44 years (Rossen et al., 2020).

GLOSSARY

Excess deaths: the number of deaths from all causes, in excess of what is normal for a country and time period, based on historic averages.

The picture according to income group

The World Bank classifies countries into four main income groupings according to their **gross national income (GNI) per capita**. In July 2020:

- Low-income economies were those with a GNI per capita of US$1036 or less.
- Lower middle-income economies were those with a GNI per capita between US$1036 and US$4045.
- Upper middle-income economies were those with a GNI per capita between US$4046 and US$12 535.
- High-income economies were those with a GNI per capita of US$12 535 or more.

GLOSSARY

Gross national income (GNI) per capita: a country's final income in a year (before tax), divided by its population, reflected in US dollars. GNI is said to be a good reflection of the general standard of living enjoyed by the average citizen in a country.

Table 2.2 Main differences between low- and high-income countries in terms of causes of death, 2015/2016

Low-income countries	High-income countries
• Nearly 4 in every 100 deaths are among children under 15 years • 2 in every 10 deaths are among people aged 70 years and older	• 7 in every 10 deaths are among people aged 70 years and older • 1 in every 100 deaths is among children under 15 years
Group 1 conditions (communicable diseases) accounted for 52% of all deaths (lower respiratory infections; HIV/AIDS; diarrhoeal diseases; malaria; TB; complications of childbirth due to prematurity, birth asphyxia and birth trauma, and maternal deaths)	Group 1 (lower respiratory infections) accounted for 7% of all deaths
Group 2 conditions (NCDs) accounted for 37% of all deaths (up from 23% in 2000)	Group 2 conditions accounted for 88% of all deaths (including cardiovascular diseases; cancers; dementia; chronic obstructive lung disease; and diabetes)
Group 3 (injuries and violence) accounted for 28.5 deaths per 100 000 people. About 90% of injury-related deaths occur in low- and middle-income countries (WHO, 2014a)	Group 3 (mainly suicide and homicide)

The breakdown of the top leading causes of death in low- and high-income countries is shown in Table 2.2.

Despite the global decline in death from communicable diseases up to 2019 (before the COVID-19 pandemic in the 2020s), they remain the leading cause of death in low- and middle-income countries. However, at the same time there was a rapid increase in deaths caused by NCDs and violence and injury. For this reason, many countries are described as struggling with a triple burden of disease, and some in Sub-Saharan Africa, where HIV/AIDS is still prevalent, with a quadruple burden of disease.

A NOTE ABOUT GROUP 3 CONDITIONS

In 2017, violence and injuries resulted in nearly 5 million deaths worldwide:

- Road accidents claimed 1.4 million lives, with 90% occurring in low- and middle-income countries, and the majority happening in Africa (see Figure 2.3).
- Another approximately 1.3 million deaths were due to suicide and homicide.
- Other main causes of death from injuries were burns, falls, drowning, poisoning and violent conflict.

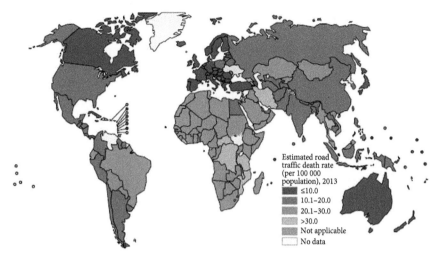

Fig. 2.3 Deaths due to road traffic accidents.
Source: WHO. (2017).

Disease in underdeveloped countries

It is important to give priority to maternal and child health and well-being when studying differences in diseases and death in poor and rich countries. Not only are children the most vulnerable age group, but also their health is important for the rest of their lives, as well as in the lives of the generation to come. Childhood mortality provides us with a good picture of child health and well-being (UNICEF, 2015b).

> In low-income countries, nearly 4 in every 10 deaths are among children under 15 years, and only 2 in every 10 deaths are among people aged 70 years and older . . . Complications of childbirth due to prematurity, and birth asphyxia and birth trauma are among the leading causes of death, claiming the lives of many newborns and infants (WHO, 2014b).

Facts and figures

According to the IHME (2019), in 1990, 12.5 million children under five years died worldwide. By 2018, this figure had dropped to 5.3 million (IHME, 2019). Clearly progress has been made in increasing child survival. On average, 15 000 children under five years still die every day (including 7000 newborns); however, regional and socio-economic inequalities remain. In 2017, it was estimated that more than 50% of under-five deaths occurred in Sub-Saharan Africa and another 30% in Southern Asia (United Nations, 2019).

The statistics remain high, especially if we take two main factors into account:

- The majority of child deaths are concentrated in the poorest countries of the world and occur within the poorest sectors within these countries (WHO, 2016). Sub-Saharan Africa has the highest **under-five mortality rate (U5MR)**, with 1 child in 13 dying before age five, followed by Southern Asia with U5MR of 1 in 24 (see Figure 2.4). These figures are stark when compared with those in high-income countries, where the U5MR is 1 in 167 and *"20 years behind the world average, which achieved a 1 in 13 rate by 1999"* (UNICEF, 2019a).
- Most child deaths are preventable or treatable, as they are mainly due to Group 1 conditions, including preterm birth complications (16%); pneumonia (15%); complications during childbirth and delivery (11%); diarrhoea (8%); and sepsis/meningitis (9%). Almost 50% of deaths are due to nutritional deficiencies—80% occurring among newborns of **low birthweight (LBW)** (UNICEF, 2019b).
- Sometimes these conditions act separately, but more often they act together (with poverty being the underlying root cause) and aggravate each other.

GLOSSARY

Under-five mortality rate (U5MR): the chances of a child dying before they reach the age of five years old.

Low birthweight (LBW): weight that is less than 2500 g in a live birth.

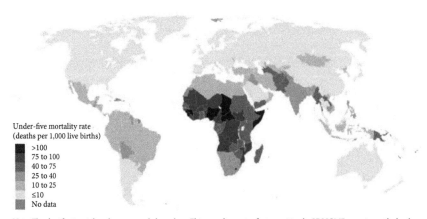

Note: The classification is based on unrounded numbers. This map does not reflect a position by UN IGME agencies on the legal status of any country or territory or the delimitation of any frontiers.

Fig. 2.4 U5MR—deaths per 1000 live births, 2018; highest risks of dying are in Sub-Saharan Africa and Southern Asia.

Source: UNICEF (2019a), p. 12.

Disease and death in the first month of life: neonatal period

The world has made substantial progress in child survival since 1990. Globally the number of neonatal deaths declined from 5.0 million in 1990 to 2.4 million in 2019. However, the decline in neonatal mortality from 1990 to 2019 has been slower than that of post-neonatal under-5 mortality (WHO, 2020b).

The first 28 days of life are when babies with LBW are most vulnerable to disease and death. In recent years, deaths of neonates (0 days to 28 days) and post-neonates (28 days to 1 year) account for a larger portion of the overall U5MR. Of the 5 million global deaths of under five year olds in 2019:

- 2.4 million occurred in the first 28 days of life, with about 1 million newborns dying in the first 24 hours.
- Main causes of neonatal deaths included preterm birth complications, intrapartum-related complications (obstructed labour, birth asphyxia or lack of breathing at birth), sepsis, pneumonia, tetanus, diarrhoea and birth defects. Many of these conditions are preventable or treatable.
- Sub-Saharan Africa had the highest neonatal mortality rate with 27 deaths per 1000 live births. This was followed by Central and Southern Asia with 24 deaths per 1000 live births. Children born in these regions of the world are 10 times more likely to die in the neonatal period than children born in a high-income country (WHO, 2020b).

The majority of neonatal deaths occur at home, among people living in poverty, and are associated with factors such as inadequate maternal health care during pregnancy and childbirth, lack of skilled birth attendants, weak health care systems, lack of immediate postnatal care and socio-cultural practices.

Children who die within the first 28 days of birth suffer from conditions and diseases associated with lack of quality care at birth or skilled care and treatment immediately after birth and in the first days of life (WHO, 2020b).

The same pattern of global inequities can be seen in the world map for maternal deaths (see Figure 2.5). The death of a mother in pregnancy or childbirth is catastrophic for an infant and society at large, but it is also an infringement of women's human rights that there should be such great inequities in their survival.

Disease and death of children aged 28 days to 1 year old: post-neonatal periods

Babies who survive the first 28 days of life often develop nutritional deficiency which makes them more vulnerable to disease and places them at increased risk of death. In

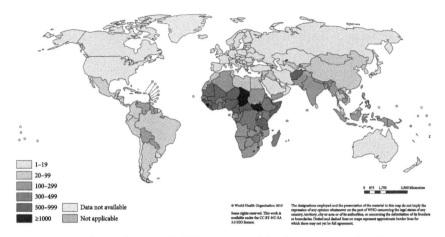

Legend:
- 1–19
- 20–99
- 100–299
- 300–499
- 500–999
- ≥1000
- Data not available
- Not applicable

© World Health Organization 2019
Some rights reserved. This work is available under the CC BY-NC-SA 3.0 IGO licence.

The designations employed and the presentation of the material in this map do not imply the expression of any opinion whatsoever on the part of WHO concerning the legal status of any country, territory, city or area or of its authorities, or concerning the delimitation of its frontiers or boundaries. Dotted and dashed lines on maps represent approximate border lines for which there may not yet be full agreement.

0   875   1,750   3,500 kilometres

Fig. 2.5 Maternal mortality ratio (MMR)—maternal deaths per 100 000 live births, 2017.
Source: WHO. (2019).

2018, 1.5 million children died in the post-neonatal period worldwide—the probability of a child dying in this period was 11 per 1000 (UNICEF, 2019a). Regional disparities and inequalities persist, with the majority of these deaths occurring in Central and Southern Asia and in Sub-Saharan Africa (UNICEF, 2019a).

Causes of disease and death of children in the first five years of life

The cycle of chronic undernutrition

Despite substantial progress in reducing global poverty and food insecurity in the past 50 years, the prevalence of maternal and child undernutrition in low-income and middle-income countries (LMICs) has remained unacceptably high … The global nutrition targets endorsed by the World Health Assembly in 2012 stress the need to reduce low birthweight, childhood stunting, and wasting and anaemia in women, and to increase exclusive breastfeeding in the first 6 months of life, yet progress has been slow in most LMICs (Victora et al., 2021).

Maternal nutritional status and low birthweight

New evidence shows that stunting and wasting might already be present at birth, and that the incidence of both conditions peaks in the first 6 months of life (Victora et al., 2021).

Nearly 15% of all babies born worldwide in 2015 suffered LBW, putting them at high risk of death in the first 28 days of their lives (UNICEF, 2019b). The **Barker hypothesis** shows the link between undernutrition in foetal life and early childhood and the propensity to develop obesity and NCDs later in life.

GLOSSARY

'Foetal origins' or Barker hypothesis: put forward in the early 1990s by epidemiologist David Barker, it shows a link between undernutrition in foetal life and early childhood and the propensity to develop obesity, cardiovascular disease, hypertension and adult-onset diabetes later in life when exposed to a calorie-rich environment (Almond & Currie, 2011).

Most LBW babies are not premature but have suffered from *in utero* undernutrition and growth restriction, usually because of the health and nutritional status of the mother before and during pregnancy (Victora et al., 2021).

Undernourished pregnant women have small, and therefore more vulnerable, babies. The mother's size and nutritional status depend on various factors including genetics, but also on her own diet in infancy, childhood and pregnancy. The age of the pregnant woman is also important. A woman's growth and maturity may not be completed until she is 18 or 19 years old; however, many women have been pregnant by this age (Save the Children, 2012).

Anaemia is common in general chronic undernutrition, recurrent infection and diseases caused by the infestation by parasites, such as malaria and hookworm. It is associated with premature labour and yet again an immature and extremely vulnerable baby.

Malaria in pregnant mothers is an acknowledged cause of infection of the placenta and thus of LBW, especially in first pregnancies. The reduction in foetal growth comes towards the end of pregnancy, when brain cells are multiplying rapidly, which means that the child's potential for intellectual development may be irreversibly impaired.

Global progress in reducing LBW babies has been slow. In 2000, globally there were 22.9 million LBW newborns; by 2015 this figure was 20.5 million. In 2015, 75% of all LBW newborns globally were born in South Asia (47%), Eastern and Southern Africa (13%) and West and Central Africa (12%) (UNICEF, 2019b).

Both alcohol and tobacco smoking during pregnancy impact on the birthweight of the baby. Evidence shows how tobacco growing and usage have become concentrated in the underdeveloped world, and that tobacco companies are specifically targeting women and children, resulting in an increase in female smoking among the urban poor population (ASH [Action on Smoking and Health], 2019). In 2016, the WHO estimated that over 1.1 billion people globally aged 15 and over smoked tobacco, with around 80% of them living in low- and middle-income countries, while tobacco demand in developed countries has fallen over time (WHO, 2018).

The cycle of chronic undernutrition (see Figure 2.6) amplifies the risks to the child's health and increases the likelihood of damage to future generations through further foetal undernutrition.

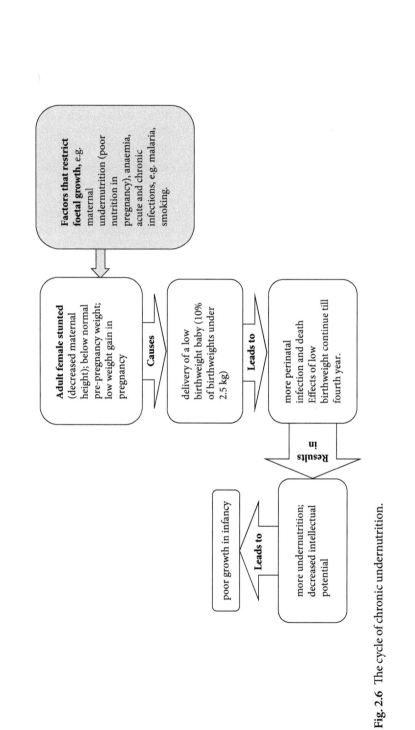

Fig. 2.6 The cycle of chronic undernutrition.

Factors that restrict foetal growth, e.g. maternal undernutrition (poor nutrition in pregnancy), anaemia, acute and chronic infections, e.g. malaria, smoking.

Adult female stunted (decreased maternal height); below normal pre-pregnancy weight; low weight gain in pregnancy

Causes

delivery of a low birthweight baby (10% of birthweights under 2.5 kg)

Leads to

more perinatal infection and death Effects of low birthweight continue till fourth year.

Results in

more undernutrition; decreased intellectual potential

Leads to

poor growth in infancy

Table 2.3 Classification of most communicable diseases in the underdeveloped world

Means of transmission	Examples of disease/illness it causes
Airborne: Disease spread by breathing airborne, respiratory secretions of infected persons	
Viral	Influenza
	Pneumonia
	Measles
	Chickenpox
Bacterial	Whooping cough
	Diphtheria
	Meningitis
	TB
Water- and/or faecally transmitted	
Waterborne: Disease transmitted when pathogen is in water which is then drunk by person who may then become infected	Cholera
	Typhoid
	Diarrhoeas, dysenteries
Water-washed: (see below)	Amoebiasis, infectious hepatitis, poliomyelitis, intestinal worms
Water-washed: Disease where prevalence will fall when increased quantities of water are for drinking and hygienic purposes (the water should be clean, but need not be pure) • Skin and eye infection • Skin infestation	Trachoma Skin infection Leprosy Scabies Louseborne typhus
Water-based: Disease where pathogen spends a part of its life cycle in an intermediate aquatic host or hosts • Penetrating skin • Ingested	Schistomiasis (bilharzia) Guinea worm
Water-related insect vectors • Biting near water • Breeding in water	Sleeping sickness Malaria Yellow fever Onchocerciasis (river blindness)
Animal vector: Zoonotic diseases are infectious diseases of animals that can cause disease when transmitted to humans. Then humans can transmit to each other, e.g. COVID-19 by droplets	
	Ebola
	Rabies
	Tetanus
	Zika
	COVID-19
Contact: Diseases transmitted from human to human via bodily fluids, e.g. blood, semen, mucus	
	Sexually transmitted diseases (STDs)
	HIV/AIDS

Source: Adapted from Bradley (1974).

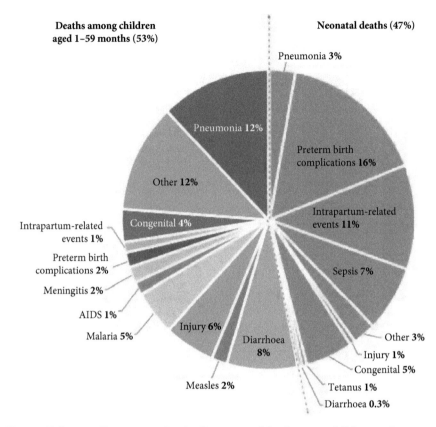

Deaths among children aged 1–59 months (53%)

Neonatal deaths (47%)

Pneumonia 3%

Pneumonia 12%

Preterm birth complications 16%

Other 12%

Intrapartum-related events 11%

Intrapartum-related events 1%

Congenital 4%

Preterm birth complications 2%

Sepsis 7%

Meningitis 2%

AIDS 1%

Malaria 5%

Injury 6%

Diarrhoea 8%

Other 3%

Injury 1%

Congenital 5%

Measles 2%

Tetanus 1%

Diarrhoea 0.3%

Fig. 2.8 Infectious diseases remain a leading cause of death among children under age five, 2018.

Source: UNICEF. (2020), p. 16.

Communicable diseases are a leading cause of death in children under five years—in 2018, 47% of the neonatal deaths and 53% of the deaths of children between one and five years globally (UNICEF, 2020). As shown in Figure 2.8, most of these deaths were from the following three preventable and treatable diseases: pneumonia (15%), diarrhoea (8%) and malaria (5%).

In addition to causing deaths, communicable diseases are among the leading causes of **disability-adjusted life years (DALYs)** in children under 10 years compared to older-age groups. For example, in 2019, globally, six infectious diseases were among the top 10 causes of DALYs: lower respiratory infections, diarrhoeal diseases, malaria, meningitis, whooping cough and sexually transmitted infections (which, in this age group, is fully accounted for by congenital syphilis) (GBD 2019 Diseases and Injuries Collaborators, 2020).

GLOSSARY

Disability-adjusted life years (DALYs): a summary measure that combines the following:

- YLL – number of years of healthy life lost due to premature death.
- YLD – number of healthy years of life lost due to time lived with disease or disability.

One DALY is generally thought of as one healthy year of life lost.

Interaction of poverty, nutritional deficiency and communicable diseases

Child mortality in developed countries is declining rapidly and the gap between high-income and low- and middle-income countries is widening, with Sub-Saharan Africa and Southern Asia accounting for a disproportionate share of child deaths.

According to UNICEF (2016), children in the following contexts are at highest risk of dying before the age of five:

- Children from the poorest households (across regions and countries) are nearly twice as likely to die as children from the richest households.
- Children from rural areas are 1.7 times as likely to die as children from urban areas.
- Children of uneducated mothers are 2.8 times as likely to die as children whose mothers are educated.
- Children in **fragile contexts** are twice as likely to die as children in non-fragile contexts.

GLOSSARY

Fragile context: fragility is assessed along five dimensions, which can affect all countries, not only those traditionally seen as 'fragile' or affected by conflict: violence, access to justice, accountable and inclusive institutions, economic inclusion and stability, and capacities to prevent and adapt to social, economic and environmental shocks and disasters (OECD, 2015).

Poverty, nutritional deficiency and communicable diseases are interrelated, interact with one another and can generate a lethal cycle (see Figure 2.9). Undernutrition is a

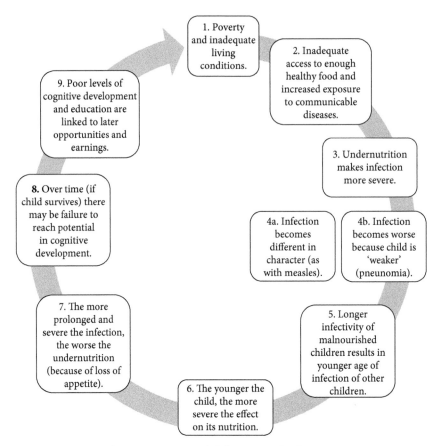

Fig. 2.9 Interaction of poverty, nutritional deficiency and infection.

major contributing factor in communicable disease. It impairs normal body responses to disease and reduces any immunity created by infections. Disease and infections, in turn, inhibit the uptake of scarce nutrients, impair appetite and hunger and cause nutritional deficiency. In this way, the vicious circle is complete.

As an example, severely undernourished children experience more severe, prolonged and frequent episodes of diarrhoea (Iskandar et al., 2015). The frequency and severity of diarrhoea attacks are exacerbated by lack of access to safe drinking water; unsanitary environments; inadequate hygiene practices; poor overall health and nutritional status; and lack of access to adequate and affordable health care. Repeated episodes of diarrhoea impair appetite and make it more difficult for the body to absorb food. They also increase the body's metabolism, causing nutritional deficiency. Thus, the vicious circle is complete (Disease Control Priorities Project, 2006).

Over time, undernutrition and micronutrient deficiencies result in impaired intellectual development, lost wages, and increased health care costs, all exacerbating the cycle of poverty (Leon et al., 2001).

Measles is especially severe in malnourished children who live in conditions where there is poor sanitation and inadequate health care, and may have a mortality rate 200–400 times greater than in well-nourished children (Bystrianyk, 2014). Measles in turn has a more severe adverse effect on the nutritional state of children than any other communicable disease, and undernutrition follows more frequently after measles than after any other infection.

A complication of measles and other severe infections, which is also associated with poverty and undernutrition, is the disfiguring affliction of cancrum oris—a gangrenous stomatitis beginning in the mucous membrane of the corner of the mouth or cheek and progressing rapidly to the lips and cheeks. Similarly, measles is the main catalyst of xerophthalmia, a progressive eye disease linked with undernutrition (PEM) and with acute and chronic infections of childhood that cause low vitamin A levels (Morley & Woodland, 1979).

TB is both more common and more severe in malnourished populations, and children in these populations are especially vulnerable. The TB infection aggravates the undernourished state, and this leads to a more rapid spread of the disease. Yet again, there is a vicious cycle.

Where are we now?
In the past few decades, there has been considerable progress in world health. The global U5MR has declined by 53%, as has the prevalence of underweight among children under five years, from 25% to 14%. There have also been large reductions in child deaths due to pneumonia, diarrhoea, malaria, HIV/AIDS and measles (UNICEF, 2019a).

However, inequity across and within rich and poor countries is growing and is a major contributing factor for the concentration of the majority of global deaths in children under five years in the poorest countries of the world and within the poorest sectors within these countries (WHO, 2016).

Sub-Saharan Africa remains the region with the highest U5MR globally. Today, over half the people in the world who live in extreme poverty, come from Sub-Saharan Africa (56%), and many are children under five years. Due to the slow decline in poverty rates and the failure to address the social, environmental, economic or political causes of ill-health, the total number of people living in poverty in this region is not expected to fall significantly (World Bank, 2018).

… the question of why children are dying cannot be answered through medical explanations alone. Many factors … increase a child's risk of early death—including low maternal education, early childbearing, limited access to water, sanitation and hygiene, and undernutrition … These risk factors, like child mortality itself, do not affect all children equally. Families in rural areas are less than half as likely to have piped water at home as families in urban areas. Children in conflict-affected countries are more likely to be out of school than their counterparts in countries not affected by conflict. Children from the poorest families are more than twice as likely to be stunted as children from the wealthiest. The list goes on, but the conclusion is clear: Children are dying not just because of sepsis, malaria or other official causes of death listed here. They are also dying because the families they are born into are poor, from a historically marginalized group, live in a rural area, or suffer other forms of social exclusion (UNICEF, 2015a).

Diseases in nineteenth-century Europe

Descriptions of the public health problems in Europe during the nineteenth century are surprisingly similar to those of today's poorest countries. And so, it is instructive to put these patterns of disease in historical perspective to understand how the problems of undernutrition and communicable diseases were overcome in the developed world.

The material conditions of people's everyday lives

Britain was the first country to industrialise and transition from a predominantly agricultural and rural society to an urbanised one. Hamlin and Sheard, in describing public health in England and Wales in the nineteenth century, explain:

*Unless we are familiar with some of the cities of the developing world, most of us are probably unable to fathom the enormity of the unplanned urbanisation of the 19th century: roughly 3 million people (slightly over 30%) were urban in 1801 in England and Wales, compared with 28.5 million (almost 80%) in 1901. Growth rates in some textile boom towns, like Bradford from 1811 to 1831, exceeded 60% per decade; this despite the fact that towns were acting as a sink for human life. In Liverpool average **life expectancy** by class ranged from 15 years for the unemployed or poor to 35 years for the well to do* (Hamlin & Sheard, 1998).

GLOSSARY

Life expectancy: The expected average number of years of life remaining at a given age. Various factors affect life expectancy, including where you were born, when, how you live, income, living conditions, gender, diet, life events and so on.

In London, half the infants baptised in the period 1770–1789 were dead before the age of five years (*The Health of Towns Magazine and Journal of Medical Jurisprudence*, 1847–48). At different times in the first half of the nineteenth century, the infant mortality rate was twice as high in the new towns that were rapidly developing. The following extract describes the slum known as Snow's Rents in Westminster:

On entering these houses you have a fine specimen of the manner in which the lower orders of Westminster live. Living by day and night in one wretched room, with scarcely any light—an intermittent supply of water, and a shocking faetid atmosphere—full of rags and filth—it is dreadful! In the corner of the room may be seen what may be termed an apology for a bed and bedding, being a mass of rags piled together, in the midst of which are the poor sickly children, whose very countenance bespeak that they will soon cease to trouble their parents; with hair uncombed, barefooted, and in rags—with their skin unwashed—the majority of them never live to manhood, while one third of them

die before they attain the age of 5 years. The adult inhabitants, also, have all the ap-
pearance of being always in a typhoid state. The courts and alleys in this colony of filth
and fever are chiefly unpaved and undrained, and mostly with but one privy for one
court, which contains, sometimes, upwards of twenty houses ... (The Health of Towns
Magazine and Journal of Medical Jurisprudence, 1847–8).

Similar conditions prevailed in all the new towns of the Industrial Revolution. Dr
G.C. Holland of Sheffield explained that social class had a lot to do with it:

We have no hesitation in asserting, that the sufferings of the working classes, and con-
sequently the rate of mortality, are greater now than in former times. Indeed, in most
manufacturing districts the rate of mortality in these classes is appalling to contemplate,
when it can be studied in reference to them alone, and not in connexion with the entire
population. The supposed gain on the side of longevity, arising chiefly from ... a relatively
much more numerous middle class than formerly existed (cited in Thompson, 1968).

Friedrich Engels described the dangerous working and living conditions of workers
and their families in the mid-1800s—malnutrition, inadequate housing, contaminated water supplies and overcrowding—which resulted in diseases like TB, typhoid
and typhus.

The great mortality among children of the working class, and especially among those
of the factory operatives, is proof enough of the unwholesome conditions under which
they pass their first years. These influences are at work, of course, among the children
who survive, but not quite so powerfully as upon those who succumb ... How is it pos-
sible ... for the lower classes to be healthy and long-lived? What else can be expected
than an excessive mortality, an unbroken series of epidemics, a progressive deterioration
in the physique of the working population? (Engels, 1845/1987).

Rudolf Virchow, a German physician who was greatly influenced by the work of
Engels, was sent by the Prussian government in 1847 to study a typhus epidemic rav-
aging a desperately poor area. Virchow's report concluded that the epidemic was due
to poor living conditions, including poor hygiene and diet, and that it could not be
controlled by treating individual patients with drugs, or with more clinics or hospitals,
but required a radical change in the conditions that permitted epidemics to occur. He
wrote that the most important causative factors of disease are the material conditions
of people's everyday lives; and that improvements in health care must correspond with
fundamental economic, political and social changes (Ponnampalam, 1992).

This population had no idea that the mental and material impoverishment to which
it had been allowed to sink, were largely the cause of its hunger and disease, and that
the adverse climatic conditions which contributed to the failure of its crops and to
the sickness of its bodies, would not have caused such terrible ravages, if it had been
free, educated and well-to-do. For there can now no longer be any doubt that such
an epidemic dissemination of typhus had only been possible under the wretched
conditions of life that poverty and lack of culture had created in Upper Silesia.

If these conditions were removed, I am sure that epidemic typhus would not recur. Whosoever wishes to learn from history will find many examples (Virchow & Reinhardt, 1848, p. 248).

Disease pattern

It is possible to classify disease in Europe in the nineteenth century in much the same way as we did for today's poor countries. Communicable diseases, whether air-, water- or food-borne, were common causes of death (see Table 2.4). The following were most commonly responsible for death:

- Airborne diseases of TB, the bronchitis–pneumonia–influenza group and the diphtheria–scarlet fever group. In children, measles and whooping cough were particularly common causes of death.
- Waterborne diseases in the diarrhoeal group of diarrhoea–dysentery–enteritis and cholera.
- Non-respiratory TB (bovine TB) was often contracted from drinking infected milk.
- Typhoid and typhus (louseborne) were often confused and grouped together.
- Most deaths from 'other conditions' were in fact due to conditions such as convulsions, now known to be mostly due to airborne infections.
- The major conditions not attributable to micro-organisms were 'old age' and 'prematurity, immaturity and other diseases of infancy'.

Table 2.4 Death rate (per million) in the 1845/1854 period, and in 1971 in England and Wales

Causes of diseases	1848/1854	1971	Percentage of reduction attributable to each category
Conditions attributable to micro-organisms (communicable)			
– Airborne diseases	7259	619	40
– Water- and food-borne diseases	3562	35	21
– Other conditions	2144	60	13
Total	12 965	714	74
Conditions not attributable to micro-organisms	8891	4070	26
Total of all disease	21 856	4784	100

Source: McKeown. (1976a).

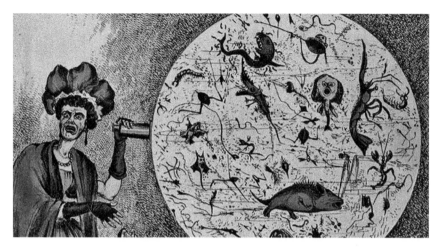

Fig. 2.10 A monster soup, commonly called Thames Water. A woman dropping her porcelain tea-cup in horror upon discovering the monstrous contents of a magnified drop of Thames water, revealing the impurity of London's drinking water.
Source: Wellcome Library. Coloured etching by W. Heath, 1828.

In the nineteenth century, sewage and waste contaminated the River Thames in London, making it a prime source of waterborne diseases such as cholera and typhoid (see Figure 2.10).

Nutritional deficiency

Although nutritional state is not mentioned as a cause of death in the classification in Table 2.4, we know that it was often an important contributing factor and that it prepared the way for the disastrous effects of infections especially among people living in poverty. Communicable disease acting in the presence of undernutrition caused most ill-health and death, particularly among infants and children. For example, descriptions of 'frightful swelling' of the bodies of children in Ireland in the potato famine of 1847 are likely to have been kwashiorkor (Morley, 1973) (see Figure 2.11). Records of heights in the nineteenth century suggest that mothers and children—and therefore fathers too—were not nearly as well nourished as in Britain today. In other words, disease and death in Europe in the not-too-distant past was strikingly similar to that in most of today's poorest countries.

Communicable diseases

In the mid-nineteenth century, TB was the largest single cause of death. Although the bacterium causing TB was identified in 1882, we now know that all the medical treatment practised before 1947 was ineffective in treating TB. Effective medical treatment began with the use of streptomycin in 1947 and immunisation with Bacillus

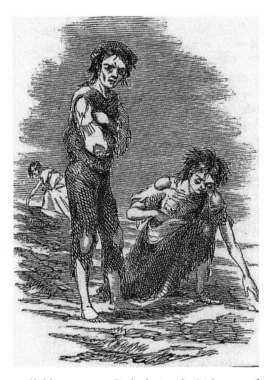

Fig. 2.11 The scene at Skibbereen, west Cork, during the Irish potato famine, in 1847.

Source: From a series of illustrations by Cork artist James Mahony (1810–1879), commissioned by *Illustrated London News*, 1847.

Calmette–Guérin (BCG) vaccine started in 1954. *Importantly, by these dates, mortality from TB had fallen to a small fraction of its level in 1848–1854.* Drug treatment is responsible for the *more rapid* fall of mortality since 1950, but the substantial reduction occurred before the era of antibiotics (see Figure 2.12).

Similarly, deaths from the major childhood killers—scarlet fever, diphtheria, measles and whooping cough—had fallen to almost their present level *before* any effective medical treatment had been developed (see Figure 2.13).

Smallpox was responsible for only a small proportion of deaths due to airborne infections, but it is the one disease in which a specific medical measure—vaccination—appears to have contributed to its decline.

The pattern for airborne disease is repeated with water-related infections (see Figure 2.14). Ninety-five percent of the decline in deaths had occurred before the 1930s, when intravenous therapy was first used. The decline was due to protected water supply, proper sewage disposal and improved nutrition.

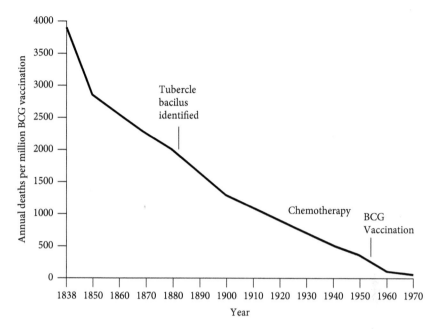

Fig. 2.12 Decline in TB before drugs.

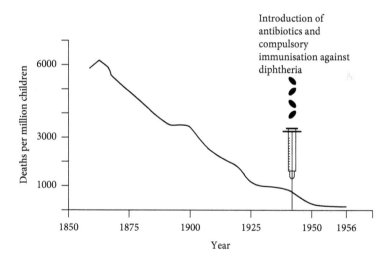

Fig. 2.13 Deaths of children under 15 years attributed to scarlet fever, diphtheria, whooping cough and measles in England and Wales.

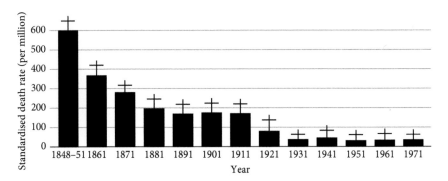

Fig. 2.14 Diarrhoea and dysentery: death rates at age five and over, England and Wales, 1848–1971.

Source: McKeown. (1976).

Cause of the decline of mortality

Changes in two factors were responsible for the fall in deaths due to infections: (a) reduced exposure to infection; and (b) a stronger response to infection. The two are interrelated: the weaker your response to infection, the longer you carry the infection and therefore you have longer to spread it to others—who therefore experience greater exposure to infection. This is true of TB, measles and gastroenteritis, for example. If many people have a weak response to infection, then that infection will be more common in the population as a whole.

Reduced exposure to infection

In England, reduced exposure to water-related infections has occurred since 1850 with the introduction of the purification of water, efficient disposal of sewage, provision of safe milk and improved food hygiene.

In the case of airborne infections, reduced exposure has resulted mainly from fewer people carrying infection because of improved nutrition. Less cramped housing conditions have reduced the spread. Exposure to TB has also been reduced by improved living conditions and less polluted working conditions (see Figure 2.15).

Stronger response to infection

Alongside reduced exposure to infection, people also became better able to resist infection. There was a large increase in food supplies in Europe between the end of the seventeenth and the middle of the nineteenth centuries and *improved nutrition* coincided with a large fall in mortality from communicable diseases.

Already by the beginning of the eighteenth century a revolution in agriculture had transformed food production in England. In the two centuries leading up to the Industrial Revolution, England did not experience the famine that continued to plague continental Europe with its largely feudal agriculture. Packard provides an example of how this transformation in agriculture was linked to the history of malaria in England:

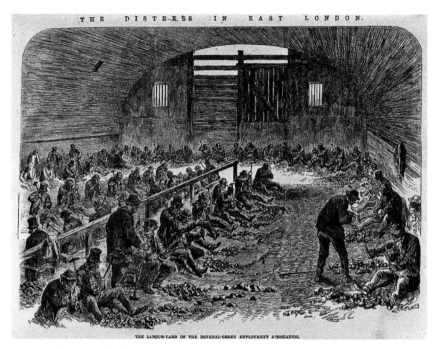

Fig. 2.15 Labour yard of the Bethnal Green Employment Association, London, 1860s.
Source: Wellcome Trustees.

During the 13th and early 14th century, the Fenlands had a large population that was decimated by the plague and other epidemics. When the population of England began growing again in the 16th and 17th centuries, the Fenlands were drained for pasturage and grain. The drainage was done poorly, leaving standing water for mosquitoes to breed abundantly. Malaria started to ravage the local population. So many people died that labor became short and wages high, which led people from outside the area without any acquired resistance to keep migrating in ... but the continued capitalization of agriculture in England led to the gradual disappearance of malaria in the Fenlands. Drainage improved, housing became better and more mosquito resistant, nutrition improved, agriculture became more efficient and the need for labor dropped (Packard, 2011).

The physician and demographic historian Thomas McKeown (1976) studied mortality records for England going back to the first half of the nineteenth century. He argued that the substantial decline in illness and death from major infectious diseases was not due to advances in the medical field, but rather due to improvements in *economic conditions*—rising real wages—which enabled rising standards of living, improved nutrition and social conditions.

McKeown's thesis challenged *"public health professionals to view targeted interventions and social change, not as dichotomous or opposing choices, but rather as essential complements to each other, and to find ways to integrate technical preventive and curative measures with more broad-based efforts to improve all of the conditions in which people live"* (Colgrove, 2002).

So, since the early nineteenth century, the huge fall in illness and death resulted from the following, in order of importance:

1. Improved conditions of living, especially in diet and nutritional status (which in turn resulted from better economic conditions).
2. Improved hygiene, such as safe drinking water and sewage disposal systems (public health interventions and the political will of the State).
3. Specific preventive measures, such as the smallpox vaccination.
4. Much later, curative measures, such as antibacterial drugs.

A similar trend towards steep reduction in deaths was seen for maternal mortality, which had rates comparable to many underdeveloped countries up to the early twentieth century and then declined due to changes in maternal nutritional status, general asepsis measures and programmes to improve antenatal care and care around birth (see Figure 2.16).

As mentioned on page 38, most of the urban living conditions and public health problems in nineteenth-century England were not that different to those found in urban areas in today's poorest countries. The description earlier in this chapter from

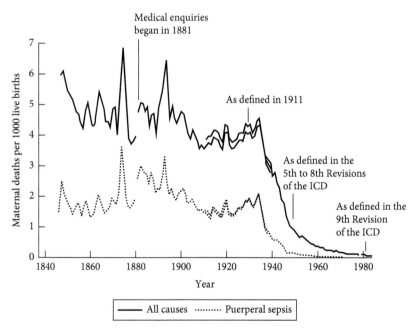

Fig. 2.16 Maternal mortality, England and Wales, 1847–1984. ICD, International Statistical Classification of Diseases and Related Health Problems.

Source: Macdonald & Johnson. (2017). General Register Office, OPCS and ONS mortality statistics, p. 16.

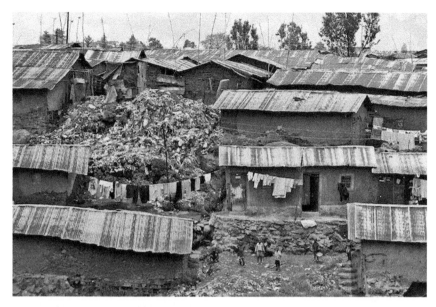

Fig. 2.17 Kibera Slum, Nairobi, Kenya. Garbage removal services are typically unavailable, so solid waste piles up in different corners. Major wind or floods wash these away into rivers and natural ecosystems.

Source: Colin Crowley. (2008). Flickr: Kibera_photoshow01.

The Health of Towns Magazine and Journal of Medical Jurisprudence (1847–8) is almost perfectly echoed in this account of Kibera in Kenya in 2008 (see Figure 2.17):

> *In Kibera, a massive slum of rusty tin roofs and makeshift homes spreading out from the southwest of the city, the rain is turning the twisting dirt roads and alleyways to thick red mud. Here in one of largest slums in the world … the rain is causing open sewers to swell and uncollected garbage to rush in rivers of tattered plastic and human waste through backyards.*
>
> *Potable water is one of the hardest resources to secure in Kibera and the torrents now being unleashed will offer no relief to the estimated 1 million people here who must use their meagre wages—usually less than a dollar a day—to buy water for drinking and cleaning.*
>
> *Tahir raised her children on the expensive and dirty water of Kibera. She tells of regular illnesses in her family due to waterborne diseases and late nights agonizing over whether or not she could afford even the transportation costs of getting an ailing child to Kenyatta Hospital a few miles down the road* (Stuteville, 2008).

If the conditions in underdeveloped countries are so similar to those in nineteenth-century Europe, does this mean that they will follow the same transition in disease pattern experienced by the developed world? To answer this question, we need to explore the transition or changes in disease patterns in different societies.

Epidemiological transition

Researchers have spent years trying to explain the tremendous differences in the disease patterns between developed and underdeveloped countries. By studying the changes in health and disease over extended periods of time, they have managed to identify a pattern that was followed in developed countries as their social, economic and demographic structures changed.

Omran (1971) was the first to describe this as an epidemiological transition. He outlined a sequence of events that occur in this transition, beginning with the predominance of infectious or communicable diseases, followed by a period when NCDs dominate. Initially these NCDs were seen among the wealthier sectors of developed countries as they adopted a more urbanised and 'western' lifestyle that included a diet of ultra-processed food products and sugary beverages, smoking tobacco and engaging in little physical activity. Omran predicted that as urbanisation increased, there would be a decline in deaths due to communicable diseases and an increase in deaths due to NCDs. It was anticipated that poor countries would also follow this disease pattern as they developed, industrialised and adopted 'western lifestyles'.

Based on observations from some large middle-income populations, Frenk et al. (1989) proposed a modification to Omran's theory, which was called the protracted-polarised model. According to this model, communicable diseases and NCDs exist in the *same* population at the *same* time, and persist over a long, protracted period.

In the protracted-polarised model more affluent sections of the population would have completed the transition, while economically disadvantaged groups continue to suffer from pre-transitional pathologies. This epidemiological pattern reflects an economic and social situation of juxtaposition within the same society of a developed and an underdeveloped sector. In short, it is an expression, in terms of morbidity and mortality, of 'combined and uneven development' (Chopra & Sanders, 2004).

Another kind of transition

There is not just one kind of epidemiological transition (from underdeveloped to developed) that can happen slower or faster. Other transitions are possible—even regression is possible. Since the 1990s, for example, Eastern Europe and the former Soviet Union have been the scene of another kind of transition: morbidity and mortality have changed dramatically during the 'transition' from 'socialism' to capitalism.

Figure 2.18 shows the widening gap in adult mortality in the Russian Federation in men who had different levels of education. This gap has been growing since the collapse of the Soviet Union in the 1990s and the transition in the economy (Murphy et al., 2006). Men with little education seemed to be more vulnerable to societal changes and had higher mortality than those with higher educational levels. This inequality in health status was related to inequalities in social status due to various rapid interrelated changes in Russian society. Two main factors were identified: lower living standards and social disorganisation.

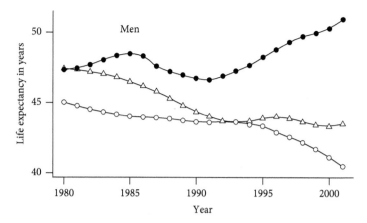

Fig. 2.18 Smooth trends in life expectancy at age 20 by educational level among Russian men. Men with elementary (open circles) and intermediate (triangles) education were more vulnerable to societal changes and showed increasing mortality and decreasing life expectancy than those with university education (filled-in circles).

Source: Data from Murphy et al. (2006).

The double and triple burden of disease

Another disease pattern that is emerging in many underdeveloped countries is referred to as the 'double burden of disease'. NCDs (sometimes called 'diseases of affluence') occur at the *same time* as communicable diseases ('diseases of poverty'), *although underdeveloped countries have not yet completed the epidemiological transition* (Frenk et al., 1991; Beaglehole & Yach, 2003). In some cases, NCDs are responsible for more deaths than communicable diseases, and these deaths occur at younger ages than the NCD deaths in rich countries (Ezzati et al., 2005). In 2000 NCDs accounted for 23% of deaths in underdeveloped countries; by 2015/2016 they accounted for 37% of deaths.

A series in *The Lancet* focusing on India gives us an insight into the leading causes of death and disability in India—chronic diseases (including cardiovascular and respiratory diseases, mental health disorders, diabetes and cancer) and injuries, usually associated with high-income countries. Chronic diseases kill more than 5 million people in India every year (half of the country's total deaths), including the urban middle class, those living in poverty, and those living in rural areas. The number of YLL due to deaths caused by coronary heart disease before the age of 60 years increased from 7.1 million in 2004 to 17.9 million in 2010, and it has been projected that by 2030 more life years will be lost as a result of this disease in India than is projected for China, Russia and the USA combined (Patel et al., 2011).

So-called diseases of affluence do not have anything to do with affluence after all. Recent research suggests that although cardiovascular risks rise with increasing affluence up to a certain point, they eventually decline as national incomes continue to rise. However, increasingly, NCDs and specifically cardiovascular disease risks are shifting to low- and middle-income countries, as well as to the least affluent in developed countries, and *"together with the persistent burden of infectious diseases, further increase global health inequalities"* (Ezzati et al., 2005).

We also saw earlier in this chapter on page 24, how violence and injury-related deaths (Group 3 conditions) have added to the pattern of disease particularly in low- and middle-income countries, so that many of these countries are now described as struggling with a 'triple burden of disease'. Add to this the burden of HIV/AIDS that Sub-Saharan African countries also face and you have a 'quadruple burden of disease'—all four groups occurring at the same time. The impact of the COVID-19 pandemic from 2020 added to the first burden, due to the major disruptions of health systems and household incomes.

These developments indicate that there are serious limitations to the epidemiological transition model. At the very least we can conclude that the reality is much more complicated, and the odds are always against people living in poverty. The growing gap between those who are rich and those who are poor—across and within countries—has made people ask whether it wouldn't be better to talk about an 'epidemiological polarisation'.

Epidemiological polarisation

Within-country disparities: underdeveloped countries

Of course, not all parts of underdeveloped countries are underdeveloped and poor; and disparities between people who are rich and those who are poor also exist in developed countries. In fact, the general pattern the world over is one of very uneven development, with grotesque inequalities across and within countries. These inequalities are obvious to health workers who see and treat the *effects* of inequalities.

South Africa is an example of a middle-income country in Sub-Saharan Africa in which the distribution and pattern of morbidity and mortality have been shaped by persistent inequalities in the personal and household resources of the four main population/'racial' groups—African, White, Coloured and Indian.

In 1998, child mortality was higher in urban settings, and four times higher among Africans than Whites. Undernutrition is also associated with poor socio-economic status, with stunting rates six times higher in the poorest quintile compared with the richest (38% vs. 6%) (Sanders et al., 2009).

The mother's educational level and her socio-economic status is often used as an indicator of under-five mortality. In Tanzania, for example, in 2004/2005, the U5MR was approximately 160 deaths per 1000 live births for mothers with no education; 140 deaths per 1000 live births for mothers with some primary education; 120 deaths per 1000 live births for mothers who had completed primary education or had some secondary education; and about 55 deaths per 1000 live births for mothers who had completed secondary education or had some higher education (see Figure 2.19).

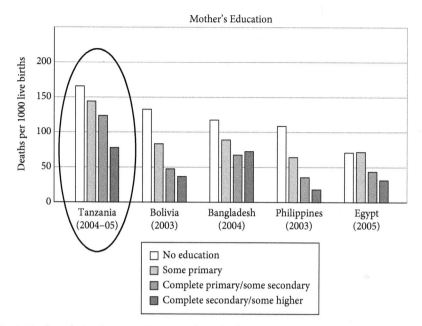

Fig. 2.19 Correlation between U5MR and mother's education.

Source: World Bank. (2007). *World Development Indicators 2007*. World Bank: Washington, DC, p. 119. Reprinted with permission.

In the rest of Africa and in Asia there were striking differences in health between poor and rich groups, with U5MR among elite groups in these regions being similar to rates for the developed world—approximately 6 per 1000 live births (UNICEF, 2013).

Within-country disparities: developed countries

Navarro (1976) studied health problems in the USA and concluded that lifestyle was not the most important indicator of mortality. Rather, ill-health was linked to the unequal distribution of economic and political power in society and the "*absence of control by the majority of the U.S. population—the working and lower-middle classes—over the work process with which they are involved, the economic wealth that they produce, and the political institutions that they pay for.*"

A study on the relationship between social status and health in the USA and the UK showed that within each country, lower socio-economic status meant worse health. Furthermore, the greatest health inequalities were among those of lowest socio-economic status who had the least education and income (Banks et al., 2006) and who lived in more precarious circumstances, experiencing less healthy conditions. Berkman and Epstein (2008) studied socio-economic inequalities in health in 22 European countries and concluded that there is a universal link across countries between social class and mortality, no matter the differing disease prevalence or risk factors in each country.

NOTE: We will discuss this in more detail in Chapter 3. Of note, inequities in health outcomes are not only a direct consequence of socio-economic inequalities, but also due to poorer communities having lesser access to effective health care.

Figure 2.20 shows that although the infant mortality rate in the USA decreased between 2007 and 2017 (from 6.75 per 1000 live births in 2007 to 5.79 in 2017), there were disparities by race and Hispanic origin. In 2017, the highest rate was 10.88 per 1000 live births for infants of non-Hispanic Black mothers and 8.90 per 1000 live births for infants of non-Hispanic American Indian or Alaska Native women. This was twice the rate for non-Hispanic Asian or Pacific Islander women (4.03 per 1000 live births). Infant deaths of non-Hispanic white women were 4.69 per 1000 live births (Chartbook, 2018).

Social status is an important factor in mortality, even among people in relatively affluent societies. Studies demonstrate that around the world, those in the higher income bracket are better able to avoid premature death, and this advantage is not linked to any known precise diseases and risk factor (Marmot & Shipley, 1996):

- In 2006 in the USA, the difference in life expectancy between Black men who were poor in downtown Washington, DC and White men who were well-off in Montgomery County, Maryland was 20 years, and yet, the two areas are just a short metro ride away from each other (Marmot, 2006).

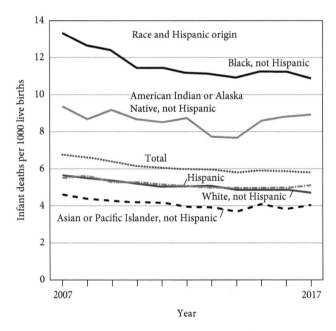

Fig. 2.20 Infant mortality rates by race and Hispanic origin of mother, USA, 2007–2017.
Source: National Center for Health Statistics. (2019). *Health, United States, 2018*. NCHS: Hyattsville, MD, p. 7.

- In 2008 in London, UK, in less than half an hour you could go from the relatively affluent area of Westminster, where male life expectancy was 78 years, to the poorer area of Canning Town, where male life expectancy was 72 years—a difference of six years (Cheshire, 2012).

NOTE: We will discuss these differences in life expectancy and social status in greater detail in Chapter 3.

Interestingly, **social exclusion** also seems to influence life expectancy. For example, Yearby et al. report that:

During the 1918 flu pandemic, 'American Indians experienced a disease specific mortality rate of four times that of other ethnic groups', whereas during the 2009 H1N1 pandemic American Indian and Alaska Natives' mortality rate from H1N1 was four times that of all other racial and ethnic minority populations combined. During the COVID-19 pandemic, although Native Americans are only 11% of the population in New Mexico, they account for nearly 37% of the COVID-19 infections and 26% of the deaths. Racial and ethnic minorities are disproportionately impacted during pandemics, not due to any biological difference between races, but rather as a result of social factors (Yearby et al., 2020).

GLOSSARY

Social exclusion: not having access to the same rights and privileges as the dominant social group, as a result of belonging to a minority social group.

In the UK, the risk factors for COVID-19 deaths are much higher for those living in deprived and overcrowded housing, as well as for key workers who are in close contact with others, for those from Black, Asian and minority ethnic (BAME) groups, and for those who are older, male and living with co-morbidities or underlying health conditions. In addition, "*living outside the South of England is also a higher risk. And the risks are cumulative*" (Marmot et al., 2020).

What lies behind this social gradient in mortality? According to Marmot (2006), the gradient is broader than that of poverty and health. It is related to where people stand in the social hierarchy and what this means in terms of their social exclusion and their access (or lack of access) to opportunity, empowerment, security and dignity.

After 30 years of research into the relationship between health and social problems and average income and inequality in 23 of the world's richest countries and within US states, epidemiologists Wilkinson and Pickett (2009) found that there is only a weak relationship between average income and social and health problems, but that health and social problems increase with greater inequality. Those countries with more equality do better than those with the greatest levels of inequality:

> *The problems in rich countries are not caused by the society being rich enough (or even being too rich) but by the scale of material differences between people within each society being too big. What matters is where we stand in relation to others in society* (Wilkinson & Pickett, 2009, p. 25).

They conclude that inequality is what makes countries sick, and as such it is a public health issue.

> *... as well as health and violence, almost all the problems that are common at the bottom of the social ladder are more common in more unequal societies—including mental illness, drug addiction, obesity, loss of community life, imprisonment, unequal opportunities and poorer wellbeing for children. The effects of inequality are not confined to the poor. A growing body of research shows that inequality damages the social fabric of the whole society. When he found how far up the income scale the health effects of inequality went, Harvard professor Ichiro Kawachi, one of the foremost researchers in this field, described inequality as a social pollutant* (Wilkinson & Pickett, 2009).

Conclusion

The disease patterns and living conditions in industrialised countries of the nineteenth century were similar to those we see today in underdeveloped countries.

The improvement of health conditions in industrialised countries was not so much a matter of advances in medical science. Instead, improvements in social and economic conditions and public health interventions were crucial to this improvement.

Instead of poor countries following the same epidemiological transition as rich countries, the current evolution is towards a growing epidemiological polarisation between rich and poor—not only between rich and poor countries but also between people who are rich and those who are poor within all countries.

Poverty is an important underlying factor for health problems in poor countries. However, social status seems to be the determining factor in this growing polarisation.

Inequities in health are attributed to a social gradient: with people with lower social status living in more precarious circumstances and experiencing less healthy conditions and less access to effective quality health care. This phenomenon can be observed on a global scale across the developed and underdeveloped world, as well as within individual countries.

References

Almond, D. & Currie, J. (2011). Killing me softly: the fetal origins hypothesis. *Journal of Economic Perspectives*, 25(3):153–172. doi:10.1257/jep.25.3.153.

ASH (Action on Smoking and Health). (2019). *ASH Fact Sheet: Tobacco and the Developing World*. ASH: London.

Banks, J., Marmot, M., Oldfield, Z. & Smith, J.P. (2006). Disease and disadvantage in the United States and in England. *JAMA*, 295:2037–2045.

Beaglehole, R. & Yach, D. (2003). Globalisation and the prevention and control of non-communicable diseases: the neglected chronic diseases of adults. *The Lancet*, 362:903–908.

Berkman, L. & Epstein, A. (2008). Beyond health care—socioeconomic status and health. *The New England Journal of Medicine*, 5:358(23):2509–2510. doi:10.1056/NEJMe0802773.

Bradley, D.J. (1974). *In Human Rights in Health. CIBA Foundation Symposium 23*. Elsevier: Amsterdam.

Chartbook. (2018). Health, United States, 2018. https://www.ncbi.nlm.nih.gov/books/nbk551097/pdf/bookshelf_nbk551097.pdf. Accessed 10 January 2021.

Cheshire, J. (2012). Lives on the line: life expectancy and child poverty as a tube map. https://jcheshire.com/featured-maps/lives-on-the-line/.

Chopra, M. & Sanders, D. (2004). From apartheid to globalisation: health and social change in South Africa. *Hygiea Internationalis—An Interdisciplinary Journal for the History of Public Health*, 4(1), Special Issue.

Colgrove, J. (2002). The McKeown thesis: a historical controversy and its enduring influence. *American Journal of Public Health*, 92(5):725–729.

Davey Smith, G. & Lynch, J. (2004). Commentary: social capital, social epidemiology and disease aetiology. *International Journal of Epidemiology*, 33(4):691–700; discussion 705–709.

Disease Control Priorities Project. (2006). Disease Control Priorities in Developing Countries (DCP2). The World Bank and Oxford University Press.

Engels, F. (1845/1987). *The Condition of the Working Class in England in 1844*. First published Germany, 1845. English translation first published 1886. Republished with some revisions and edited by Victor Kiernan. Penguin Books: New York, pp. 171–184.

Ezzati, M., Vander Hoorn, S., Lawes, C.M.M., et al. (2005). Rethinking the 'diseases of affluence' paradigm: global patterns of nutritional risks in relation to economic development. *PLoS Med* 3:e133.

FAO, IFAD, UNICEF, WFP & WHO. (2019). *The State of Food Security and Nutrition in the World 2019. Safeguarding Against Economic Slowdowns and Downturns*. FAO: Rome. https://docs.wfp.org/api/documents/wfp-0000106760/download/?_ga=2.28862268.1865697046.1610094946-1568228876.1610094946. Accessed 10 January 2021.

Frenk, J., Bobadilla, J.L., Sepúlveda, J. & Cervantes, L.M. (1989). Health transition in middle-income countries: new challenges for health care. *Health Policy and Planning*, 4(1):29–39.

Frenk, J., Bobadilla, J.L., Stern, C., Frejka, T. & Lozano, R. (1991). Elements for a theory of the health transition. *Health Transition Review: The Cultural, Social, and Behavioural Determinants of Health*, 1(1):21–38.

GBD 2019 Diseases and Injuries Collaborators. (2020). Global burden of 369 diseases and injuries in 204 countries and territories, 1990–2019: a systematic analysis for the Global Burden of Disease Study 2019. *The Lancet*, 396:1204–1222.

Hamlin, C. & Sheard, S. (1998). Revolutions in public health: 1848, and 1998? *BMJ*, 317:587–591.

IHME. (2019). Tackling inequality could save millions of children. http://www.healthdata.org/news-release/tackling-inequality-could-save-millions-children.

Iskandar, W.J., Sukardi, W. & Soenarto, Y. (2015). Risk of nutritional status on diarrhea among under five children. *Paediatrica Indonesia*, 55(4):235–238.

Leon, D.A., Walt, G. & Gilson, L. (2001). International perspectives on health inequalities and policy. *BMJ*, 322:591–594.

Macdonald, S. & Johnson, G. (eds.). (2017). Mayes' Midwifery E-Book, Elsevier Limited.

Marmot, M. (2006). Health in an unequal world. *The Lancet*, 368:2081–2094.

Marmot, M. & Shipley, M.J. (1996). Do socioeconomic differences in mortality persist after retirement? 25 years follow up of civil servants from the first Whitehall study. *BMJ*, 313:1177–1180.

Marmot, M., Allen. J., Goldblatt, P., Herd, E. & Morrison, J. (2020). *Build Back Fairer: The COVID 19 Marmot Review. The Pandemic, Socioeconomic and Health Inequalities in England, Executive Summary*. Institute of Health Equity: London.

McKeown, T. (1976). The Modern Rise of World Population. Edward Arnold: London.

Morley, D. (1973). *Paediatric Priorities in the Developing World*. Butterworths: London.

Morley, D. & Woodland, M. (1979). *See How They Grow: Monitoring Child Growth for Appropriate Health Care in Developing Countries*. Macmillan: London.

Murphy, M., Bobak, M., Nicholson, A., Rose, R. & Marmot, M. (2006). The widening gap in mortality by educational level in the Russian Federation, 1980–2001. *American Journal of Public Health*, 96:1293–1299.

National Center for Health Statistics. (2019). *Health, United States, 2018*. NCHS: Hyattsville, MD.

Navarro, V. (1976). The underdevelopment of health of working America: causes, consequences and possible solutions. *American Journal of Public Health*, 66(6):538–547.

OECD. (2015). Conflict, fragility and resilience. http://www.oecd.org/dac/conflict-fragility-resilience/.

Omran, A. (1971). The epidemiologic transition: a theory of the epidemiology of population change. *Millbank Memorial Fund Quarterly*, 49(1971):509–538.

Packard, R.M. (2011). *The Making of a Tropical Disease: A Short History of Malaria (John Hopkins Biographies of Disease)*. Johns Hopkins University Press: Baltimore.

Patel, V., Chatterji, S.L., Chisholm, D., et al. (2011). Chronic diseases and injuries in India. The Lancet, 377(9763):413–428.

Ponnampalam, M. (1992). *Fourth World: The Third World Within the First World—Implementing Racial Hygiene in the Late Twentieth Century*. United Kingdom Council for Human Rights: London.

Rossen, L.M., Branum, A.M., Ahmad, F.B., Sutton, P. & Anderson, R.N. (2020). Excess deaths associated with COVID-19, by age and race and ethnicity—United States, January 26–October 3, 2020. *MMWR Morbidity and Mortality Weekly Report*, 69:1522–1527.

Sanders, D., Bradshaw, D. & Ngongo, N. (2009). The status of child health. In: Kibel, M., Lake, L., Pendlebury, S. & Smith, C. (eds). *South African Child Gauge 2009/2010*. Cape Town: Children's Institute, University of Cape Town.

Save the Children. (2012). Nutrition in the first 1,000 days—state of the world's mothers 2012. https://reliefweb.int/report/world/nutrition-first-1000-days-state-worlds-mothers-2012.

Stuteville, S. (2008). Kenyans tap sun to make dirty water sparkle. https://womensenews.org/author/sarah-stuteville/.

The Health of Towns Magazine and Journal of Medical Jurisprudence. (1847–48). [RCSE] v.1-v.2 [1847-48]. W. Fletcher: London. https://wellcomecollection.org/works/r2s9q8wa.

Thompson, E.P. (1968). *The Making of the English Working Class*. Pelican: London, p. 359.

UN-Habitat. (2021). Housing. The challenge. https://unhabitat.org/topic/housing. Accessed 10 January 2021.

UNICEF. (2013). *Levels and trends in child mortality. Report 2013. Estimates developed by the UN Inter-Agency Group for Child Mortality Estimation.* UNICEF: New York. https://data.uni cef.org/resources/levels-trends-child-mortality-report-2013/.

UNICEF. (2015a). *Committing to Child Survival: A Promise Renewed. Progress Report 2015.* UNICEF: New York. https://www.unicef.org/health/index_maternalhealth.html.

UNICEF. (2015b). *Levels and trends in child mortality. Report 2015. Estimates developed by the UN Inter-agency Group for Child Mortality Estimation United Nations.* UNICEF: New York. https://data.unicef.org/resources/levels-and-trends-in-child-mortality-2015/.

UNICEF. (2016). Levels and trends in child malnutrition UNICEF/WHO/World Bank Group Joint Child Malnutrition Estimates Key findings of the 2016 edition.

UNICEF. (2019a). Levels and trends in child mortality. Report 2019. Estimates developed by the UN Inter-agency Group for Child Mortality Estimation United Nations. https://www.unicef.org/reports/levels-and-trends-child-mortality-report-2019. Accessed 10 January 2021.

UNICEF. (2019b). Low birthweight. https://data.unicef.org/topic/nutrition/low-birthweight/ Accessed 10 January 2021.

UNICEF. (2020). Malnutrition. https://data.unicef.org/topic/nutrition/malnutrition/. Accessed 10 January 2021.

UNICEF & WHO. (2019). Progress on household drinking water, sanitation and hygiene: 2000–2017: special focus on inequalities. https://www.who.int/water_sanitation_health/publicati ons/jmp-2019-full-report.pdf. Accessed 10 January 2021.

Victora, C.G., Christian, P., VIdaletti, L.P., Gatica Domínguez, G., Menon, P. & Black, R.E. (2021). Revisiting maternal and child undernutrition in low-income and middle-income countries: variable progress towards an unfinished agenda. Maternal and Child Undernutrition Progress 1. *The Lancet*, 397(10282):1388–1399.

Virchow, R. & Reinhardt, B. (1848). Reports about the typhus epidemic in Upper Silesia, 1848. *Archiv für Pathologische Anatomie und Physiologie und für Klinische Medicin*, 2(2):248.

WHO. (2014a). *Injuries and Violence: The Facts 2014.* WHO, Geneva.

WHO. (2014b). Social determinants of health: Differences in causes of death between rich and poor countries. https://www.who.int/news-room/questions-and-answers/item/what-are-the-main-differences-between-rich-and-poor-countries-with-respect-to-cau ses-of-death.

WHO. (2017). *Ten Years in Public Health 2007–2017: report by Dr Margaret Chan, Director-General.* WHO, Geneva.

WHO. (2018). *WHO Global Report on Trends in Prevalence of Tobacco Smoking 2000–2025*, 2nd edn. WHO, Geneva.

WHO. (2019). *Trends in Maternal Mortality 2000 to 2017: Estimates by WHO, UNICEF, UNFPA, World Bank Group and the United Nations Population Division.* WHO: Geneva.

WHO. (2020a). The Global Health Observatory. Global health estimates: Leading causes of death, Cause-specific mortality, 2000–2019. https://www.who.int/data/gho/data/the mes/mortality-and-global-health-estimates/ghe-leading-causes-of-death. Accessed 10 January 2021.

WHO. (2020b). Newborns: improving survival and well-being. https://www.who.int/news-room/fact-sheets/detail/newborns-reducing-mortality. Accessed 10 January 2021.

WHO. (2021). WHO Coronavirus (COVID-19) Dashboard. https://covid19.who.int/. Accessed 3 May 2021.

Wilkinson, R. & Pickett, K. (2009). *The Spirit Level: Why Equality Is Better for Everyone.* Penguin: London.

World Bank. (2007). World Development Indicators 2007. Washington, DC. https://openkn owledge.worldbank.org/handle/10986/8150.

World Bank. (2018). Where do the world's poorest people live today? https://datatopics.worldb ank.org/world-development-indicators/stories/where-do-the-worlds-poorest-people-live-today.html. Accessed 10 January 2021.

Yearby, R. & Mohapatra, S. (2020). Law, structural racism, and the COVID-19 pandemic. *Journal of Law and the Biosciences*, 7(1):lsaa036.

3

Health, Population and Inequality

Chapter 2 highlighted how rather than following the same epidemiological transition as wealthy countries, the current evolution of poor countries is towards a growing epidemiological polarisation between people who are rich and those who are poor—*between* and *within* both the low-income and high-income countries of the world.

What historical factors and events explain this widening inequality and its consequences for the health of populations? What lessons can we learn by looking back at the measures taken by developed, industrialised countries to promote the health of their populations? Can these measures be used in poor, underdeveloped countries today?

To explore the answers to these questions, it is first worth looking at why and how nutrition and general living conditions improved in Europe in the nineteenth and twentieth centuries, resulting in a decline in many diseases. Circumstances in England and Wales for this period are particularly well documented (see Figure 3.1 as an example), and so they will be used as the main source of information.

The developed world: a historical perspective

The Agricultural Revolution

The long, slow improvement in English living standards started around the early to mid-eighteenth century, with a revolution in agricultural production. This fulfilled two important requirements of the subsequent Industrial Revolution: adequate food supplies and an increasingly urban population.

During feudal times, most of the population was engaged in agriculture, with 90% of food being home produced. The British revolutionary Parliament of the 1640s abolished the last legal remains of the old feudal tenures, clearing the way for more efficient, capitalist, profit-oriented agriculture. Parliament ordered that common land that had long been used for semi-communal pasture and cultivation be enclosed or fenced off into larger units, which could then be taken over by large private landlords. Between 1761 and 1801, over 3 million acres of land were enclosed and used for crops, particularly corn (Hobsbawm, 1969).

The main effect of this enclosure was to dispossess peasants and **cottagers** of their land, bringing mass poverty to rural England. Some peasants and cottagers became farm labourers; others relied on **Poor Law** relief. By far the largest part of the rural population was driven to the cities to become the factory fodder for the Industrial Revolution (see Figure 3.2).

The Struggle for Health. David Sanders with Wim De Ceukelaire and Barbara Hutton, Oxford University Press.
© Oxford University Press 2023. DOI: 10.1093/oso/9780192858450.003.0003

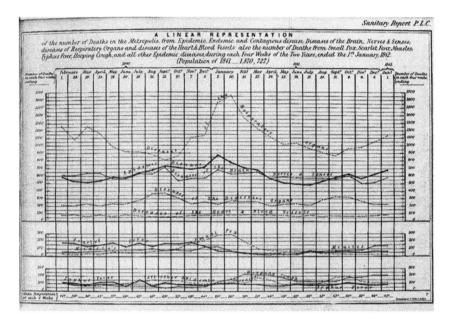

Fig. 3.1 Sanitary Report, 1842: Report to Her Majesty's principal secretary of state for the Home Department from the Poor Law Commissioners, on an inquiry into the sanitary condition of the labouring population of Great Britain; with appendices. Presented to both Houses of Parliament, by command of Her Majesty, July 1842 (by Edwin Chadwick).

Source: Wellcome Collection. Attribution 4.0 International (CC BY 4.0).

https://wellcomecollection.org/works/rjddxkae.

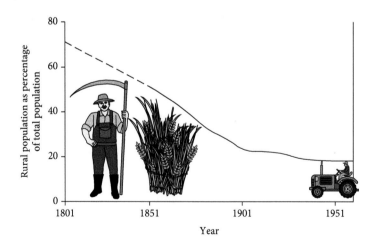

Fig. 3.2 Urbanisation of the English population.

GLOSSARY

Cottagers: from the 1600s most production was done at home in cottage industries. Whole families worked together to produce cloth for the cities.

Poor Laws: a system of poor relief for older adults, people who were destitute, sick or living with a mental health condition. In the nineteenth century they could only receive assistance if they entered a workhouse, where conditions were deliberately harsh so as to discourage people from claiming assistance.

The agrarian revolution had dire social consequences for many, but it undoubtedly brought about a qualitative rise in efficiency. Market gardening and intensive fruit farming date from the mid-seventeenth century and *"brought about a minor revolution in the diet of ordinary citizens"* (Hill, 1967).

The Industrial Revolution

The Industrial Revolution radically transformed the way production was organised. Small farmers and self-employed spinners and weavers were unable to compete with large capitalist industries and were forced into factories in the towns. Production became increasingly centralised, using modern technology like steam power, which made production cheaper and more efficient and led to a massive expansion of output.

Much of the necessary capital came from private landlords and farmers who ploughed their profits back into their industries. Another important supply of capital was from overseas trade. But the single most important source of English trade revenue was the barbarous traffic in human beings from Africa to the Americas. Hardly a voice was raised in protest against the slave trade until English merchants ceased to profit by it. This will be discussed later in this chapter in the section, 'Colonialism and the slave trade'.

Without the exploitation of the non-European world, the Industrial Revolution could not have happened in the form or in the place that it did. For decades, cotton imported from slave production in the USA and from plantations in India was the spearhead of industrialisation and the manufacturing of cotton cloth products. Until 1770 more than 90% of British cotton exports went to colonial markets. Even much later, in the second quarter of the nineteenth century, cotton products accounted for half of British exports. The cotton industry, based on colonial imports and exports, in turn stimulated industry in other sectors.

Effects of the Agricultural and Industrial Revolutions

For most people, the consequences of the Agricultural and Industrial Revolutions were profound. The rapid movement of the rural population to towns and cities that had limited facilities gave rise to horrific conditions, with dire consequences for people's health. Overcrowding, filth and squalor existed on a scale seen today only in the towns of the underdeveloped world (see Figure 3.3A and B).

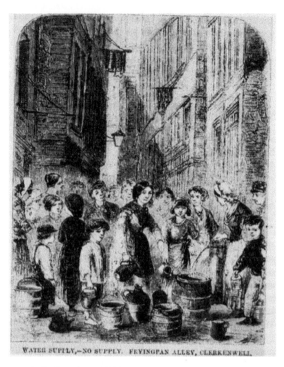

Fig. 3.3A Water supply in London, 1862.
Source: Wellcome Trustees.

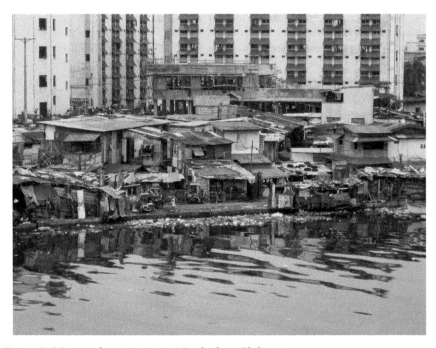

Fig. 3.3B Water and sanitation in a Manila slum, Philippines.
Source: Wim De Ceukelaire.

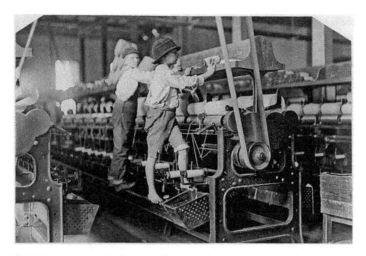

Fig. 3.4 Child labourers worked 14 to 15 hours a day.
Source: Lewis Hine (Public domain), via Wikimedia Commons.

Massive unemployment of the urban poor allowed employers to exploit workers cruelly. Even young children were forced to perform heavy manual work for 14–15 hours a day and were whipped if they faltered. Conditions were so harsh that eventually the Cotton Mills and Factories Act was passed, forbidding the employment of children younger than nine years and limiting daily working hours of 9-year-olds to 16-year-olds to 'only' 12 hours (see Figure 3.4).

Popular pressure: the emerging social movements

There was widespread discontent among the masses of the people who had been dispossessed of land or displaced from individual domestic production and forced into industry, particularly when it was difficult to get jobs. This discontent caused riots and strikes, which often provoked brutal repression. However, it also resulted in more organised forms of popular pressure, such as the formation of trade unions and other workers' movements, which together with social reformers forced certain concessions and reforms. Pressure from labour organisations and social reformers resulted in higher wages and improvements in the appalling working conditions.

The high death rates from infectious diseases, and particularly from four major cholera epidemics between 1830 and 1866, created public unrest, illustrated by the poster of 1832 (see Figure 3.5).

As these cholera epidemics affected the middle class (who had the vote) as well as the working class (who did not), Parliament reluctantly passed the 1848 Public Health Act. This provided for a General Board of Health and Local Boards of Health. However, both these bodies remained steeped in the punitive Poor Law outlook towards health care. But even these bodies were too much for Parliament, which first reduced the powers of the General Board and then dissolved it altogether. The Local

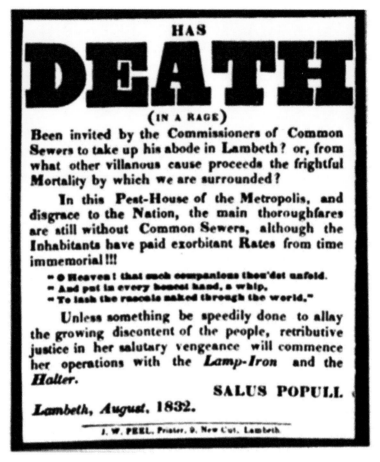

Fig. 3.5 An 1832 poster on sanitary conditions.
Source: Wellcome Trustees.

Boards remained, and in 1870 Parliament passed new reforming legislation, which finally meant that every local area was covered by some type of body that was responsible for sanitary measures.

It was a decade that saw several important environmental provisions which all resulted in health improvements—water supply, sewage disposal, control of slaughtering of animals, development of parks and open spaces, isolation hospitals and the beginning of housing control—as well as the beginning of compulsory education.

The Long Depression

Ironically, the Long Depression—a worldwide price and economic recession that began in the 1870s—meant an improvement in some working-class living standards, with the rise of the value of **real wages**. Eating habits underwent a further important transformation. Meat and tea consumption rose significantly, and working-class people began to eat fruit. The decade even saw the first appearance of that great British institution—the fish and chip shop!

GLOSSARY

Real wages: wages adjusted for inflation; or wages in terms of the amount of goods and services that can be bought.

However, public expenditure on social services other than education was minimal. It was, in fact, the increasing polarisation of wealth and living conditions between people who were rich and those who were poor that led to a revival of militant trade unionism in the 1880s and the formation of a mass independent working-class party—the Labour Party—at the turn of the century.

In short, *health promotion* was the result of improvements in living conditions. These improvements did not always come about *automatically* with economic progress. People had to fight for them. Health promotion was by far the most important component in the major improvements in the health of the population of Britain and in other industrialised countries since the eighteenth century.

Living conditions in England today

As we saw in Chapter 2, even today living conditions in England (as in most developed countries) are not uniformly good across the population. As an example, in the financial year ending 2016, the wealthiest fifth of the population (top income quintile group) had an average income of £85 000 per year compared with £7000 for the poorest fifth, before direct taxes and cash benefits. This is a ratio of nearly 12:1 (see Figure 3.6) (Office for National Statistics, UK, 2017).

GLOSSARY

Equivalisation: the process of accounting for the fact that households with many members are likely to need a higher income to achieve the same standard of living as households with fewer members (Office for National Statistics, UK).

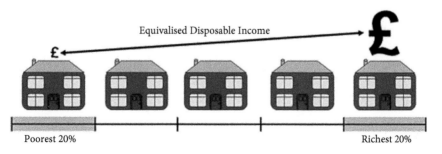

Equivalised Disposable Income

Poorest 20%   Richest 20%

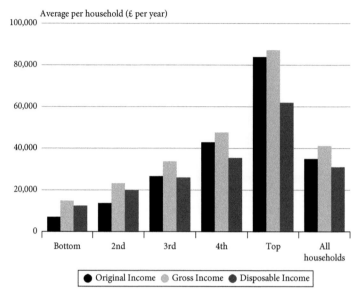

Fig. 3.6 Original (includes earnings, private pensions and investments), gross and disposable income by quintile group, all households, in the financial year ending 2016. **Note:** Households are grouped into quintiles (or fifths) based on their equivalised disposable income. The richest quintile is the 20% of households with the highest equivalised disposable income. Similarly, the poorest quintile is the 20% of households with the lowest equivalised disposable income.
Source: Office for National Statistics, UK licensed under Open Government Licence v.1.0.

Inequalities in health and wealth

Physician and epidemiologist Michael Marmot established a strong link between social class and mortality in the famous 1967–1977 Whitehall study of British male civil servants between 20 and 64 years old. He found that:

- The lower a civil servant's position in the hierarchy, the higher their risk of disease and death from all causes, but specifically from coronary heart disease.
- Men in the lowest grade (messengers, doorkeepers, etc.) had a mortality rate three times higher than those in the highest grade (administrators).
- Everyone who was not at the top of the hierarchy had worse health than those at the top of the hierarchy (see Figure 3.7).

There were clear employment grade differences in health-risk behaviours including smoking, diet, and exercise, in economic circumstances, in possible effects of early-life environment as reflected by height, in social circumstances at work (e.g. monotonous work characterised by low control and low satisfaction), and in social supports (Marmot et al., 1991).

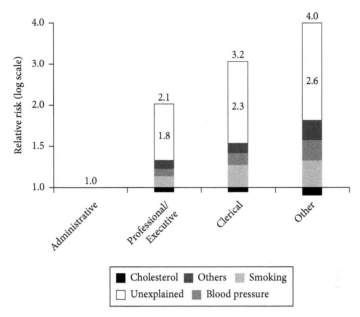

Fig. 3.7 Relationship between job grade and mortality – congestive heart disease (CHD). *Source*: Marmot et al. (1978).

In 2008, the London Health Observatory used the London tube (underground train) as a way of illustrating the link between wealth and health. It showed that if you caught the Jubilee tube line, more than a year of life expectancy was lost for every tube station between the wealthy Westminster area travelling eastwards to the poorer area of Canning Town.

In 2012, James Cheshire created a tube map for the London network called *Lives on the Line*. He explained:

The map shows two key statistics: 1) the life expectancy at birth of those living around each London Underground, London Overground and Docklands Light Railway (DLR) station; and 2) the rank of each London ward on the spectrum of Income Deprivation Affecting Children Index (IDACI). The inclusion of the IDACI rank highlights the linkage between deprivation and life expectancy, which is especially poignant in this context as it demonstrates that, without significant social change … the fates of many children living in the poorest parts of London are seemingly already sealed (Cheshire, 2012).

So, for example, newborns near Oxford Circus were predicted to live on average for 96 years, while those around Kentish Town were predicted to live on average for 76 years—a 20-year difference in life expectancy (see Figure 3.8).

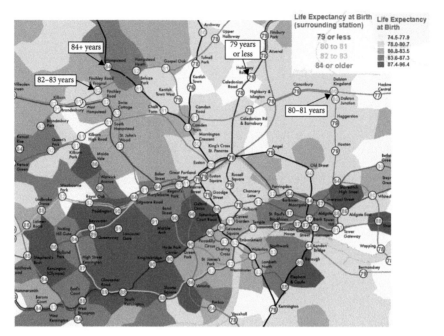

Fig. 3.8 Life expectancy (in years) mapped by London Tube stops.

Source: Created by James Cheshire (2012).

https://jcheshire.com/featured-maps/lives-on-the-line/.

Marmot's research on life expectancy in Britain and other areas of the world corroborates this 'ridiculously large' gap in life expectancy. In Glasgow, Scotland, for example:

> *If a man dies in his prime in Calton, a down-at-heel part of Glasgow, it may be a tragedy, but it's not a surprise. Actually, the question of what constitutes his 'prime' in Calton is moot. Life expectancy for men, when I first looked at figures from 1998–2002, was fifty-four. In Lenzie, a much more upmarket place a few kilometres away, 'in his prime' has an altogether different meaning: life expectancy for men was eighty-two. That converts to a twenty-eight-year gap life expectancy in one Scottish city (Marmot, 2015).*

The 28-year gap that Marmot refers to in the above quote was taken from data in the 1970s and 1980s. Today the figure is probably closer to 20 years, which is the same as that between women in India and women in the USA.

> *The social gradient in life expectancy runs all the way from top to bottom. It doesn't just feel better at the top. It is better. At the top, not only do you live longer but the quality of life is better—you spend more years free from disability ... 'Disability' here is quite broadly defined: any limiting long-standing illness ... (Marmot, 2015).*

These major differences in social status and disease and death occur across the British population—both in the cities and smaller communities.

> There is ample evidence that social factors, including education, employment status, income level, gender and ethnicity have a marked influence on how healthy a person is. In all countries—whether low-, middle- or high-income—there are wide disparities in the health status of different social groups. The lower an individual's socio-economic position, the higher their risk of poor health (WHO, 2018a).

This reinforces the conclusion *that it is living and working conditions that are most important in determining the health of populations*. The material conditions in which people "*are born, grow, live, work and age*" make them more, or less, vulnerable to germs, diseases and health conditions (Marmot, 2005). These conditions are called the social determinants of health (see Figure 3.9).

GLOSSARY

Social determinants of health: "*The conditions in which people live and die, [which] are in turn shaped by political, social and economic forces*" (Marmot, 2005).

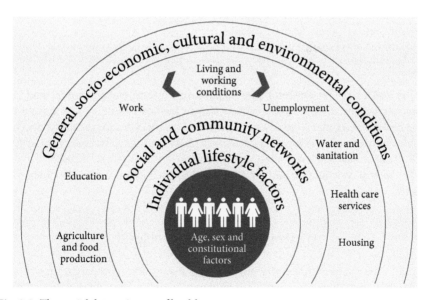

Fig. 3.9 The social determinants of health.
Source: Dahlgren, G. & Whitehead, M. (1991). *Policies and Strategies to Promote Social Equity in Health*. Institute of Future Studies: Stockholm.

What of the medical contribution?

The decline in death rate from the mid-nineteenth century onwards was overwhelmingly due to a reduction in the prevalence and effects of communicable diseases. Most of this was achieved through social change and an improvement in living standards and hygiene—*health promotion*. Considerably less of this mortality reduction was because of specific preventive and curative medical measures.

Different theorists attribute the fall in mortality to either rising living standards and improved diet and nutrition (McKeown & Lowe, 1974) or to "*the public health movement working through local government*" (Szreter, 1988). According to Szreter, improvements in working and living conditions during the economic, social and political transitions in nineteenth-century England were due to increasing state intervention in social provisioning, "*albeit differentially for different social groups—and with that the long, slow and substantial improvement of the health of their populations*" (Chopra & Sanders, 2004).

Before the twentieth century, it is unlikely that immunisation or therapy had a significant effect on mortality from infectious diseases, apart from the smallpox vaccination, compulsorily enforced in 1871. Rather, between 1900 and 1935 the following measures contributed to the prevention or cure of some diseases:

- Antitoxin in treatment of diphtheria.
- Surgery in appendicitis, peritonitis and ear infections.
- Salvarsan in the treatment of syphilis.
- Intravenous therapy in diarrhoea.
- Immunisation against tetanus.
- Improved hygiene in obstetric care resulting in prevention of puerperal fever.

After 1935, the first powerful chemotherapeutic agents, sulphonamides and later antibiotics were used, as well as improved vaccines. Medical care only became accessible to the broad masses after World War II, when modern social security was introduced in Europe. In Britain, the National Health Service (NHS) was set up in 1948, making good medical care available to everyone instead of only to those who could afford it.

The medical contribution and the NHS are discussed in more detail in Chapters 4, 5 and 6.

What of the 'population problem'?

Britain in the nineteenth century also gives an insight into population growth and composition, which will be considered later in relation to the underdeveloped world in the section, 'The underdeveloped world: a historical perspective'.

When it was first recorded in 1086 in the *Doomsday Book*, the population in England and Wales was 1.5 million. In the next six centuries it more than trebled, to 4.5 million. The population increased from 9 million in 1801 to 33 million in 1901. So, it seems that the English too have experienced a 'population explosion'!

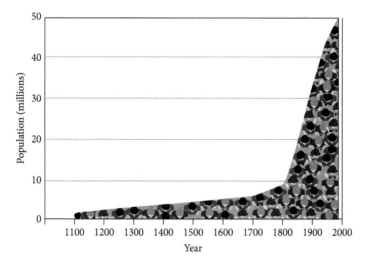

Fig. 3.10 Growth of population of England and Wales (1100 to 2000).
Source: Blackwell Scientific Publications, Oxford.

It is possible to interpret the causes of the rise in the population using the information available since 1838, when births and deaths were first registered. Mortality remained fairly constant between 1838 and 1870 and then began to decline.

The continuous growth of population since 1838 and the particularly rapid growth between 1840 and 1910 were because of more births than deaths (see Figure 3.10). After 1838 there was a decline in the very high death rate, but the birth rate remained high. At first, this decline in the death rate was small, and up to 1900 only dropped significantly in the 2- to 34-age group. After 1900, death rates in the very young and old also fell.

As we have seen, most of the decline in the death rate was due to a decrease in deaths from infectious diseases (see Figure 3.11), mainly due to social changes and health promotion.

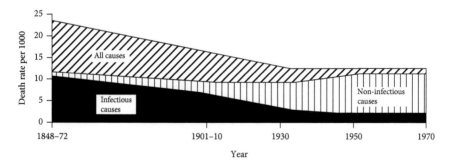

Fig. 3.11 Mean annual death rates (males) and causes, England and Wales (1848 to 1970).
Source: Blackwell Scientific Publications, Oxford.

The fall in the very high birth rate only began in about 1880. It was in the period between 1840 and 1880 that the most rapid population growth occurred. This makes sense, because when both death rates and birth rates are high, only a small fall in the death rate is necessary to cause a rapid increase in population.

Death rates in all age groups, particularly in young children, continued to fall until the mid-twentieth century, with a parallel fall in the birth rate. This meant that the rate of population growth began to slow down.

This change from high death rates matched by high birth rates, to low death rates with still high birth rates, then finally to low death rates with low birth rates, is called the demographic transition. A similar process occurred in all the now developed countries, which are said to be in the late phase of this demographic transition, while underdeveloped countries are in the early phase.

Today, some developed countries are experiencing a negative or zero natural population growth—where there are more deaths than births, or an even number of deaths and births (the figures do not include the impact of immigration or emigration). Among those with the highest decrease in natural birth rate are Ukraine, Russia, Germany and Greece. The only non-European country on the list is Japan, where it is expected that there will be a 21% decrease in the population size by 2050.

Typically, there is a decline in the high death rate, followed by a lag period and then a slower decline in the high fertility. The length of this lag period varies from country to country, one factor being the size and variability of the country (see Figure 3.12).

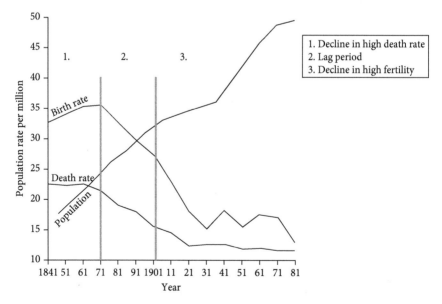

Fig. 3.12 Birth rates, death rates and population, England and Wales (1841 to 1981).
Source: McKeown & Lowe (1974).

Population pyramid

Another important factor in the growth of populations is their *structure*. In 1841, when the UK was in the early phase of the demographic transition, approximately half its population was under 20 years of age. By 2020, it had an ageing population, with 70.88% being over 24 years (see Figure 3.13A). Compare this with the population of Malawi in 2020, which was in a relatively early phase of the demographic transition, where 66.38% of the population was under 24 years of age and approximately 34% was over 25 years (see Figure 3.13B).

We will discuss these differences later in the section, 'The underdeveloped world: a historical perspective'.

GLOSSARY

Population pyramid: the age and gender structure of a country's population. It can be represented as a graph, with the population distributed along the horizontal axis, with males shown on the left and females on the right, represented as horizontal bars along the vertical axis. The youngest age groups are at the bottom and the oldest at the top. The shape of the population pyramid gradually evolves over time based on fertility, mortality and international migration trends.

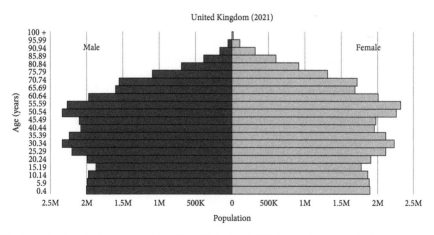

Fig. 3.13A Population pyramid of the UK in 2021 (70.88% of the population over 24 years).

Source: US Census Bureau, International Data Base.

https://www.census.gov/data-tools/demo/idb/#/country?COUNTRY_YEAR=2021&COUNTRY_YR_A NIM=2021&FIPS_SINGLE=UK.

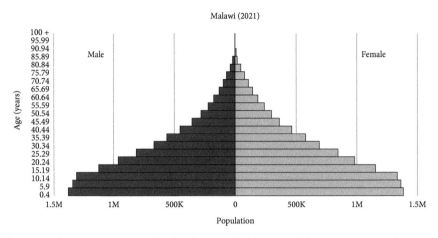

Fig. 3.13B Population pyramid of Malawi, 2021 (66.31% of the population under 24 years of age).

Source: US Census Bureau, International Data Base.

https://www.census.gov/data-tools/demo/idb/#/country?COUNTRY_YEAR=2021&COUNTRY_YR_A NIM=2021&FIPS_SINGLE=UK.

The underdeveloped world: a historical perspective

With the transformation of social, economic and demographic structures, the epidemiological transition in England and Wales from the nineteenth century onwards followed a linear movement away from the dominance of undernutrition and communicable or infectious diseases linked to poverty, to a profile of predominantly NCDs. (See Chapter 2 for more on the epidemiological transition.)

Underdeveloped countries have not followed the same epidemiological pattern. Instead, in many countries 'combined and uneven development' exists, where a highly developed, technologically advanced and wealthy sector lives alongside a large, poor population who live in squalor (Chopra & Sanders, 2004).

This dual socio-economic situation is reflected in the double, or triple, burden of disease, where people living in poverty simultaneously have a high burden of morbidity and mortality from infectious diseases, NCDs, and trauma and violence and where people who are wealthy being mainly affected by NCDs. As we saw in Chapter 2, this growing epidemiological polarisation exists between people who are rich and those who are poor both *across* and *within* countries.

Why does 'combined and uneven development' exist across all countries and why is it most stark in the underdeveloped world? Why have substantial and sustained improvements in living conditions and thus health promotion not occurred for most people in Africa, Asia and Latin America? Why are underdeveloped countries underdeveloped?

Once again, a historical perspective can help us understand the processes that have occurred in underdeveloped countries which have impacted on the health status of their populations.

Colonialism and the slave trade

Before the sixteenth century, contact between Europe and other continents was limited mostly to trade with the Middle and Far East and to a lesser extent with Africa in such goods as spices, precious metals and ivory. This changed with the discovery expeditions of the sixteenth century which significantly altered international relations between the continents. **Colonialism** became the main feature.

GLOSSARY

Colonialism: the domination of one people or power over other people or areas, generally with the aim of economic and political control. Typically, it involves the transfer of population to the new territory where they become settlers but remain loyal to their country of origin (adapted from *Stanford Encyclopedia of Philosophy*, 2017).

After Columbus accidentally 'discovered' the Americas in 1492 for the Spanish Crown, Spain and Portugal colonised Central and South America. They plundered treasure, usually gold and silver, and sent it back to Europe.

By the sixteenth century, the Spanish had established mining centres in Mexico and Peru to supply them with raw materials, and farms and ranches to supply them with food. They channelled the precious metals back to Spain to be used in manufactured goods. The impact of colonisation on the indigenous Indian population was disastrous. Millions died as they fought to resist the forced labour imposed on them. Or they were struck down by diseases introduced from Europe to which they had no resistance—smallpox, measles and typhus. Similar conquests of parts of Africa and the East occurred with similar effects on the indigenous populations (Doyal & Pennell, 1976).

In the late sixteenth century, trade in people began. Over the next 200 years, the slave trade flourished. One hundred million people captured in West Africa were transported under the most inhumane conditions to the Americas, where they were forced to work on English- and French-owned sugar, cotton and tobacco plantations (see Figure 3.14). Not only did many slaves die as a result of the brutal exploitation they suffered, but also communicable diseases such as yellow fever, hookworm, leprosy and yaws were carried to the Americas (Doyal & Pennell, 1976).

By the end of the sixteenth century, Britain, France and Holland had started to develop their industries and needed the raw materials and mineral wealth that Spanish America could provide. At the same time, the Spanish American colonies had begun to struggle for freedom from ruthless Spanish domination. Wars of Independence broke out and, with assistance from Britain, between 1808 and 1826, all Latin America, except for the Spanish colonies of Cuba and Puerto Rico, grabbed their independence.

Over the next 50 years, Latin America supplied Europe and America with raw materials at very low prices. The surplus goods produced in Europe were sold in Latin America, enabling a small group of European capitalists to accumulate further wealth and cement their domination of agriculture and industry in their own countries.

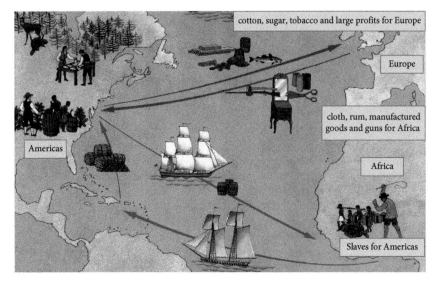

Fig. 3.14 The classical model of the triangular slave trade.
Source: http://i0.wp.com/hylbom.com/family/wp-content/uploads/2013/05/triangular-trade-map.jpg.

A similar process occurred in Asia, where spices, tea and rubber were the main spoils of the East India Company, whose exploitative operations were ended after the Indian Mutiny of 1857–1858. Trade, however, continued with the colonies of the East. Some indigenous industry was even developed—as in China, where the very low wages paid to workers in the textile mills made such foreign operations exceedingly profitable.

More often though, indigenous industry was destroyed. This happened in India, where the British used a combination of administrative and economic measures to extinguish the prosperous cotton textiles industry.

Imperialism

Colonial trade relations paved the way for **imperialism**—the extension of the colonial government's power. Raw materials for industry were easily available from current colonies, as well as from former colonies in Asia and the Americas. Capitalism—the economic system that marked off the nineteenth century from earlier times—became widespread in industrialised countries.

GLOSSARY

Imperialism: "*comes from the Latin term* imperium, *meaning to command. Thus, the term imperialism draws attention to the way that one country exercises power over another, whether through settlement, sovereignty, or indirect mechanisms of control*" (*Stanford Encyclopedia of Philosophy*, 2017).

The colonies of the European powers expanded until the system reached its limits in the 1800s. Every significant territory was now part of the global capitalist system.

By the 1860s, unregulated **free competition** on which capitalism is based reached a zenith and led competing industrialists to produce a surplus of goods. They then had to lower their prices to sell their products. Lower prices meant less profits and many of the smaller and less efficient industries were forced to cut labour costs by firing their already poorly paid workers.

GLOSSARY

Free competition: a system in which industries operate without much government regulation or control. Prices are determined by the relationship between the amount of goods for sale and the amount that people want to buy, i.e. supply and demand.

Thus, the 1870s saw an economic crisis of overproduction and in 1873 there was a serious depression throughout Europe. Millions were out of work and by the end of the 1800s emigration from Europe to North and South America and Australia was swelled by this surplus labour force. Between 1853 and 1880 Britain alone sent almost 2.5 million emigrants abroad (Thomson, 1950). Many small businesses went bankrupt and only the larger, more efficient ones survived, especially in those industries where machinery was more complex and more expensive.

By the early twentieth century important sectors of industry were dominated by a few large firms owned by a very small number of people. In other words, free competition was being transformed into **monopoly**.

Already by the 1970s in the USA, only 500 companies were responsible for nearly 70% of industrial output. The top 50 companies had sales revenue amounting to nearly a quarter of the US's **gross national product (GNP)**. General Motors alone had an annual sales revenue of more than US$35 billion—more than the total GNP of countries like South Africa, Denmark, Austria, Yugoslavia, Turkey and Norway. By 2017, the top 500 US companies represented two-thirds of the US gross domestic product (GDP) with US$12 trillion in revenues and US$890 billion in profits. Top on the list was the retail giant Walmart, with total net sales in the USA amounting to approximately US$480 billion and its international net sales amounting to US$116.12 billion (Statista, 2017).

GLOSSARY

Monopoly: a single seller controls the market and sets prices of goods because there is no competition.

Gross national product (GNP): *"an estimate of total value of all the final products and services produced in a given period by the means of production owned by a country's residents"* (Investopedia). Anything produced by foreign residents in the country's borders is excluded. Anything produced by the country's residents outside its borders is counted.

The consequences of the transformation to a monopoly for the underdeveloped world were important. For the companies in the developed world, further investment in their own countries would have simply led to overproduction and the lowering of prices. To maintain their profits, they began to export capital to the non-industrialised world. They set up in countries where capitalism had not yet emerged and where monopolies were not yet entrenched. This is how at the turn of the century, colonisation in all its varieties managed to spread like wildfire, eventually embracing the whole world. Every country on the map was transformed into a 'sphere of influence' and a field of investment for capital.

This 'capturing' of most of the world's population was not because the imperialists were particularly inherently malicious, although the methods they used were often extremely brutal. It was because the concentration of capital that had resulted from unrestrained free competition pushed them to invest abroad to maintain their profits.

Frequently, competition reached its natural conclusion in wars. In the eighteenth century, Britain launched a series of wars for export markets. With the colonial division of the world, such pressures were exacerbated, culminating in the horrors of the World War I.

Creating a labour force

Earlier it was shown that the two conditions that facilitated the growth of agricultural and industrial capitalism in Britain were:

- Dispossessing peasants and cottagers of their land and replacing them with more efficient farming of consolidated areas.
- Displacing individual producers of manufactured goods by mechanised industry, concentrated in factories.

Thus, a permanent workforce was created in the towns, and agricultural and industrial production was concentrated in the hands of a few. This process was repeated in the colonised countries. It was especially stark in Africa in the nineteenth and early twentieth centuries. Here most people were stock breeders and primitive cultivators but always had a relative abundance of land. Without a transformation in land administration, both a labour force and a market in which manufactured goods could be sold were unrealisable. So:

- Large areas of what was often the best land were taken by foreign companies or the colonising State and used for the production of cash crops—tea, coffee, cotton, sugar, cocoa, tobacco, jute, rubber and so on—rather than food. The Black African population was forced into small areas called 'reserves'.
- A head-tax—and often a hut tax and cattle tax—was imposed. People had to produce crops for sale in order to be able to pay this.

In other words, people were forced to work for money.

Neocolonial State

Imperialism was only ever able to carry out this process with the help of local rulers. In the early colonial days, a class of local agents was created which owed its wealth to the foreign coloniser and could be trusted to defend its interests. In Bengal, for example, the *zamindari* were transformed from tax collectors for the Mogul emperors into landlords with a vested interest in British rule.

As colonial countries gained independence, a new alliance emerged between foreign capitalists, the small class of local industrial capitalists and the top bureaucrats of the newly independent State. This neocolonial State could be relied upon to protect the interests of foreign capital. Often, of course, it was the army that formed the government.

But the capitalist economic system is unstable. Contractions and expansions follow each other periodically, so a reserve workforce is necessary to keep wages stable. In some countries, the 'reserves' literally became labour reserves—the 'bantustans' serving South Africa's needs, North Yemen serving Saudi Arabia, Mexico serving the USA, Turkey serving primarily West Germany, Portugal and North Africa mostly serving France, Ireland serving England. Within certain countries, underdeveloped regions supplied developed regions with labour—southern Italy supplied the north, south-western France provided the north-west, the southern states in the USA supplied the north-eastern. Even within certain towns, the underdeveloped served the developed (see Figure 3.15). And in underdeveloped countries, the countryside supplied the towns.

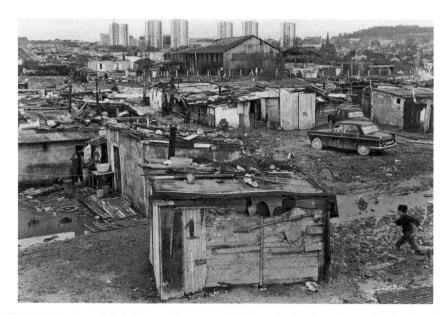

Fig. 3.15 Region of Ile de France, France, 1968. The underdeveloped serve the developed.
Source: https://farm2.static.flickr.com/1727/41762804664_49bbe75cdb_b.jpg.

The impact on health

The creation of a workforce was only achieved at the most appalling cost to the health of workers. For example, the growth of roads in Africa helped spread the tsetse fly, which carries sleeping sickness; and food production dropped because of the concentration on the export of raw materials and the production of manufactured goods, rather than food.

Africa, once self-sufficient in food, in 2017 had an annual food import bill of US$35 billion, which was estimated to rise to US$110 billion by 2025, and still starvation is on the increase (President of the African Development Bank, 2017).

Pre-colonial life was no idyll, but it did not compare with the perils of the modern neocolonial world. The Tonga people in Zimbabwe were displaced from their home in the Bumi River area to make way for the artificial Lake Kariba. This forced removal destroyed their traditional sources of food and created widespread malnutrition. When the government provided a grain store it was sited in a place that became a transmission site for sleeping sickness (Hughes & Hunter, 1971).

Contemporary globalisation

Let us return to the question posed earlier: Why are underdeveloped countries underdeveloped? The question can be extended and made more precise: Why are all countries unevenly developed and why is this uneven development most stark in the underdeveloped world?

As mentioned earlier, competition between enterprises in the advanced capitalist countries has resulted in large monopolies, which need to expand abroad so as to maintain their profits. Throughout the twentieth century and into the twenty-first, immense **transnational corporations** (TNCs) strengthened their monopolies and grip on the world markets; and this has resulted in what is called contemporary globalisation—essentially a continuation of imperialist political and economic relations, with poverty, underdevelopment and health and wealth inequalities as the logical consequences.

GLOSSARY

Multinational corporations (MNCs)/Transnational corporations (TNCs): 'stateless companies' that operate, produce goods, deliver services or have investments in more than one country. Most are the result of mergers of companies based in different countries. They usually have management headquarters in one country (the home country) but operate in a variety of other countries (host countries), either in their own name or through subsidiaries.

TNCs are the *apex predators of the global economy* (Öney, 2017). They tend to pro-duce where raw materials are cheap and wages are lowest—the underdeveloped world. They sell where prices are high; juggle profit and loss figures between subsidiaries and so declare minimal profits; and funnel their profits to their shareholders—most of whom are from developed countries.

They shape the ecosystems in which others seek their living. They direct the flows of goods, services and capital that brought globalisation to life. Though multinationals ac-count for only 2% of the world's jobs, they own or orchestrate the supply chains that account for over 50% of world trade; they make up 40% of the value of the West's stock markets; and they own most of the world's intellectual property (Öney, 2017).

Globalisation has accelerated the growth and domination of TNCs both inter-nationally and regionally, so that many are more economically powerful than some states. For example, according to Oxfam:

- In 2017, 69 of the 100 largest economic entities in the world were TNCs, not countries.
- Ten of the largest TNCs had a combined revenue that was greater than the com-bined revenue of 180 of the poorest countries.
- The 10 most profitable TNCs in the USA *"made a collective US$226 billion in profit in 2015 or US$30 for every person on the planet"* (Oxfam, 2017).
- By 2017, collectively just eight men owned the same amount of wealth as the poorest half of humanity. They were, in order of net worth:
  o Bill Gates: American founder of Microsoft (US$75 billion)
  o Amancio Ortega: Spanish founder of Inditex which owns the Zara fashion chain (US$67 billion)
  o Warren Buffett: American chief executive officer (CEO) and largest share-holder in Berkshire Hathaway (US$60.8 billion)
  o Carlos Slim Helu: Mexican owner of Grupo Carso (US$50 billion)
  o Jeff Bezos: American founder, chairman and CEO of Amazon (US$45.2 billion)
  o Mark Zuckerberg: American chairman, CEO and co-founder of Facebook (US$44.6 billion)
  o Larry Ellison: American co-founder and CEO of Oracle (US$43.6 billion)
  o Michael Bloomberg: American founder, owner and CEO of Bloomberg LP (US$40 billion).

Commenting on these figures, Winnie Byanyima, Executive Director of Oxfam International, said:

It is obscene for so much wealth to be held in the hands of so few when 1 in 10 people survive on less than $2 a day. Inequality is trapping hundreds of millions in poverty; it is fracturing our societies and undermining democracy (Oxfam, 2017).

Globally, the wealth of billionaires increased by $US3.9 trillion through the COVID-19 pandemic in 2020, as they were able to buy more company shares when markets around the world were crashing (Oxfam, 2021). On the other hand, according to the Oxfam (2021) report, *The Inequality Virus*, it could take more than a decade for the world's poorest people to recover from the economic impacts of the pandemic.

Increased TNC domination and concentration of power has led to growing inequalities both between and within developed and underdeveloped countries. Governments of underdeveloped countries have become interconnected with corporate strategies in ways that make them dependent and subordinate, resulting in the surrender of strategic sectors, such as food and agriculture. Being transnational, with headquarters usually in developed countries, it becomes difficult for trade unions within individual countries to protest for fairer working conditions.

How global economic policies have developed to maintain globalisation

Rennen and Martens (2003) highlight key landmarks that have shaped the evolution of globalisation, including in the economic, political, technological, social-cultural and environmental domains. These multiple domains continuously interact and impact each other, and it is through this dynamic that globalisation, underpinned by the ideology of **neoliberalism**, has evolved (see Table 3.1 for a brief overview of the development of contemporary globalisation).

GLOSSARY

Neoliberalism: "*new political, economic and social arrangements within society that emphasize market relations, re-tasking the role of the state, and individual responsibility*" (Springer et al., 2016, in Labonté & Sanders, unpublished paper).

Some elements of neoliberalism include:

- **Privatisation**: reduction in government spending and increase in private ownership.
- **Market deregulation**: reduction in government control over private industry.
- **Government deficit reduction**: leading to cuts in health and other public services.
- **Trade and finance liberalisation**: removal or reduction of restrictions on barriers (especially taxes on imports and exports) that prevent free trade between nations. In a free market economy, prices for goods and services are set freely by the forces of supply and demand, without intervention by government policy.
- **Individual responsibility**: this replaces the concepts of public goods and services—which are administered by the government and paid for collectively through taxation.

Table 3.1 Key landmarks in the development of contemporary globalisation

1940s	1950s	1960s	1970s	1980s	1990s	2000s	2010	2020
The Bretton Woods Conference: post World War II (1940s–1960s)		First global oil supply crisis/loans to underdeveloped countries (1960s–1970s)		• The mounting burden of debt • Structural Adjustment Programmes (SAPs) • Enhanced SAPs and Heavily Indebted Poor Countries Initiative (HIPC)	• The World Trade Organization (1995) • The 'Battle of Seattle' (1999)	• Doha Development Agenda (2001–2016) • Agricultural subsidies • Global financial crisis (2007) • Financialisation (neoliberal rollout) • Food price hikes (2008)	• The neoliberal austerity agenda (2013) • Changes in geopolitics (2016) • Sidelining multilateralism in favour of multistakeholderism	

The Bretton Woods Conference: post World War II (1940s–1960s)

The era of contemporary globalisation is usually dated from the mid-1940s when most of the industrialised nations signed the Bretton Woods Agreement and the United Nations (UN) was founded (in 1945).

The Bretton Woods Agreement (so-called because the 1944 Monetary and Financial Conference was held in Bretton Woods, New Hampshire, USA) led to the international monetary system that is still in place today. The Conference focused on establishing a stable exchange rate; discussing the rebuilding of the war-ravaged economies of Europe; and negotiating a system of rules, procedures and institutions to regulate international commercial and financial relations. The 44 allied nations present at the Conference adopted a monetary policy that tied their national currencies to the US dollar.

The outcomes of the Conference were the setting up of the following:

- The International Monetary Fund (IMF) aimed at maintaining global economic stability, especially by assisting those countries with **balance of payment (BOP)** deficits.
- The General Agreement on Tariffs and Trade (GATT), an international trade agreement, aimed at reducing **tariffs** as a financial barrier to trade.
- The International Bank of Reconstruction and Development (the World Bank) aimed at providing low-interest loans and grants for development.

GLOSSARY

Balance of payment (BOP): a record of all the financial transactions between countries—for exports, imports, loans and investments. Ideally the BOP should balance to zero, with no surplus or deficit. A negative imbalance means that the country is in deficit—it has imported more than it has exported. It would need to counterbalance the shortfall by trying to earn foreign capital, through, for example, attracting foreign investments or receiving loans from other countries or institutions. The latter usually means that the deficit country becomes increasingly indebted to the countries or institutions it has borrowed from. In many cases, loans are provided by the IMF or World Bank.

Tariffs: taxes on imports and exports between independent nations.

Loans to underdeveloped countries (1960s–1970s)

In the 1970s, the **Organization of the Petroleum Exporting Countries (OPEC)** quadrupled the price of oil, resulting in the first global oil supply crisis. OPEC deposited the excess 'petrodollars' in commercial banks in high-income, developed countries. These banks, in turn, invested the money in high-risk loans to underdeveloped countries, earmarked for large-scale **agribusiness** and industry. It was anticipated that the goods that the underdeveloped countries would produce for export would generate the foreign exchange they needed to service their debts and repay the loans (Werner & Sanders, 1997).

GLOSSARY

Organization of the Petroleum Exporting Countries (OPEC): established in 1960 to unify and coordinate the petroleum policies of oil-rich nations. Member states include (inter alia) Iran, Iraq, Kuwait, Saudi Arabia, Venezuela, Algeria, Ecuador, Gabon, Libya, Qatar, Nigeria and the United Arab Emirates.

Agribusiness: a large-scale business that earns most or all of its revenue from agriculture, including from the production, processing, manufacturing, packaging and distribution of products.

The mounting burden of debt (1980s)

By the early 1980s, the world was in a major economic recession. In an important policy shift, the USA tightened its monetary policies to control inflation, and reversed the flow of petrodollars. The consequence was an increase in interest rates on loans worldwide. At the same time, underdeveloped countries were not getting the expected returns on their exports because of reduced demand. The overall result was a reversal of flow of capital between the developed and underdeveloped world, trapping underdeveloped countries in a mounting burden of debt that they could not repay.

Figure 3.16 shows the rate at which the external debt of underdeveloped countries increased in the period 1970–2014. After 2000, the growth increased and debt accumulated much faster. According to Alves and Topoowski (2019), between 1970 and 1980, *"external debt accumulation was mainly through the public sector, in the early 1990s the private sector gradually began to borrow, and since the mid-2000s, has done so at a rapid pace."*

Structural Adjustment Programmes (SAPs) (1980s)

At the height of this debt crisis the IMF and World Bank came to the rescue of the commercial banks by offering bail-out loans to underdeveloped countries to prevent them from defaulting on their loan repayments (Werner & Sanders, 1997). However, these loans were accompanied by the conditionalities of the SAPs. The main condition

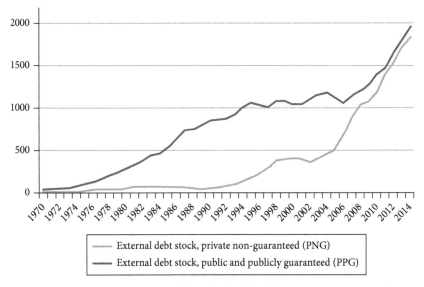

Fig. 3.16 Total external debt stocks of all underdeveloped countries, 1970–2014 (current US$ in billions).

Source: World Bank's international debt statistics, cited in Alves & Topoowski (2019).

was that underdeveloped countries needed to fundamentally restructure their economies so that they could service their foreign debts. This meant:

- Devaluing the local currency.
- Trade liberalisation—opening borders to foreign trade and investors with incentives and the lowering of tariffs and other barriers to imports.
- Deregulating markets and prices—removing restrictions that could prevent free trade.
- Privatising public enterprises and removing state subsidies especially on food.
- Reducing public sector employment and lowering real wages.
- Slashing budgets for public health, education and other social services.
- Introducing cost recovery measures (user fees) in health and education (Werner & Sanders, 1997).

A major consequence of SAPs, specifically of trade liberalisation, was to accelerate the integration of the economies of underdeveloped countries into the global economy. This, together with other conditions in each country, gave rise to the extremely unequal distribution of income and wealth across both the developed and underdeveloped world (Labonté & Schrecker, 2007). The austerity packages also impacted access to health care and health outcomes (Bilamarghus et al., 1998).

Once import tariffs, which had protected domestic producers from international competition, were removed, foreign companies could flood local markets with cheap goods. Many domestic producers lost their livelihoods. What is more, the conditions attached to SAPs meant that the ability of many nations to redistribute resources to meet the basic needs of their populations was reduced or diminished. This contributed to the rapid escalation of poverty.

A change of name, but the same conditions remain

Over time, the IMF and World Bank transformed or incorporated SAPs into other programmes, for example, Enhanced Structural Adjustment Programmes (ESAPs) and the Heavily Indebted Poor Countries Initiative (HIPC). However, the conditions remained essentially the same, with the main condition being that underdeveloped countries prioritise their export markets.

The problem, according to Rudin and Sanders (2011), was that most of these countries relied on mining and agriculture and thus would have been exporting similar products to the same markets. It was inevitable that this would result in the market being flooded, with increased competition between countries and prices falling because of overproduction of these commodities, resulting in further debt.

The World Trade Organization (1990s)

On 1 January 1995, the World Trade Organization (WTO) replaced GATT, which had been set up after the Bretton Woods Conference. GATT was essentially an international trade agreement, regulating the trade in goods only; the WTO was a permanent global body which regulated trade in goods, services and some aspects of **intellectual property rights (IPRs)** between member nations. By 2016 it had 164 members—the bulk of the world's trading nations.

GLOSSARY

Intellectual property rights (IPRs): owners/creators of discoveries, inventions, formulas, designs, etc. are granted certain exclusive rights of ownership over their intellectual property for a period.

Today, the WTO oversees a range of trade agreements (both tariff and non-tariff) entered into by individual member states. Many of these trade agreements are skewed towards opening markets to the private sector based in the main industrialised, developed countries.

Important trade agreements that impact public health are:

- **The General Agreement on Trade in Services (GATS):** deals with minimising trade barriers to the buy and sell services, including the trade in health services and health workers—physicians, nurses, dentists and so on. The international migration of health workers (typically from underdeveloped to developed countries) results in financial loss, health workforce shortages and weaker health systems in underdeveloped countries. This has the potential to perpetuate social stratification and injustice by undermining the capacity of health systems in underdeveloped countries to address health and health inequities.

NOTE: We will look at this so-called 'brain drain' in detail in Chapter 4.

- **The Agreement on Agriculture (AoA):** deals with agricultural production and trade. By the 1980s, governments in developed countries were providing large export and producer subsidies to agricultural producers, resulting in overproduction and the flooding of global markets with surplus crops that were sold below the cost of production. The AoA targeted three sections of agricultural production:
  - o **Domestic support:** this includes domestic subsidies and other support programmes that directly increase production and may interfere with trade (financial assistance for farmers). Domestic support is divided into two categories:
    - *Trade distorting support*: directly linked to trade that increases production levels and interferes with trade. These are called 'amber box' subsidies and were marked for reduction.
    - *Non-trade or minimal trade distorting*: includes 'blue' subsidies (which limit production but distort trade) and 'green' subsidies (which lead to minimal distortion of production and trade). These subsidies did not have to be reduced and could actually be increased.
  - o **Market access:** this includes the reduction of barriers to trade by WTO members, giving greater access to markets.
  - o **Export subsidies:** developed countries had to reduce their financial assistance for food exports over 6 years (from the 1995 AoA). Underdeveloped countries had to reduce these export subsidies over 10 years.
- **Trade-Related Aspects of Intellectual Property (TRIPS):** deals with granting monopoly rights to intellectual property through a system of patents, copyright and trademarks, across national boundaries. Applies to, among others, pharmaceutical companies and large TNC agribusinesses that dominate key components of the food system—from the supply of seed through to the retail and consumption of food products. TNCs argue that without the protection of TRIPS, once its products are released for public consumption, they are easy to copy. Critics argue that TRIPS interferes with the free market because it protects the 'inventor' from competition, establishes a monopoly, pushes up prices and makes lifesaving treatment unaffordable to people who are poor.

In 2021, in response to the COVID-19 pandemic, South Africa and India proposed to the WTO that the IPR on COVID vaccines be waived so that vaccine manufacturing could be done in low- and middle-income countries. Part of the argument was that the development of the vaccines was the result of significant investments of public funds. Civil society groups have argued for public health considerations over private profits for transnational pharmaceutical companies (Legge & Kim, 2020).

- **Agreement on Technical Barriers to Trade (TBT):** ensures that technical regulations and standards do not interfere with trade.

Technical regulations and standards are important, but they vary from country to country. Having too many different standards makes life difficult for producers and exporters. If the standards are set arbitrarily, they could be used as an excuse for protectionism. Standards can become obstacles to trade. But they are also necessary for a range of reasons, from environmental protection, safety, national security to consumer information (WTO, 2017).

- **Agreement on Application of Sanitary and Phytosanitary Measures (SPS):** reduces trade barriers that arise from governments' regulations and laws regarding food safety and the safety of humans, animals and plants.

CASE STUDY: Who owns the genes that become our food?

Plant breeding

Plant breeding is the science of changing the genes of plants to determine the type of traits they have and to produce desired characteristics. Technological developments in plant breeding which occurred after World War II generated new varieties of seeds (or hybrids) for staple crops. These seeds were designed to give higher yielding crops than traditional varieties. However, there were two main threats:

- Although these hybrids did produce higher yields, the second- and third-generation seed they produced does not. This means that farmers can no longer store seed as they had traditionally done for generations, but had to keep buying more seed.
- The increasingly sophisticated technology is owned by a small number of large TNC agribusinesses ('Big Food'), who have flooded the agricultural sector with these hybrids, driving out the mainly genetically diverse varieties farmers have cultivated for generations.

Big Food also perfected a model of seed engineering and ownership, with the advent of genetically modified organisms (GMOs), i.e. genetically engineering the DNA of an organism so that its *"DNA contains one or more genes not normally found there"* (dictionary.com).

How are genetically modified (GM) seeds developed?

1. Scientists identify the desired trait in the crop that they want, for example:
   - A herbicide tolerant (HT) crop: a crop that can tolerate a specific herbicide that kills the surrounding weeds and vegetation but leaves the crop intact (see the Note on 'Roundup Ready' below).

- A Bt crop: a crop that contain the Bt (*Bacillus thuringiensis*) bacteria which is poisonous to many insects, so it acts as a 'built-in pesticide'.
2. Scientists change the genetic material (DNA) in the plants for the traits they want. They do this by, for example, taking genetic material from different species and splicing it together to get the desired traits.
3. They then transfer the genetically engineered material into the plant seed. The plant expresses the new gene in all its cells.

What is 'Roundup Ready'?

Roundup is the brand name of a herbicide produced by the agribusiness Monsanto. The active ingredient is glyphosate. Monsanto also produce GM seeds which have been genetically engineered to be resistant to Roundup and are called 'Roundup Ready'. Farmers who plant these seeds must use Roundup because the seeds are not resistant to other herbicides and will die.

Roundup Ready seeds are also known as 'terminator seeds'. This is because the crops produced from them are sterile. This means that every year, farmers must buy new seed from Monsanto. They cannot reuse seeds as they have traditionally done in the past.

(*Source*: Adapted from: Economic Justice Network of the Fellowship of Christian Councils in Southern Africa & The School of Public Health [as part of the Centre of Excellence in Food Security] at the University of Western Cape. [2016].)

The 'Battle of Seattle' (1999)

The authoritative voice of the WTO has not gone unchallenged and the process of globalisation itself has also enabled a growing transnational anti-globalisation civil society movement to emerge.

At the end of 1999, the WTO convened a ministerial conference in Seattle, USA, to discuss changes to the rules of world trade. The talks collapsed as a rift emerged between the developed and underdeveloped countries, and this culminated in African countries walking out. This began a historic chapter in WTO multilateral trade negotiations which involved questions about the legitimacy of the trading system itself.

The collapse of the Seattle ministerial conference exposed significant differences among member countries concerning what should be on the WTO agenda as well as shortcomings in the manner in which the WTO conducts its business and interacts with other international and nongovernmental organisations (NGOs) (Schotte, 2000).

Large civil society protests also highlighted how global trade agreements were biased in favour of developed countries (see Figure 3.17). Protesting directly against TRIPS, this growing civil society movement argued that the patenting system was

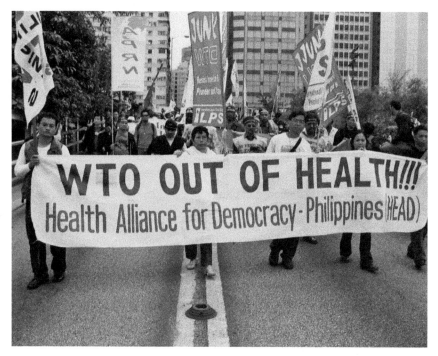

Fig. 3.17 Health Alliance for Democracy (HEAD): the Philippines protests WTO interference in health.

Source: Wim De Ceukelaire—Viva Salud.

abusive as it enabled pharmaceutical corporations to jeopardise equitable access to life-saving medicines, such as antiretrovirals (ARVs) for treating HIV in the 1990s, and that it skewed research and development in favour of more lucrative markets, rather than meeting the health needs of people living in poverty. Overall, it was argued, TRIPS reinforced disparities by denying underdeveloped countries access to knowledge, health care, seeds for crops and technology.

The Doha Development Agenda

In 2001, a WTO meeting was held in Doha, Qatar to negotiate lower trade barriers and modify trade rules. The round of talks was called the Doha Development Agenda, because improving trade with underdeveloped countries was one of its main objectives. At least 20 areas of trade were on the agenda, including agriculture, services and intellectual property. However, the talks were stalled on several occasions (between 2001 and 2008) because of major disagreements between developed and underdeveloped nations on issues related to agriculture and non-agriculture market access and services.

In 2013, a WTO ministerial conference concluded with an agreement called the Bali Package, which dealt with some of the agricultural issues from the Doha round of negotiations (WTO, 2013). However, in 2016 members of the WTO ended the 14-year Doha Round of Negotiations because it was clear that, *"neither developed economies like the United States and the European Union nor developing countries like China and India were willing or able to make fundamental concessions"* (*New York Times*, 2016).

Agricultural subsidies

Areas of disagreement in the Doha Round of Negotiations were to do with the following:

- Distortions in agricultural trade caused by domestic agricultural support and subsidies.
- How the AoA categorises domestic support into 'amber box' (trade distorting), which must be reduced, and 'blue' and 'green boxes' (non-trade distorting subsidies), which do not have to be reduced and could be increased.

These different categories:

> *... allowed the rich countries to maintain or raise their very high subsidies by switching from one kind of subsidy to another ... This is why after the Uruguay Round the total amount of subsidies in OECD countries have gone up instead of going down, despite the apparent promise that Northern subsidies will be reduced* (Third World Network, 2003).

Subsidised agriculture (including 'green box' subsidies) distorts world trade and undercuts agricultural producers in underdeveloped countries who cannot compete with these subsidies. It leads to **dumping** or undercutting, which occurs when a product is exported to another country at below the normal price. The aim is to increase sales in the foreign market and drive out competition and create a monopoly in which the exporter can dictate the price and quality of the product.

GLOSSARY

Dumping: when a company sets the price of an exported product or service lower than the price it normally charged in its own home market.

As an example, the African Growth and Opportunity Act (AGOA) is a US Trade Act aimed at allowing certain products from eligible Sub-Saharan countries to be imported into the USA duty free. In 2015, the USA gave South Africa until 15 March 2016 to remove trade barriers that were preventing US meat from being imported into

South Africa. The consequence of not removing these barriers was that the duty-free import of South African agricultural products like wine, citrus and macadamia nuts into the lucrative US market would be cancelled. On 16 March 2016, for the first time in 15 years, US frozen chicken pieces were sold in South Africa at 'dumping prices' with which South African chicken farmers—who unlike US farmers do not receive a government subsidy—could not compete.

> *American chicken producers prefer chicken breast meat and wings and regard the leg quarter, i.e. the thigh and the drum as by-products. They are exporting these pieces to South Africa at 'dumping' prices. This means that for many South African chicken farmers it is a threat to their livelihoods and those of their employees* (Farming News, 2016).

According to Borders and Sterling Burnett (2006):

> *Subsidized agriculture in the developed world is one of the greatest obstacles to economic growth in the developing world . . . Countries with unsubsidized goods are essentially shut out of world markets, devastating their local economies.*

In addition to distorting world trade, many 'green box' subsidies damage the environment, because they encourage an intensification of agricultural production, causing habitat destruction, exposing the environment to pesticides and fertilisers, and ultimately lead to land degradation.

Figure 3.18 shows the estimated domestic support in US$ billions that agricultural producers in countries belonging to the **Organization for Economic Co-operation**

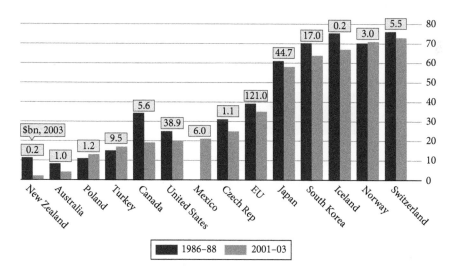

Fig. 3.18 Agricultural subsidies—producer support estimate (PSE) as a percentage of gross farm output (US$ billions), 1986–1988 and 2001–2003.

Source: Vogeler, I. (2005). *Food Security, Agriculture Policies and Globalization: Lessons from USA and India*. Institute for Social and Economic Change: Bengaluru, India.

and Development (OECD) received to artificially reduce the costs of production, in 1986–1988 and 2001–2003. Although Switzerland has the highest per capita subsidy at US$5.5 billion (predominantly for dairy farmers), the EU has the largest aggregate subsidy (US$121 billion), followed by Japan (US$44.7 billion) and then the USA (US$39.9 billion).

GLOSSARY

Organization for Economic Co-operation and Development (OECD): an intergovernmental economic organisation founded in 1960 to stimulate economic progress and world trade. Its 35 member countries have high-income economies and are regarded as developed countries.

From 1993 to 2008 the average per capita income of Sub-Saharan African economies barely budged—it increased from US$742 to US$762 per year (measured in 2005 purchasing-power parity-adjusted dollars). If we exclude South Africa and the Seychelles, we see a decline from US$608 to US$556 over the period. In 2008, Switzerland's annual dairy subsidy per cow was approximately US$1600, begging the question raised in Figure 3.19: Why should a Swiss cow enjoy a higher income than an African citizen?.

By 2013, support to agricultural producers across the OECD amounted to US$258 billion. In the EU, these subsidies go to 1% of producers, while in the USA 70% of subsidies go to 10% of its producers, mainly agribusinesses. From 1996 to 2000 the national median farm subsidy in the USA was US$4695. Some wealthy recipients received up to 20 times more than this (see Figure 3.20).

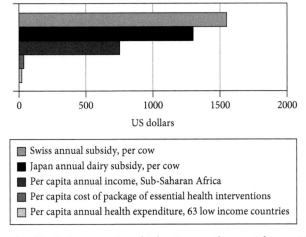

US dollars

☐ Swiss annual subsidy, per cow
■ Japan annual dairy subsidy, per cow
■ Per capita annual income, Sub-Saharan Africa
■ Per capita cost of package of essential health interventions
☐ Per capita annual health expenditure, 63 low income countries

Fig. 3.19 Why should a Swiss cow enjoy a higher income than an African citizen?

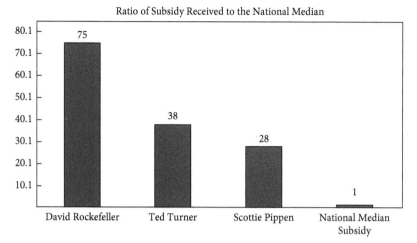

Fig. 3.20 Some wealthy recipients receive more than 20 times the median farm subsidy, 1996–2000.

Source: Frydenlund, J. & Riedl, B. (2001). *At the federal trough: farm subsidies for the rich and famous.* Environmental Working Group.

https://www.heritage.org/agriculture/report/the-federal-trough-farm-subsidies-the-rich-and-famous.

… once again confirms that the lion's share of farm subsidies for 'covered commodities' like corn and soybeans are flowing to the nation's largest and most successful farm operations. Between 1995 and 2016, the top 10 percent received 77 percent of all 'covered commodity' subsidies … The top 1 percent received 26 percent of all subsidies, or $1.7 million per recipient … The top recipient of 'covered commodity' subsidies was Deline Farms Partnership, which received more than $4 million in 2016. By contrast, the median household income in Charleston, Mo., where Deline Farms is based, is $27,000 (Environmental Working Group [EWG], 2017).

Global financial crisis (2007–2011)

The global financial crisis of 2008 began within a specific sector of the American mortgage market called **sub-prime loans**. These are a type of loan offered above prime interest rate to people who are not eligible for ordinary loans, for example because of their low credit rating. In other words, they were high-risk loans because financial institutions understood that many borrowers could not repay them. Financial institutions packaged these sub-prime loans into a financial product called securities, which were then sold on to other financial institutions across the globe. In this way, they spread the risk of default among several creditors.

By 2008, 20% of people who had the original sub-prime loans had defaulted, putting many financial institutions on the brink of bankruptcy. American authorities decided to rescue some of these institutions with bail-out loans. However, when they decided not to bail out the investment bank Lehman Brothers, this destabilised the global financial market.

GLOSSARY

Sub-prime loan: a type of loan offered at a rate above prime to individuals who do not qualify for prime rate loans—the interest rate that banks charge most credit-worthy customers.

Towards the end of 2008, the economies of the developed countries began to reduce their credit, especially to small and medium enterprises, and this resulted in many companies closing, with massive job losses. America's demand for imports fell and this affected international trade. Those countries that were mostly export-oriented suffered. In the light of this global financial crisis, many countries cut their spending on public services, including their health budgets.

Food price hikes

Financial institutions have always helped farmers and those involved in the production of food to cope with the uncertainty of growing crops by offering them a type of contract called a **futures contract (futures)**. These allow farmers to sell their crops at a future date at a guaranteed price.

Futures worked well until the global financial crisis of 2008 and the deregulation of the **commodities derivatives market**, allowing **speculators** and large institutional investors to enter the market and begin betting on the price of food. There was so much money being invested in these commodities that it pushed up the already high prices and created what is called 'a speculative bubble'. Speculators—who have no connection to food—now dominate the agricultural goods market. Higher food prices lead to increases in the percentage of families suffering from hunger.

GLOSSARY

Futures contracts (futures): a forward contract or agreement to buy or sell something—a commodity like crops—in the future at a predetermined price agreed today.

Commodities derivatives market: a market that trades in the primary economic sector, e.g. in agricultural products (maize, wheat, soy, coffee, sugar, fruit) and mined commodities like gold and oil.

Derivative: a contract that derives its value from the performance of the underlying asset or commodity (e.g. crops).

Speculators: people or institutions whose objective is to make a profit based on the future difference in the prices of assets, rather than to invest in and add value to a commodity or asset.

According to Wahl (2008), there is no one factor that on its own determines the increase in food prices. The following factors are frequently cited:

- The increasing demand for a food commodity.
- The decline of the dollar.
- The decline of agricultural productivity in underdeveloped countries due to, for example, SAPs and the imposition of an export orientation instead of a focus on national food security.
- WTO trade agreements and deregulation.
- The large-scale cultivation of agricultural commodities, like rape and sugar cane to produce biofuels like ethanol and diesel as an alternative to oil.
- The increase in oil and fertiliser prices.
- Bad harvests.
- Restrictions on export on food by countries that want to guarantee food self-sufficiency due to rising food prices.
- In 2006, Merrill Lynch, the wealth management division of Bank of America, estimated that speculation was causing commodity prices to trade at 50% higher than if they were based on fundamental supply and demand.

Prior to 2007, food prices showed a modest increase on the global market. Thereafter, prices soared. Figure 3.21 shows the fluctuation in food price indices of some of the most important food commodities between 1990 and 2014. You can see that from late 2006 to early 2008 there was an overall food price increase of 71% for the most essential foodstuffs. This rapidly declined after mid-2008 to the 2006 level and rose once again in 2011 (Wahl, 2008). Note how the price of sugar was particularly volatile—rising to a 30-year high at the beginning of 2011 and then falling just as rapidly, only to increase again in 2012.

Food speculation is contributing to higher and more volatile food prices. Higher prices force millions of people into poverty and hunger, and drive land-grabs in developing countries. All while banks, life insurers and pension funds reap huge profits (Friends of the Earth Europe, 2012).

Rising food prices affect people who are poor the hardest and are a threat to food security. In a developed country, a typical household spends about 10%–20% of their household budget on food. In an underdeveloped country, this percentage is between 60% and 80%. This means:

... a 50% price increase on basic food leads to a mere 6% rise in expenditure for a high-income country, but it amounts to 21% for a food importing country of low income (People's Health Movement, Medact, Global Equity Gauge, 2008).

The global economic crisis of 2008 did not affect all countries in the same way, and in some **emerging markets**, such as China and India, there was in fact a growth in their GDP (see Figure 3.22).

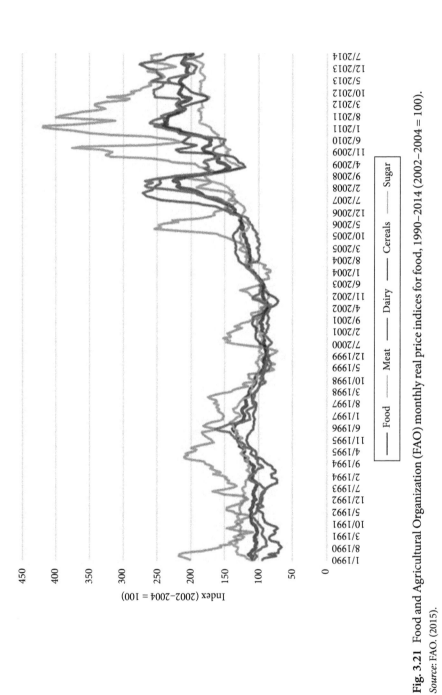

Fig. 3.21 Food and Agricultural Organization (FAO) monthly real price indices for food, 1990–2014 (2002–2004 = 100).
Source: FAO. (2015).

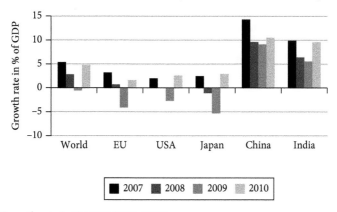

Fig. 3.22 Growth rate in % GDP, 2007–2010.

Source: Paulo, S. (2011). *Europe and the Global Financial Crisis: Taking Stock of the EU's Policy Response.*
Foundation Robert Schuman: Paris.

GLOSSARY

Emerging markets: 'newly industrialised' countries which are rapidly developing
economically due to growing their manufacturing capabilities and increasing their
export trade.

Financialisation (neoliberal rollout)

The period of neoliberalism leading up to the global financial crisis is referred to as
the 'financialisation' of the economy, whereby the financial sector, including banks,
investment funds, insurance companies, real-estate agencies, the stock market and
wealthy elites, began to acquire greater control over economic policies and outcomes
(Palley, 2007). The main impacts of financialisation have been to:

- Elevate the importance of the financial sector in relation to the real economy—
  that part of the economy that is concerned with producing goods and services.
- Transfer money from the real economy to the financial sector.
- Increase income inequality.

The Great Recession has led to the following health costs, felt especially by low- and
middle-income countries:

- A further increase in poverty.
- Rising unemployment, especially among young adults.

- Increasing child deaths as a result of increased food prices, falling incomes, reduced public health expenditure and reduced usage of health care services.
- Decreasing development aid, overall financial flows and remittances (people living in a foreign country sending money back to their home country).

However, while the majority of the world's population descended into the cycle of poverty, the gap between them and the super-wealthy elites grew (as mentioned previously in this chapter).

> ... the 24 million people whom investment banks refer to as 'high- and ultra-high net worth individuals' saw their balance sheets decline for a year or two, but then increase by over 20% (Baxter, 2011, cited in People's Health Movement, ALAMES, Health Action International, Medico International, Third World Network, & Medact, 2014).

Once again, many countries relied on IMF and World Bank loans with their conditionalities, and the world moved into a new phase of neoliberalism with its agenda of 'austerity'.

The neoliberal austerity agenda

Neoliberal austerity policies operate in much the same way as SAPs, with the main difference being that these policies have also affected developed countries. Greece, for example, cut its hospital budget by more than 40%, despite demand increasing by an estimated 25% (Kentikelenis et al., 2011, cited in People's Health Movement, ALAMES, Health Action International, Medico International, Third World Network, & Medact, 2014). In 2013, it was estimated that globally 80% (5.8 billion) of people were affected by the austerity agenda and this was expected to increase to 90% by 2015 (People's Health Movement, ALAMES, Health Action International, Medico International, Third World Network, & Medact, 2014).

The global economic crisis affected the lives and livelihoods of almost everyone in our increasingly interconnected world, with people living in poverty being the hardest hit because of rising food prices, among other adverse effects such as droughts, floods and cyclones due to climate change.

Changes in geopolitics (2016)

The 2016 election of Donald Trump as President of the USA and the UK Brexit decision ushered in changes in **geopolitics** with consequences for global health. **Multilateralism** was beginning to break down, bolstered by the Trump administration pursuing national interests and withdrawing from international agreements (Labonté & Sanders, unpublished paper).

GLOSSARY

Geopolitics: how geography, economics and demography influence the politics and foreign policies of states (Labonté & Sanders, unpublished paper).

Multilateralism: alliances between multiple countries; intergovernmental platform.

As an example, the Trans-Pacific Partnership (TPP) Agreement was entered into in 2005 by a small group of Pacific Rim countries (Brunei, Chile, New Zealand and Singapore). In 2008, the USA, Australia, Vietnam and Peru joined the group and then as talks proceeded so did Canada, Japan, Malaysia and Mexico. In 2011, then-Secretary of State Hillary Clinton announced that the TPP would be at the heart of the USA's trade agreement with the Asia-Pacific region, opening trade and investment in this region by removing trade obstacles like tariffs and import quotas. Negotiations took place in secrecy and outside of the checks and balances that operate at traditional multilateral treaty-making organisations such as the WTO.

The TPP was eventually signed in early 2016 and was set to become the world's largest free trade deal, covering 40% of the global economy. It included IPR laws and rules of enforcement that were far more restrictive than those required by other multilateral agreements. Countries that were not TPP members would have to comply with it as a condition of bilateral trade agreements with TPP members.

However, in 2017, the Trump administration withdrew the USA from the TPP Agreement, claiming that it would accelerate the US decline in manufacturing, lower wages and increase inequality. The remaining 11 TPP countries signed a new version of the Agreement in 2018, called the Comprehensive and Progressive Trans-Pacific Partnership (CPTPP), which kept most of the original agreement intact.

Economic protectionism, whereby countries restrict imports through methods like tariffs and quotas, increased, although the volume of global trade continued to rise. But as we can see from the example of the TPP Agreement, negotiations occurred outside the global economy's traditional multilateral treaty-making organisations, indicating:

> … a weakening of international law and norms (notably human rights), and the global economy's institutional anchors, the IMF, WTO, and World Bank, struggling for legitimacy in a less predictable global environment (WEF Global Risks Report, cited in Labonté & Sanders, unpublished paper).

How will the changes in geopolitical global order impact the health of people and the planet? Labonté and Sanders (unpublished paper) argue that health outcomes will largely reflect the same trends of the past 40 years, with important differences:

- Climate change and the depletion of environmental resources will continue to endanger human health, especially the health of people who are poor.

- The breakdown in multilateralism will increase the risk of global conflict and war.
- The increase in **autocracy** and nationalism will intensify the risk of domestic conflicts and the suppression of people's political rights and civil liberties.
- The widening gap between the people who are rich and those who are poor will lead to a continuing decline in inequitable health outcomes between and within countries.

GLOSSARY

Autocracy: power is concentrated in the hands of one person whose decisions are not subject to legal restraints or other regulations.

Efforts to promote health equity based on policies enacted solely within national borders are unlikely to be optimally effective, with national governments being increasingly reliant on placating global capital for their own survival and thereby often allowing the intrusion of commercially damaging industries and commodities (Labonté & Sanders, unpublished paper).

Sidelining multilaterialism in favour of multistakeholderism

In 2018, the UN-Forum Partnership, a new partnership agreement, was quietly signed by the World Economic Forum (WEF) and the United Nations (UN), giving TNCs a place inside the UN, thus giving them influence over global governance matters (Gleckman, 2019). The agreement bypassed the UN member states' review process, established multistakeholder partnerships as the solution to the problems with the multilateral system, and proposed that these partnerships do not need to be governed by the system of democracy, i.e. the one-country-one vote system (Gleckman, 2019).

The agreement includes new multistakeholder partnerships to deliver public goods in six fields—education, health, gender equality, financing, climate change and digital cooperation. Critics warn that the goal of each seems to be less in line with intergovernmentally agreed goals and more consistent with the business interests of WEF members (Gleckman, 2019).

By 2020, the COVID-19 pandemic saw a transformation in multilateralism in global health forever, although it is unclear whether it has in fact strengthened it. On the one hand, countries did join in solidarity during this crisis; however, it is unclear whether this international cooperation can address the question of equitable access to medical products for people throughout the world (Patnaik, 2021a). The Biden administration (2021) is more committed to multilateralism.

In April 2020, the European Union (EU), more than a dozen countries, the Bill & Melinda Gates Foundation, key Gates-funded global health actors, the World Bank Group and the World Health Organization (WHO) established a multistakeholder initiative, the ACT-Accelerator. The aim was to collaborate around hastening the process of COVID-19 diagnostics, therapeutics and vaccine development and production.

Concerns have been raised around the governance structure of the ACT-Accelerator, with decision-making power being removed from the multilateral WHO platform to a multistakeholder partnership of self-appointed rich and powerful donors and excluding the majority of countries and people's voices. It is feared that as we move forward, multistakeholder partnerships in global health governance will be formalised and will ultimately impact on equitable access to health and quality health care for all.

The pandemic illustrates how private partners in global health have come to assume more space even as smaller countries have been edged out of the table and their populations pay the price for the lack of transparency and equity in global health governance (Patnaik, 2021a).

Notwithstanding the health and economic shocks and setbacks of the global COVID-19 pandemic, on average human health has improved over the past few decades. However, these gains have not been equitably shared between or within countries, and in the poorest regions there have been reversals as well as persistent high rates of maternal and child mortality. This leads back to the question posed at the beginning of this chapter: Why are underdeveloped countries still underdeveloped today?

Is overpopulation a cause of underdevelopment?

Is poverty and underdevelopment not merely a matter of scarce resources? Is the cake too small and there are too many mouths to feed? This idea is not new. It was Thomas Malthus (1766–1834) who was the first to refer to overpopulation as the reason for hunger in England in the early nineteenth century, asserting that the number of people will always exceed the amount of food available and the 'natural' result was poverty and starvation. The solution, according to Malthus was 'sexual restraint'—the only escape from this threat of overpopulation of the Earth by people living in poverty. He was proven wrong by historical developments. After a period wherein both death rates and birth rates were high, birth rates started to fall after 1880. As living standards improved, mortality declined. Subsequently fertility also declined, and the rate of population growth slowed down and eventually turned into a decline in some countries.

However, since the 1960s, when 'population explosion' hysteria was at its peak, *overpopulation* has once again been persistently mentioned as one of the reasons for underdevelopment. Robert McNamara, a past President of the World Bank, for example, stated that, "*the greatest single obstacle to the economic and social advancement of the peoples in the underdeveloped world is rampant population growth ... *" (quoted in *New Internationalist*, May 1974, p. 11). This argument has given rise to family planning and population control programmes in poor countries.

During the twentieth century, the global population grew from 1.65 billion to 6 billion. The annual growth rate reached its peak in the late 1960s, when it was growing at around 2%. Since then, the rate of increase has almost halved and has continued to decline. By 2017 it was around 1.12% (Worldometer, 2017).

We will discuss population growth in more detail in the next section.

It is easy enough to show that Malthus was quite wrong in terms of his prediction about inevitable food shortage due to the number of people exceeding the amount of food available:

- Comparing 1830 with 1750, *fewer* food producers were producing *more* food, for *more than double* the population.
- By 1850, *four* farmers could produce enough food to feed *five* people.
- By 1940, *one* farmer could produce enough food to feed 10 people.
- By 1960, *one* farmer could produce enough food for 24 people (cited in Hansen, 1970).
- By 2012, *one* farmer could produce enough to feed 160 people worldwide (*The Gazette*, 2017).

The real problem is *not* inadequate food production. It is *inappropriate production* and *inequitable distribution*. The impact of capitalism on traditional societies has been greatest in terms of land ownership and food production. The dispossession of peasants and cottagers of their land and the replacement of them with capitalists, which occurred during England's agricultural revolution, has been repeated in an exaggerated way in the twentieth century.

Large agribusiness has not only expanded onto the most arable farming land in underdeveloped countries, but has also promoted **cash-crop production** at the expense of traditional subsistence farming, so that underdeveloped countries now rely on meagre payments for their cash crops—which people can't eat—and other industrial production, to buy the excess grain that the developed countries produce.

GLOSSARY

Cash-crop production: an agricultural crop which is grown for sale to make a profit rather than used to feed the producer's own family or livestock. It includes, for example, plants grown for animal feed or biofuels, coffee, cocoa, tea, sugarcane, cotton and spices, as well as non-food crops like fresh cut flowers.

The means of, and the control over, the production of food are shifting from the farmers in the South to big agri-food businesses and transnational retail companies based mainly in the North, removing power from local producers, consumers, and, in many instances, policy-makers. Liberalised trade regimes, food price speculation in the global market and land grabs are contributing to this shift. The Agreements of the World Trade Organization (WTO) have moved control over the right to food and food security to the global market. Human-induced climate change plus other forms of environmental degradation are also affecting the food system, contributing to the impaired quantity, quality and affordability of food in countries (People's Health Movement, ALAMES, Health Action International, Medico International, Third World Network, & Medact, 2014).

Land ownership/inequitable distribution

Giant foreign and local TNCs have penetrated countries where subsistence agriculture predominated. They now control the best land, as well as the most technologically advanced production, processing and manufacturing, procurement, storage and transportation, and retailing and marketing methods.

Underdeveloped countries are unable to develop their agricultural potential because of grossly unfair land distribution. In Latin America, for example, which has the most unequal distribution of land in the world, 1% of the largest farms control more than 50% of the region's productive land (Oxfam, 2016). The most extreme case is in Colombia, where 0.4% of the largest farms control over 67% of productive land and 84% of the smallest farms occupy less than 4% of productive land. Women are particularly marginalised in terms of access to land (Oxfam, 2016).

According to the Secretary General of the Ports Management Association of Eastern and Southern Africa, although Africa has the potential to feed itself and export surplus food to the rest of the world, over the past few decades its agricultural imports have far exceeded its exports. Apart from now importing grain from developed countries, Africa even imports products that compete with its own products, such as meat, dairy products, cereals and oils.

Africa accounts for 47 percent of the total land area transferred to foreign owners worldwide, followed by Asia at 33 percent. The United States is the largest land purchaser, although large purchases are made by China, India, Israel, the United Arab Emirates (UAE) and the United Kingdom (UK). Africa is now estimated to account for about 560 000 km² of 830 000 km² of land transferred to foreign ownership globally since 2000 (Maoulidi, 2015).

The developed world has not escaped the reach of large agribusiness, and agricultural production is concentrated on a small number of large farms. For example, in the USA:

- In the 1930s there were 6.8 million farms; by 2016, this had decreased to an estimated 2.06 million (USDA, 2017).
- In 1870, almost 50% of the US population was employed in agriculture. By 2008, this was down to less than 2% of the population (Bureau of Labor Statistics, US Government, 2013).
- In the past, most farms were owned by small property owners. By 2017, it is estimated that 30% of American farmland was owned by institutional investors and foreign corporations who leased it out to farmers (Keiffer, 2017).

According to the agricultural census 2010, there were 186 660 farms in the UK, with 1.4% of the British active population working on farms, which produce less than 60% of the food the UK eats.

Vast areas of the world are potentially able to produce food crops. It has been calculated that only 11% (1.5 billion hectares) of the world's land surface (13.4 billion hectares) is used in crop production. A further 2.7 billion hectares have the potential to be used for crop production (FAO, 2015). Most commercial agriculture today uses intensive farming or industrial agriculture, which is heavily reliant on industrial methods designed to increase crop yields or output per unit land area. This means:

> Concerning the future, a number of projection studies have addressed and largely answered in the positive the issue as to whether the resource base of world agriculture, including its land component, can continue to evolve in a flexible and adaptable manner as it did in the past, and also whether it can continue to exert downward pressure on the real price of food (see, for example, Pinstrup-Andersen, Pandya-Lorch and Rosegrant, 1999). The largely positive answers mean essentially that for the world as a whole there is enough, or more than enough, food production potential to meet the growth of effective demand, i.e. the demand for food of those who can afford to pay farmers to produce it (FAO, 2015).

Inappropriate crop production

Most agricultural production in the underdeveloped world is by peasant farmers. With their small plots of land, they are economically vulnerable to large-scale producers who control productive technology, storage and marketing facilities. This threatens the very survival of the peasants.

India is the third largest agricultural producer globally by value, after the USA and China. Agriculture is the primary means of livelihood for more than 50%–60% of India's population, although India is also home to a quarter of the undernourished people globally and almost 50% of the children under five years old are stunted and 20% are wasting (People's Health Movement et al., 2014). In 2020, according to the Global Hunger Index, India ranked 94th among 107 hunger-afflicted countries globally (Patnaik, 2021b). See Chapter 1 for more information on wasting.

According to Patnaik (2021b) the government-run Food Corporation of India (FCI) holds massive food grain stocks. However, this does not mean that India grows enough food grains to meet its requirements. Patnaik argues that the stock buildup is not caused by people having more food than they need, but by the majority of people having less income because "whenever the amount of purchasing power in the hands of the people has increased, stocks have tended to dwindle."

> The fall in per capita consumption of food grain can be explained only by a decline in income and purchasing power for a majority of the population, and is a symptom of general rural distress, combined with acute distress in specific regions. Rural distress is apparent from the recurrent and widespread incidence of farmers' suicides. Over 270 000 farmers are estimated to have committed suicide between 1995 and 2011 (People's Health Movement et al., 2014).

Before World War II, the underdeveloped countries as a whole were net exporters of cereals, but they have subsequently become net importers, while coffee, cocoa, tea and sugar are being exported to the developed world in increasing amounts. In Senegal, desert has been irrigated so that TNCs can grow eggplant and mangoes for Europe's wealthy elites, while some Senegalese starve. In Costa Rica, the beef export business expands as local consumption of meat and dairy products declines. In Colombia, wheat production declines as cut flowers destined for the USA bring 80% greater returns per acre.

Further challenging the Malthusian argument (that the number of people will always exceed the amount of food available and the 'natural' result is poverty and starvation) are the great disparities that exist across the world today. For example, according to the Worldwatch Institute (2017):

- 12% of the world's population who live in the USA and Western Europe consume 60% of the world's total resources, while the one-third living in underdeveloped countries consume 3.2%.
- The USA, "*with less than 5% of the world's population, uses about a quarter of the world's fossil fuel resources—burning up nearly 25% of the coal, 26% of the oil, and 27% of the world's natural gas.*"

So, we have a situation where hunger abounds in the underdeveloped world, while grain, beef, butter and milk accumulate in the developed world. And to complete this incredible picture, in 2019, 34 million Americans or 10.5% of the population was living in poverty and struggled to put food on the table (see Figure 3.23) (Semega et al., 2020). In 2018/2019 more than 14.5 million people or 22% of the population in the UK were living in poverty (Francis-Devine, 2020). It was predicted that a further 700 000 would be pushed into poverty due to the COVID-19 pandemic.

Population growth, mortality and underdevelopment

The world's population doubled from about 500 million in the 1600s to 1 billion in 1804 and doubled again to 2 billion in 1930. In 1959, the world population was 3 billion; 4 billion in 1974; 5 billion in 1987; and 6 billion in 1999—this is a 100% increase in just 40 years (see Figure 3.24). It is estimated that the world population will continue to grow into the twenty-first century but at a much slower rate; for example, it will take another 40 years to increase by another 50% to become 9 billion by 2037 (Worldometer, 2017).

GLOSSARY

Population growth rate: the difference between birth rates and death rates.

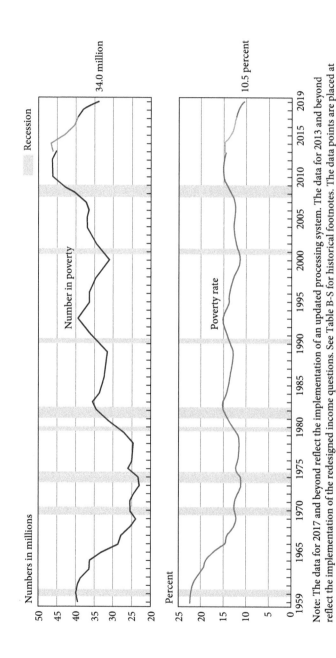

Fig. 3.23 Number in poverty and poverty rate, 1959–2019. **Note:** Median household income was US$68 703 in 2019.

Note: The data for 2017 and beyond reflect the implementation of an updated processing system. The data for 2013 and beyond reflect the implementation of the redesigned income questions. See Table B-S for historical footnotes. The data points are placed at the midpoints of the respective years. For information on recessions, See Appendix A. For information on confidentiality protection, sampling error, nonsampling error, and definitions, see <http://www2.census.gov/programs-surveys/cps/techdocs/cpsmar20.pdf>.

Source: Semega et al. (2020). *Income and Poverty in the United States: 2019.* US Census Bureau.

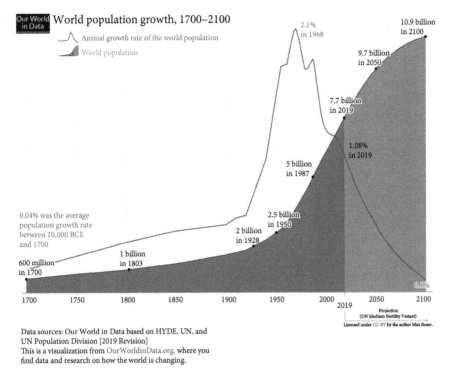

Fig. 3.24 World population growth, 1700–2100.

Source: Roser, M. (2014b). Future population growth. OurWorldInData.org.
https://ourworldindata.org/future-population-growth.

Previously we saw that in the nineteenth century, a disproportionate share of the population growth occurred in the now developed countries. In England and Wales, improved social, economic and demographic structures led to a sustained drop in mortality from undernutrition and infectious disease. This was followed by a sustained decline in fertility. The overall effect was a continuous but decelerating growth of population, which has only recently ceased.

Since the mid-twentieth century, most of the increase in population occurred in the underdeveloped world. This was partly as a result of an unexpected rapid decline in death rates due to the reduction of famines and because of specific medical measures being transferred to the underdeveloped world for the control of epidemic and endemic diseases. These factors helped to bring about a small drop in death rates, but fertility remained high, allowing for a rapid, short-lived population growth. The relatively small decline in mortality, however, was *not* sustained, because the nutritional and environmental improvements that accompanied these medical measures in nineteenth-century England did not occur.

Globally, child mortality was still high in the twentieth century. In 1960, almost 20 million children under the age of five years died each year. Since then, this number has decreased, mostly due to preventable causes in underdeveloped countries. Since the 1990s, there has been a declining population growth rate in all countries at all stages of development (see Figure 3.25) (Roser, 2014a).

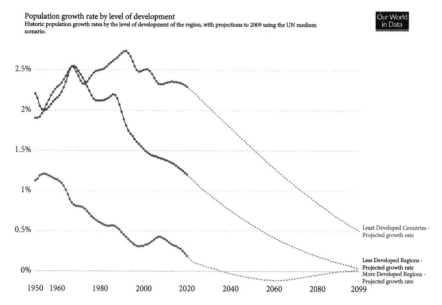

Fig. 3.25 Population growth rate by world region, 1950–2020 and projections through 2099.
Source: United Nations—Population Division. (2017 Revisions). World Population Growth. OurWorldInData.org.
https://ourworldindata.org/world-population-growth.

Population growth, fertility and underdevelopment

Today, changing fertility is determining what happens to population growth. Fertility in poor countries, especially in Africa, remains higher than the world average (see Figure 3.26). Why is this so? One of the most important factors influencing fertility is high infant and child mortality. There is also a relationship between parental educational levels (especially that of mothers) and children's health. Children who live in poorer households in rural areas and whose mothers have less education have a higher risk of dying before the age of five (UNICEF, 2010).

Having many children increases the chances that some will become adults. And for families living in poverty, in a subsistence economy, adult children are one of the only means of support for the elderly. Without further nutritional and environmental improvements, as happened in the developed world, it will be impossible to ensure a lasting reduction of child mortality and fertility.

According to Roser, from 1975 to 1980 some countries were able to substantially reduce their fertility rate. For example, India's fertility rate fell to 4.9 children per woman and China's to 3 children per woman. However, in other countries, like Yemen, the fertility rate was still very high at 8.6 children per woman. Since then, globally the fertility rate has halved, with 80% of the world population living in countries with a fertility rate below 3 children per woman; 10% living in countries with a fertility rate of more than 5; and 40% living in countries where each woman has on average fewer than 2 children (Roser, 2014a).

Total fertility rate (TFR) is the number of children that would be born to a woman if she were to live to the end of her childbearing years and bear children in accordance with age-specific fertility rates of the specified year.

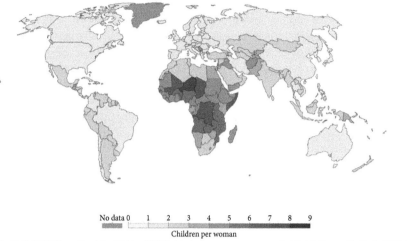

Source: United Nations – Population Division (2017 Revision)   OurWorldInData.org/fertility/ • CC BY-SA

Fig. 3.26 Children per woman (total fertility rate), 2015.
Source: Roser, M. (2014a). Fertility. OurWorldInData.org.
https://ourworldindata.org/fertility/.

*Global fertility is barely higher than the **global replacement fertility** .... With the current level of mortality, the global replacement fertility is 2.3—the narrow gap between the current global fertility and the global replacement rate means that the increase of the world population is due to the increasing length of life and population momentum. Population momentum occurs—as the World Bank explains, "when a large proportion of a country's population is of childbearing age. Even if the fertility rate of people in developing countries reaches replacement level, that is if couples have only enough children to replace themselves when they die, for several decades the absolute numbers of people being born still will exceed the numbers of people dying.*

We also see convergence in fertility rates: the countries that already had low fertility in the 1950s only slightly decreased fertility, while many of the countries that had the highest fertility back then saw a rapid reduction of the number of children per woman" (Roser, 2014a).

GLOSSARY

Total fertility rate (TFR): the number of children born per woman.

Global replacement fertility: *"The total fertility rate at which the population size stays constant. If there were no mortality in the female population until the end of the childbearing years, the replacement fertility would be exactly 2"* (Roser, 2014a).

Beijing and Cairo Declarations against population control

As a result of the above theories on population growth, together with advocacy by development theorists and women's groups, two global meetings—the International Conference on Population Development in Cairo, Egypt in 1994 and the Fourth World Conference on Women in Beijing, China in 1995—ratified a developmental approach and argued against the population control arguments of the mid-1950s–1980s.

In summary, although the conditions into which people are born, live, work, age and die look similar to those of nineteenth-century Europe, the political, social and economic forces at play in the twenty-first century are extremely different. 'Overpopulation' and limited resources are not the real causes of underdevelopment. They are the consequences of the global economic system that underdeveloped countries have been subjected to since the era of colonisation, which perpetuates uneven development. Contemporary approaches promote social and economic development, female education and providing women with safe choices to control their fertility, as well as improved child survival. These strategies are meant to replace the population control ideologies of the mid-1950–1980s, although implementation has been very uneven, especially for underdeveloped countries.

Contemporary globalisation directly and indirectly affects health and development in the following ways:

- It *directly* affects health through its impact on a country's health system, health policies and other policies that impact on health. We will explore this further in Chapter 4.
- It also *indirectly* affects health by impacting on the economic policies of a nation. These policies in turn have an impact on the economic climate, employment, livelihoods, food security and general health and well-being. These policies also influence budget allocations, including the health budgets and the budgets of other public-sector departments which might address the social determinants of health, for example access to water and sanitation.

As an example, we turn to the role of the main institution that has come to dominate the global food system—the 'Big Food' TNCs.

CASE STUDY: Big Food TNCs

> ... *global public health problems take on different forms, [but] they are all linked to the production and consumption of food. And while what we eat is ultimately affected by what we do or do not place in our own mouths, there are far larger forces at work. One of these is 'globalization', a process promoted as the solution to world food problems* (People's Health Movement, Medact, Global Equity Gauge, 2008).

In Chapter 2 we saw that diet-related illnesses are among the top 10 leading risk factors for the global burden of disease. While there are multiple causes of this, they

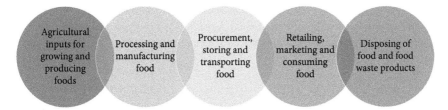

Fig. 3.27 The food value chain.

can ultimately be linked to the global food system, which includes all the processes, inputs and outputs that are involved in providing food or food-related products, such as growing, producing, processing, manufacturing, procuring, storing, transporting, advertising, marketing, selling, consuming and disposing of food and food waste products (see Figure 3.27).

In today's globalised world, each node in the food chain is dominated by the same small group of very large TNCs—Monsanto, Cargill, Syngenta, Nestlé, Coca-Cola, Walmart and McDonald's, among others. These 'stateless' corporations operate across borders, organise the system in their own favour and control the flow of food through the food value chain. They influence what food people have access to and eat, with implications for public health, hunger and nutrition. They potentially undermine the development agendas of many countries and contribute to aggregate wealth but also to poverty and inequality.

The impact of Big Food dominance on agricultural inputs and production
In 2016, six mega-TNCs controlled 75% of the global seed and agrochemical market. It was expected that they would rapidly be reduced to three or four, which would then control 60% of the seed and 70% of the agrochemical market worldwide.

> *The most recent large-scale merger proposal was that of Dow Chemical Co. and DuPont Co. This merger would create the single largest biotechnology and seed firm in the United States, controlling 76% of the market for corn and 66% of the market for soybeans. This would only further thin a market most recently hit with a round of mergers that resulted in the existence of only six large biotechnology firms; Monsanto, Syngenta, Bayer, DuPont, Dow, and BASF* (National Farmers Union, 2016).

The impact of TNC dominance on small-scale farmers and producers
Big Food TNCs impact most harshly on small-scale farmers around the world, but especially in underdeveloped countries. Small-scale farmers are being forced off their land to make way for large-scale commercial farming activities. Today, although over 90% of all farms globally are 'small' (being an average of 2.2 hectares), they have less than 25% of the world's farmland (GRAIN, 2014). However, they still focus on food production, while Big Food TNCs tend to focus on producing commodities and export crops, many of which people cannot eat.

Small or peasant farms prioritise food production. They tend to focus on local and national markets and their own families. Much of what they produce doesn't enter into national trade statistics, but it does reach those who need it most: the rural and urban poor (GRAIN, 2014).

While mega-TNCs are enriched, small farmers are marginalised and large sections of the global population are rendered poorer, more dependent and thus more vulnerable. Those small farmers that manage to survive are being diverted away from the genetically diverse crops that they have cultivated for generations and towards a smaller variety of tightly controlled seed. This is expensive for small farmers and reduces genetic diversity in seed stock.

The impact of TNC dominance in processing and manufacturing

TNCs use their power as the main buyers of crops (such as grains and sugar) to fix at low levels direct purchasing prices from producers and to impose high sales prices on consumers. Their dominance in the food system and in specific commodity chains contributes towards creating an 'abnormal' food environment, which has implications for public health (Swinburn et al., 2011).

Their monopoly over agricultural inputs and production has destroyed nutrients and has removed much of the taste and colour from food. The global food industry compensates by adding artificial flavourings, colourings and chemical preservatives to extend the shelf-life that foods destined for the global marketplace require. TNC monopoly in the sugar milling sector and in the manufacturing of processed products has the following effects:

- It displaces healthy calories, both in terms of the kind of nutritious crops farmers can grow and in terms of consumption, where people eat these 'dead calories' instead or nutrient-rich ones. This in turn contributes to the increase we are seeing in illnesses like diabetes, heart disease and certain cancers.
- Growing sugar uses up farmland, as well as valuable environmental resources needed to grow it, which could otherwise be used to grow nutrient-dense foods, i.e. foods that provide a high amount of nutrients but have relatively few calories (e.g. vegetables and fruit).

And yet the demand for sugar means that how it is grown, traded, processed into foods and consumed has a knock-on effect through the whole food system.

Agribusiness has been involved in industrial food animal production (known as 'factory farms') since just after World War II and the practice has grown exponentially since then. Addressing the 2016 World Health Assembly, the departing Director-General of WHO, Dr Margaret Chan, cautioned that the global health landscape was being shaped by '*three slow-motion disasters*', climate change, the rise in chronic non-communicable diseases and antibiotic-resistant microbes, and "*factory farming connects the dots among them*" (Weathers et al., 2017):

- Factory farms generate more greenhouse gas emissions than 'all forms of transportation combined' (Weathers et al., 2017).

- "*Livestock production* [most of which is carried out in industrial systems] *is responsible for 18% of global greenhouse gas (GHG) emissions from all human activities … This is a higher share than transport, which accounts for 14% of global GHG emissions*" (Compassion in World Farming, 2008).
- Meat consumption, especially inexpensive processed and red meats, has been linked to the growing incidence of chronic diseases.
- About 75% of the antibiotics used in the USA and EU are used on factory farm animals to prevent superbugs spreading among the densely packed animals and to speed up their growth. This leads to the breeding of antibiotic-resistant bacteria, which are passed from animals to humans in the food they eat, so that regular antibiotics may soon be rendered ineffective in treating bacterial infections.

The impact of TNC dominance in procurement, storage and transportation of food

By taking over the procurement, storage and transportation of fresh produce to capture added value, large TNCs cut out intermediaries, reduce the amount of produce going through fresh food markets and reduce the turnover and profitability of independent retailers and informal traders.

The FAO predicted that the total global bill for importing food in 2017 would be US$1.318 trillion—a 10.6% increase from 2016 (Third World Network, 2017). This is partly because of higher volumes of food, price hikes and rising freight costs. The increase in food prices leads to deepening poverty, especially for the urban poor who already live below the extreme poverty line of US$1.90 a day and who spend most of their income on staple foods (Roser, 2014a). The crisis means that the urban poor resort to eating less and to eating poorer diets, which have long-term nutritional and health consequences.

> … the global tendency for higher import costs in 2017 concerns many of the economically vulnerable nations. The food import bills of least-developed countries (LDCs), low-income food deficit countries (LIFDCs) and those geographically situated in sub-Saharan Africa (SSA) are forecast to rise by more than the global average, with the overall increase amounting to 13 percent in the case of the LDCs, the most vulnerable country group (Third World Network, 2017).

The impact of TNC dominance in retail, marketing and consumption

The increasing control of TNCs over the food environment, the unregulated operations of the fast-food sector and the extensive advertising of 'high-status' fast foods have resulted in an environment saturated with unhealthy and cheap foods, with implications for public health, hunger and nutrition.

In summary, the monopolistic control by TNCs of the global food chain threatens each country's capacity for development and the realisation of the population's right to food. For a nation, region or household to be food secure, conditions must be such that not only is food produced and available, but also that people have access to it, both financially and physically; and that food is used in a way that supports nutrition, has sufficient protein and micronutrients, and is safe to eat.

Consumption, nutrition and health

Increasing urbanisation, long working and commuting hours and less time available to shop for and cook wholesome meals push people to eat 'on the run'. These factors have led to significant market expansion of fast-food options that are cheap, highly processed, starchy, calorie-dense and nutrient-poor.

The structure of the habitual diet is altered and is characterized by increasing consumption of fats, saturated fats largely from animal sources and sugars. Lifestyle changes in an increasingly urbanized environment which occurs concurrently contributes to a reduction in physical activity levels which promotes overweight and obesity (Shetty, 2013).

The 'nutritional transition' and the 'dietary transition'

There is a direct link between the increasing sales of ultra-processed fast foods and beverages, the aggressive marketing and promotion strategies used by Big Food TNCs (to promote the perception that these products are desirable) and the global epidemic of obesity and its link to NCDs. TNCs are **commercial determinants of health (CDoH)** and drivers of these epidemics, undermining NCD prevention and control (Moodie et al., 2013; Mialon, 2020).

GLOSSARY

Commercial determinants of health (CDoH): *"factors that influence health which stem from a profit motive"* such as the marketing and promotion of harmful goods including unhealthy foods, tobacco, sugar-sweetened beverages and alcohol (Ireland et al., 2019).

A 'nutritional transition' is occurring in some underdeveloped countries, where there is the traditional shift away from undernutrition and its related diseases of poverty to an increasing prevalence of overnutrition, obesity and diet-related NCDs.

In Chapter 2, the protracted-polarised model proposed by Frenk et al. (1989) is discussed in more detail in the section 'Epidemiological transition').

However, there is a more complex picture of the nutritional status of population, showing a mixed disease pattern occurring over a protracted period of time. *At the same time,* in *other* population groups in the *same* country, there is both widespread undernutrition and poverty-related diseases *coexisting* with widespread overweight, obesity and diet-related NCDs (Frenk et al., 1989). Underlying this burden of undernutrition is a 'dietary transition'—a general move to a diet that is higher in

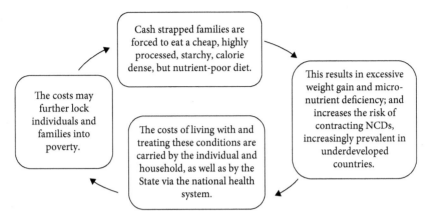

Fig. 3.28 The vicious cycle of an unhealthy diet, NCDs and poverty.

calories, less diverse and lower in fibre and made up of more highly processed, energy-dense but nutritionally poor foods.

> As a result, many low- and middle-income countries now face a growing burden from the modern risks to health, while still fighting an unfinished battle with the traditional risks to health (WHO, 2009).

An unhealthy, cheap diet, NCDs and poverty, combined with the intergenerational perpetuation of malnutrition or the 'foetal origins' hypothesis, creates a vicious cycle that further entrenches poverty and inequality, undernutrition, NCDs and so on (see Figure 3.28). (See page 29 for more information about the 'foetal origins' or Barker hypothesis.)

Writing in 2004 about the specific nature of this dietary transition in South Africa, Chopra and Sanders (2004) comment that:

> Increased exposure to fast foods, decreases in the relative cost of meat and high fat foods, and reduced time for food preparation are all changing dietary patterns in the urban setting ... Until a couple of decades ago the African population consumed a typical traditional diet, where the fat intake was only 16% of the total calories. By 1990 the fat intake in an urban African community had increased to 26% ... [In addition, those who lived most of their lives in cities] consumed a typical westernised diet with 30% of calories from total fat, while those who had spent less than 20% of their lives in the city only consumed 22.5% of calories from total fat.

A further driver of ill-health is the threat of climate change, which will disproportionally affect people living in poverty. Global economic expansion has changed the natural environment in both direct and indirect ways; and it has affected the ability of people to control these changes.

Increasing population significantly increases the pressures of climate change, and so reduction of the ecological footprint is vital, bearing in mind that rich countries have a higher footprint than low- and middle-income countries.

TNCs, climate change and ill-health

Up until the Industrial Revolution, the world's climate was relatively stable, with changes occurring so slowly that animals and human beings managed to adapt. However, researchers at the Berkeley Earth Project have concluded that over the past 250 years or so the world has warmed 1.5°C (Berkeley Earth, 2014). The Earth is now failing to regulate its temperatures or retain its temperature balance as well as it used to. In the past few decades there have been changes in the global climate that previously took millions of years to occur—more frequent extreme weather incidents and major natural disasters, like unseasonal rains, floods, hurricanes, higher global temperatures, earthquakes, volcanoes, tsunamis and wildfires.

The direct changes to the Earth's environment have occurred via some of the following human activities and processes:

- The consumption and use of fossil fuels in the form of gas, coal and oil in industrial processes or by vehicles has resulted in high concentrations of greenhouse gases being emitted into the atmosphere, resulting in global warming.
- A change in land-use, for example by mega agribusinesses, has resulted in **deforestation**, land cover change and the loss of certain species—affecting ecosystems and biodiversity. This is thought to encourage the spread of zoonotic infections (infections that pass from animals to humans), such as Ebola in West Africa and COVID-19 globally.
- The greater concentration on **monoculture** has led to extensive soil erosion and loss of soil fertility.
- The extraction and exploitation of natural resources in mining processes has resulted in **desertification**, land degradation and displacement of communities.
- The depletion and contamination of our natural resources, such as our freshwater systems, has resulted in water shortages for humans, plants and animals. Drought has multiple consequences for health: skin diseases, diarrhoeal diseases and contagious diseases.

GLOSSARY

Deforestation: the destruction of huge forests from an area of land.

Monoculture: a single crop is cultivated at a time over a wide area, again and again. This has an adverse impact on the environment as well as on agriculture.

Desertification: a process by which land becomes increasingly dry until almost no vegetation grows on it, making it a desert.

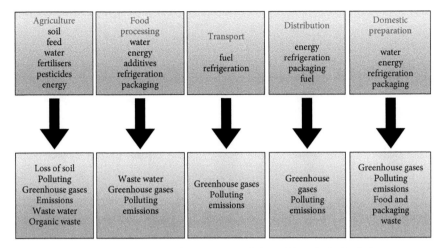

Fig. 3.29 Sustainability of food products: responsibility of the whole food chain.
Source: Data from ENEA (Iannetta, 2010).

Activities across the entire globalised food value chain play a major role in environmental degradation and in greenhouse gas emissions that impact on global warming (see Figure 3.29).

Different methods have been used to calculate the impact of the global food system on energy usage and greenhouse gas emissions. One method is to analyse the carbon footprint that can be attributed to food miles—how far food travels from where it is grown to where it is bought and consumed.

Increasingly efficient global transport networks make it practical to bring food before it spoils from distant places where labor costs are lower. And the penetration of mega-markets in nations from China to Mexico with supply and distribution chains that gird the globe—like Wal-Mart, Carrefour and Tesco—has accelerated the trend. But the movable feast comes at a cost: pollution—especially carbon dioxide, the main global warming gas—from transporting the food (Rosenthal, 2008).

However, the transportation of food is only one factor that determines its global environmental impact. How the food is produced and using what kind of energy along the entire food life cycle should be taken into account.

Climate change creates direct and indirect risks to human health, well-being and security, especially for those with the fewest resources, but ultimately for everyone (see Figure 3.30). In 2000, for example, it was estimated that approximately 150 000 deaths were as a result of climate change, with almost all these deaths being among the world's poorest populations, even though they contribute the least to the world's total carbon footprint (Marmot et al., 2008). The WHO estimates that between 2030 and 2050, climate change is expected to cause approximately 250 000 additional deaths annually, from malnutrition, diarrhoea and heat stress (WHO, 2018b). Changing temperatures

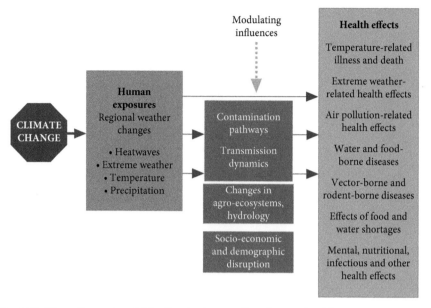

Fig. 3.30 The pathways by which climate change affects human health.

Source: WHO (2003). Summary. Climate change and human health: risks and response. https://www.who.int/globalchange/summary/en/.

accelerate transmission rates of diseases and can also allow the resurgence of previously eradicated organisms in certain areas, such as malaria mosquitoes.

Unless much stronger climate change mitigation efforts are introduced, it is highly likely that severe droughts will occur during the twenty-first century over most of Africa, southern Europe and the Middle East, and most of the Americas, Australia and South-East Asia (Dai, 2010). In addition to the effect of drought on agriculture and food production, the increase in temperature during the growing season causes additional serious problems for agricultural productivity, farm incomes and food security.

Conclusion

This chapter has provided a historical perspective to explain how imperialism is entrenched in the current world order. Debunking the myths about medical interventions and overpopulation, it explains how contemporary globalisation is a continuation of imperialist political and economic policies.

Underdeveloped countries have not always been poor. The historical context demonstrates that they were subjected to a global economic system that perpetuates an uneven distribution of resources, which explains their being 'underdeveloped'. The monopolistic control by TNCs of the global food chain (from farm to fork) threatens each country's capacity for development and the realisation of their populations' right to food, directly and indirectly affecting health and well-being and placing them in a situation of high vulnerability and dependency. Development requires that the mechanisms that keep people 'underdeveloped' are removed.

References

African Development Bank. (2017). Africa's pathway out of poverty—by Dr. Akinwumi A. Adesina, President of the African Development Bank, World Food Prize Laureate Luncheon, October 20, 2017, in Des Moines, Iowa. https://www.afdb.org/en/news-and-events/africas-pathway-out-of-poverty-by-dr-akinwumi-a-adesina-president-of-the-african-development-bank-world-food-prize-laureate-luncheon-october-20-2017-in-des-moines-iowa-17468.

Almond, D. & Currie, J. (2011). Killing me Softly: The Fetal Origins Hypothesis. *Journal of Economic Perspectives*, 25(3):153–172.

Alves, C. & Topoowski, J. (2019). Growth of international finance and emerging economies: elements for an alternative approach. Paolo Sylos Labini *Quarterly Review*, 72(288):3–26.

Berkeley Earth, 2014. Know the facts: a skeptic's guide to climate change. http://static.berkeleyearth.org/pdf/skeptics-guide-to-climate-change.pdf.

Bijlmakers, L.A., Bassett, M. & Sanders, D. (1998). Socioeconomic stress, health and child nutritional status in Zimbabwe at a time of economic structural adjustment: a three year longitudinal study. Research report, no. 105. Nordiska Afrikainstitutet: Uppsala, Sweden.

Borders, M. & Sterling Burnett, H. (2006). Farm subsidies: devastating the world's poor and the environment. National Center for Policy Analysis. Brief Analysis, no. 547. http://www.ncpa.org/pdfs/ba547.pdf.

Bureau of Labour Statistics, US Government. (2013). Employment by major industry sector. www.Bls.gov. Accessed 1 April 2014.

Cheshire, J. (2012). Lives on the line: life expectancy and child poverty as a Tube map. https://jcheshire.com/featured-maps/lives-on-the-line/.

Chopra, M. & Sanders, D. (2004). From apartheid to globalisation: health and social change in South Africa. *Hygiea Internationalis: An Interdisciplinary Journal for the History of Public Health*, 4:153–174.

Compassion in World Farming. (2008). Global warning: climate change and farm animal welfare executive summary. https://www.ciwf.org.uk/media/5161319//global_warning.pdf.

Dai, A. (2010). *Drought Under Global Warming: A Review*. National Center for Atmospheric Research: Boulder, CO.

Dahlgren, G. & Whitehead, M. (1991). *Policies and Strategies to Promote Social Equity in Health*. Institute of Future Studies: Stockholm.

Doyal, L. & Pennell, I. (1976). 'Pox Britannica': health, medicine and underdevelopment. *Race and Class, A Journal on Racism, Empire and Globalisation*, 18(2):155–172.

Economic Justice Network of the Fellowship of Christian Councils in Southern Africa & The School of Public Health (as part of the Centre of Excellence in Food Security) at the University of Western Cape. (2016). Cross-Country Research on the Role of Multinational Corporations in Food Systems: The Case of South Africa, Mexico and Brazil.

Edwards, M. (2017). The Barker hypothesis. In: Preedy, V. & Patel, V. (eds). *Handbook of Famine, Starvation, and Nutrient Deprivation*. Springer: Cham.

Environmental Working Group (EWG). (2017). Farm subsidy database. https://farm.ewg.org/.

Eurostat Statistics Explained. (2010). Agricultural census in the United Kingdom. European Commission. https://ec.europa.eu/eurostat/statistics-explained/index.php?title=arch ive:agricultural_census_in_the_united_kingdom.

FAO. (2015). World agriculture: towards 2015/2030. An FAO perspective. EARTHSCAN. http://www.fao.org/3/y4252e/y4252e00.htm#topofpage.

Farming News. (2016). *Unwanted American Chicken Dumped in South Africa.* http://farmingpor tal.co.za/index.php/farmingnews/farmer-john-says/item/6864-unwanted-american-chic ken-dumped-in-south-africa.

Francis-Devine, B. (2020). *Poverty in the UK: Statistics.* Research Briefing. House of Commons Library, UK Parliament: London.

Frenk, J., Bobadilla, J.L., Sepulveda, J. & Lopez Cervantes, M. (1989). Health transition middle income countries: new challenges for health care. *Health Policy and Planning,* 4(1):29–39.

Friends of the Earth Europe. (2012). Food speculation still a threat following vote. http://www. foeeurope.org/food-speculation.

Frydenlund, J. & Riedl, B. (2001). *At the federal trough: farm subsidies for the rich and famous.* Environmental Working Group. https://www.heritage.org/agriculture/report/the-federal-trough-farm-subsidies-the-rich-and-famous.

Gleckman, H. (2019). How the United Nations is quietly being turned into a public-private partnership. Felix Dodds, blog. https://blog.felixdodds.net/2019/07/how-united-nations-is-quietly-being.html.

GRAIN. (2014). Hungry for land: small farmers feed the world with less than a quarter of all farmland. GRAIN, 28 May 2014. https://www.grain.org/article/entries/4929-hungry-for-land-small-farmers-feed-the-world-with-less-than-a-quarter-of-all-farmland.

Hansen, J. (1970). *The Population Explosion.* Pathfinder Press: New York.

Hill, C. (1967). *Reformation to Industrial Revolution.* Weidenfeld and Nicolson: London.

Hobsbawm, E.J. (1969). *Industry and Empire.* Pelican: London.

Hughes, C.C. & Hunter, J.M. (1970). Disease and 'development' in Africa. *Social Science & Medicine,* 3(4):443–493.

Iannetta, M. (2010). Food and Energy: A Sustainable Approach. ENEA. International Scientific Symposium, Biodiversity and Sustainable Diets United Against Hunger, 3–5 November 2010. FAO: Rome.

Ireland, R., Bunn, C., Reith, G., et al. (2019). Commercial determinants of health: advertising of alcohol and unhealthy foods during sporting event. *Bulletin of the World Health Organization,* 97:290–295.

Keiffer, K. (2017). Who really owns American farmland? *The Counter.* https://thecounter.org/ who-really-owns-american-farmland/.

Labonté, R. & Sanders, D. (unpublished). *The relevance of changing geopolitics for global health.*

Labonté, R. & Schrecker, T. (2007). Globalization and social determinants of health: introduction and methodological background (part 1 of 3). *BMC. Globalization and Health,* 3(5).

Legge, D. & Kim, S. (2020). Equitable access to Covid-19 vaccines: cooperation around research and production capacity is critical. *NAPSNET Special Reports,* 29 October, 2020. https://nauti lus.org/napsnet/napsnet-special-reports/equitable-access-to-covid-19-vaccines-cooperat ion-around-research-and-production-capacity-is-critical/.

Maoulidi, M. (2015). African land is a profitable but potentially dangerous investment. http:// www.ngopulse.org/article/2015/05/27/african-land-profitable-potentially-dangerous-inv estment.

Marmot, M.G. (2005). Social determinants of health inequities. *The Lancet,* 365:1099–1104.

Marmot, M. (2015). *The Health Gap: The Challenge of an Unequal World.* Bloomsbury: London.

Marmot, M.G., Friel, S., Bell, R., Houweling, T. & Taylor, S. (2008). Closing the gap in a generation: health equity through action on the social determinants of health. *The Lancet*, 372(9650):1661–1669.

Marmot, M.G., Rose, G., Shipley, M. & Hamilton, P.J. (1978). Employment grade and coronary heart disease in British civil servants. *Journal of Epidemiology and Community Health*, 32(4):244–249.

Marmot, M.G., Smith, G.D., Stansfeld, S., et al. (1991). Health inequalities among British civil servants: the Whitehall II study. *The Lancet*, 337:1397–1393.

McKeown, T. & Lowe, C.R. (1974). *An Introduction to Social Medicine*. Blackwell: Oxford.

Mialon, M. (2020). An overview of the commercial determinants of health. *Global Health*, 16:74.

Moodie, R., Stuckler, D., Monteiro, C., et al. (2013). Profits and pandemics: prevention of harmful effects of tobacco, alcohol, and ultra-processed food and drink industries. *The Lancet*, 381(9867):670–679.

National Farmers Union. (2016). *Fact Sheet, Consolidation in Agriculture*. National Farmers Union. Washington DC.

New Internationalist. (1974). People and population. Issue 015. https://newint.org/issues/ 1974/05/01/.

New Internationalist. (1976). How can the basic needs of all the people in the world be met? Issue 042. https://newint.org/issues/1976/08/01.

New York Times. (2016). Global trade after the failure of the Doha Round, by the Editorial Board. https://www.nytimes.com/2016/01/01/opinion/global-trade-after-the-failure-of-the-doha-round.html.

Office for National Statistics, Great Britain. (2017). Statistical Bulletin, Household disposable income and inequality in the UK: financial year ending 2016. Office for National Statistics, Government, UK.

Öney, B. (2017). The retreat of the global company. Economist.com. http://barisoney.com/en/the-retreat-of-the-global-company-economist-com/.

Oxfam. (2016). *Unearthed: Land, Power, and Inequality in Latin America*. Oxfam International: Nairobi.

Oxfam. (2017). Just 8 men own same wealth as half the world. https://www.oxfam.org/en/pressr oom/pressreleases/2017-01-16/just-8-men-own-same-wealth-half-world.

Oxfam. (2021). *The Inequality Virus: Bringing Together a World Torn Apart by Coronavirus Through a Fair, Just and Sustainable Economy*. Oxfam International: Nairobi.

Palley, T.I. (2007). Financialization: what it is and why it matters. Working Papers wp153. Political Economy Research Institute, University of Massachusetts at Amherst. https://ideas. repec.org/p/uma/periwp/wp153.html.

Patnaik, P. (2021a). COVID-19 vaccine governance: sidelining multilateralism. People's Health Movement. https://phmovement.org/wp-content/uploads/2021/01/final_phm_covid-and-governance-compressed.pdf. Accessed 11 February 2021.

Patnaik, P. (2021b). Why are people going hungry in India despite a massive grain surplus? *MRonline*. https://mronline.org/2021/01/12/why-are-people-going-hungry-in-india-desp ite-a-massive-grain-surplus/.

Paulo, S. (2011). *Europe and the Global Financial Crisis: Taking Stock of the EU's Policy Response*. Foundation Robert Schuman: Paris.

People's Health Movement, Medact, Global Equity Gauge. (2008). *Global Health Watch 2: An alternative World Health Report*. Zed Books, London. https://www.ghwatch.org/ghw2.html.

People's Health Movement, ALAMES, Health Action International, Medico International, Third World Network, & Medact. (2014). *Global Health Watch 4: An alternative World Health Report*, 2014. Zed Books Ltd. https://phmovement.org/global-health-watch-4/.

Rennen, W. & Martens, P. (2003). The globalisation timeline. Integrated Assessment, 4(3):139.

Rosenthal, E. (2008). Environmental cost of shipping groceries around the world. *The New York Times*. http://www.nytimes.com/2008/04/26/business/worldbusiness/26food.html.

Roser, M. (2014a). Fertility rate. Published online at OurWorldInData.org. Retrieved from: https://ourworldindata.org/fertility-rate/.

Roser, M. (2014b). Future population growth. OurWorldInData.org https://ourworldindata.org/future-population-growth.

Rudin, J. & Sanders, D. (2011). Debt, structural adjustment and health. In: Solly, B. & Brock, G. (eds). *Global Health and Global Health Ethics*. Cambridge University Press: Cambridge.

Schotte, J.J. (2000). *The WTO After Seattle*. Institute for International Economics: Washington, DC.

Semega, J., Kollar, M., Shrider, E.A. & Creamer, J.F. (2020). *Income and Poverty in the United States: 2019*. US Census Bureau, Current Population Reports, pp. 60–270. US Government Publishing Office: Washington, DC.

Shetty, P. (2013). Nutrition transition and its health outcomes. *Indian Journal of Pediatrics*, 80:21–27.

Statista. (2017). Walmart's net sales worldwide from fiscal year 2008 to 2022, by division (in billions US dollars. Statista. https://www.statista.com/statistics/269403/net-sales-of-walmart-worldwide-by-division/.

Swinburn, B., Sacks, G., Hall, K., et al. (2011). The global obesity pandemic: shaped by global drivers and local environments. *The Lancet*, 378(9793):804–814.

Szreter, S. (1988). The importance of social intervention in Britain's mortality decline c.1850–1914: a re-interpretation of the role of public health. *Social History of Medicine*, 1(1):1–38.

The Gazette. (2017). Fact check: Reynolds says one Iowa farmer feeds 155 people worldwide. http://www.thegazette.com/subject/news/government/fact-check/fact-check-reynolds-says-one-iowa-farmer-feeds-155-people-worldwide-20140524.

Third World Network. (2003). Third World Network Statement on Agriculture at the UN ECOSOC High-Level Session. TWN: Malaysia. https://www.twn.my/title/twninfo36.htm

Third World Network. (2017). World food import bill to rise by over 10% this year. SUNS #8481, 14 June 2017. TWN: Malaysia. https://www.twn.my/title2/wto.info/2017/ti170613.htm.

Thomson, D. (1950). *England in the Nineteenth Century*. Pelican: New Orleans.

UNICEF. (2010). The state of the world's children, 2010. https://www.unicef.org/reports/state-worlds-children-2010.

US Census Bureau, International Data Base. (2021). Population pyramid of the UK in 2021. US Census Bureau, International Data Base. https://www.census.gov/data-tools/demo/idb/#/country?COUNTRY_YEAR=2021&COUNTRY_YR_ANIM=2021&FIPS_SINGLE=UK.

US Census Bureau, International Data Base. (2021). Population pyramid of Malawi in 2021. https://www.census.gov/data-tools/demo/idb/#/country?COUNTRY_YEAR=2021&COUNTRY_YR_ANIM=2021&FIPS_SINGLE=MI.

USDA. (2017). Farms and land in farms 2016 summary. National Agricultural Statistics Service. https://www.nass.usda.gov/publications/todays_reports/reports/fnlo0217.pdf.

Wahl, P. (2008). Food Speculation: The Main Factor of the Price Bubble in 2008. Briefing Paper, World Economy, Ecology & Development (WEED).

Weathers, S., Hermanns, S. & Bittman, M. (2017). Health leaders must focus on the threats from factory farms. *New York Times*. https://www.nytimes.com/2017/05/21/opinion/who-factory-farming-meat-industry-.html.

Werner, D. & Sanders, D. (1997). *Questioning the Solution: The Politics of Primary Health Care and Child Survival*. Palo Alto, CA: HealthWrights.

WHO. (2009). *Protecting Health from Climate Change: Connecting Science, Policy and People*. WHO: Geneva.

WHO. (2018a). Health inequities and their causes. https://www.who.int/news-room/facts-in-pictures/detail/health-inequities-and-their-causes.

WHO. (2018b). Climate change and health. Fact sheet. https://www.who.int/news-room/fact-sheets/detail/climate-change-and-health.

Vogeler, I. (2005). *Food Security, Agriculture Policies and Globalization: Lessons from USA and India*. Institute for Social and Economic Change: Bengaluru, India.

Worldometer. (2017). Worldometer. http://www.worldometers.info/.

Worldwatch Institute. (2017). *EarthEd: Rethinking Education on a Changing Planet (State of the World)*. Island Press: Washington, DC.

WTO. (2013). The Bali Ministerial Declaration, adopted on 7 December 2013. https://www.wto.org/english/thewto_e/minist_e/mc9_e/balideclaration_e.htm.

WTO. (2017). Standards and safety. https://www.wto.org/english/thewto_e/whatis_e/tif_e/agrm4_e.htm#trs.

4

The Medical Contribution

Chapter 3 showed how the resources needed for health promotion are inequitably distributed within and across underdeveloped and developed countries, and that this situation is worsening. What then of the medical contribution? What about disease prevention, treatment and cure? Does the medical contribution significantly counteract the imbalance in the spread of health-promoting resources?

Once again, it is useful to look at the history of medical services in those societies dominated by imperialism, because these services are the foundations of the present-day health care services, which we explore in later chapters (see Figure 4.1).

Health services in the underdeveloped world

Health care and colonisation

Before, during and after the colonial period, traditional healers—variously described as herbalists or witchdoctors—provided an alternative to western scientific medicine for the majority of people in the colonies.

In the British Empire, before the nineteenth century, formal medical facilities in the colonial territories were provided by doctors attached to trading companies and were almost exclusively for their European employees. They were joined by physicians and surgeons serving in the armed forces overseas, and in the nineteenth century medical Christian missionary work in the colonies expanded rapidly (Doyal & Pennell, 1976).

In the late nineteenth century, economic depression in Europe resulted in major emigration to the colonies. The number of fatal epidemics among the colonisers abroad and the simultaneous improvements in health conditions at home highlighted the inadequacies of medical services in the colonies. By 1903 the policy of colonising governments was firstly, to preserve the health of the European community; secondly, to keep the local labour force in good working condition, to enhance their productivity; and thirdly, to prevent the spread of epidemics. This policy resulted in selective minimal medical facilities for plantation workers, miners and railway builders. The medical problems of the majority were neglected, unless they threatened the health of the administration.

What little medical care there was for the local population generally came from the missionaries who mainly served remote rural areas and provided rudimentary curative medicine. In addition to promoting evangelism, this work was recognised as, "*most helpful to the Government in their endeavour of opening up tropical Africa*" (Beck, 1970) (see Figure 4.2). Consequently, the colonising administration granted permanent subsidies to medical missions in the colonies (Doyal & Pennell, 1976).

The Struggle for Health. David Sanders with Wim De Ceukelaire and Barbara Hutton, Oxford University Press.
© Oxford University Press 2023. DOI: 10.1093/oso/9780192858450.003.0004

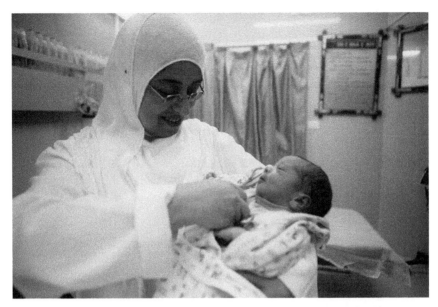

Fig. 4.1 What alternative approaches to health care are emerging to provide everyone with equal access to health care?
Source: Wim De Ceukelaire—Viva Salud.

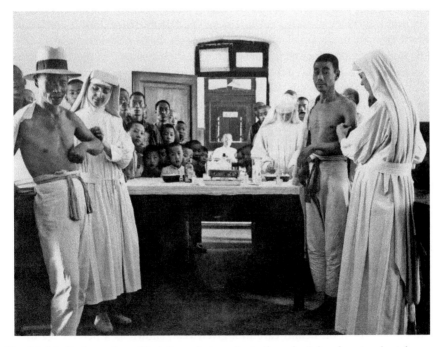

Fig. 4.2 Medical care from Christian missionaries in the colonial and post-colonial era was shaped by a complex of factors related to religion, education and politics.
Source: Alamy stock.

Later, as the colonies were increasingly viewed as potential markets for the Empire's manufactured goods, the colonising administration initiated public health activities to combat diseases that affected the European population (like malaria and sleeping sickness) or to maintain a healthier workforce and potential consumers. For example, in 1939 the Colonial Development Advisory Committee of Britain noted that:

If the productivity of the East African territories is to be fully developed, and with it, the potential capacity of those territories to absorb manufactured goods from the United Kingdom, it is essential that the standard of life of the native should be raised and to this end the eradication of disease is one of the most important measures (Meredith, 1975).

Health care in the post-colonial period

By the end of the colonial period, in the 1950s and 1960s, the organisation of health services in the underdeveloped world was largely modelled on a modified version of the system in the developed world, and this has continued with little change into the twenty-first century.

Health financing

Up until the mid-1970s, most developed countries devoted 5%–8% of their GNP to direct health service expenditure. Underdeveloped countries seldom devoted more than 2% of their much smaller GNPs to health services (World Bank, 1975). For the 65 underdeveloped countries for which data were available in the 1970s, about 40 spent less than US$3.00 per person per year on health care, with 27 spending US$2.00 or less (World Bank, 1975). Even today, most developed and underdeveloped countries still only devote on average 9.9% of their **gross domestic product (GDP)** to **total health service expenditure**, ranging from 12.3% for high-income countries to 4.5% for lower-middle-income countries (World Bank, 2017).

GLOSSARY

Gross domestic product (GDP): the total value of all the goods and services produced by all the citizens within a country's borders, usually in one year.

Average GDP per person or per capita: calculated by dividing the GDP by the total population. If, for example, two countries have the same GDP but one is twice as populated as the other, it will have a lower GDP per capita than the other country. In other words, the less populated country is more productive.

Total health service expenditure: the total amount of government and private money spent on health care in a given year, shown as a percentage of a country's GDP.

However, statistics such as these are misleading for several reasons, the most important being the inequitable access different groups of people have to health care services within most countries.

Health expenditure per capita is a particularly misleading statistic because health budgets (like any other) include capital and recurrent expenditures. Capital in the form of buildings or expensive equipment is likely to consume an appreciable proportion of the budget and yet be available to only a very limited section of the population. The running costs of health care institutions (recurrent budget) are usually at least one-third of the capital cost.

GLOSSARY

Health expenditure per capita: the amount spent on health care per person per year calculated by dividing the total health expenditure by the number in the population.

Thus, a teaching hospital built in the early 1970s might well have cost approximately US$18 million. To run such a hospital would cost approximately US$4–6 million a year.[1] This, in most underdeveloped countries, was about 25% of the total health budget, and in some it exceeded 50% of the budget (Morley, 1975). Therefore, even the small 'per capita' expenditures are exaggerations of the amount spent on the health care of most individuals.

Generally, most of the small health budget of an underdeveloped country is still spent on expensive high technology and urban-based curative services in large hospitals, with only a small proportion being allocated to health promotion and preventive activities. The needs of people living in rural areas and urban slums remain largely neglected (as an example, compare the health care facilities shown in Figure 4.3 on pages 130 and 131).

Organisation of health services

The organisation of health services in underdeveloped countries continues to be based on a modified version of the 'referral system' which evolved in the colonising countries. This system developed to different degrees in different countries. It is based on the ideal of patients being treated as close to their homes as possible in the cheapest, smallest, most simply equipped and most humbly staffed unit (King, 1975)—aid stations and dispensaries. When a unit cannot provide adequate care for a patient, the patient is referred to the health centre, then to the rural or district hospital and finally to the regional, central or teaching hospital. The capital and running costs of these different units vary enormously. The regional, central and teaching hospitals have the

---

[1] Pound Sterling Live (2022). https://www.poundsterlinglive.com/bank-of-england-spot/historical-spot-exchange-rates/gbp/gbp-to-usd-1975.

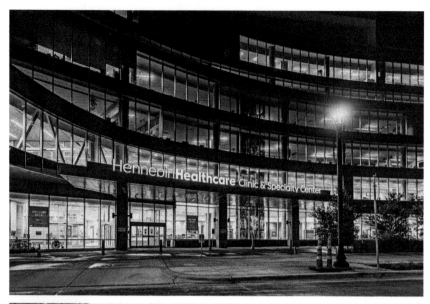

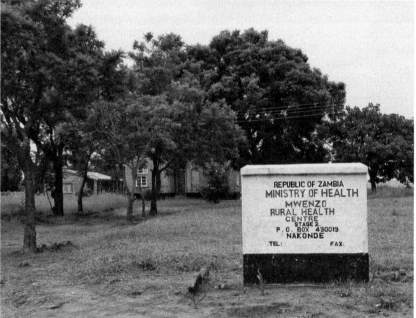

Fig. 4.3 Capital expenditure: which option? 'Disease palaces' for doctors or health centres and small hospitals for the community?

Source: Photo 1: Tony Webster. (2020). Hennepin Healthcare Clinic and Specialty Center. Flickr.

Source: Photo 2: Seyemon. (2007). Mwenzo Rural Health Clinic. Flickr.

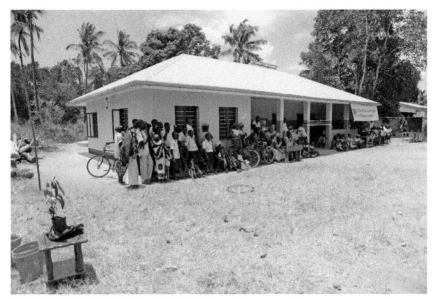

Fig. 4.3 (continued) Masaika Clinic in Tanzania
Source: Photo 3: US Army Southern European Task Force, Africa. Jonathan Kulp. (2009). Flickr.

highest running costs because of their size and higher proportion of specialist doctors, general duty doctors, and nurses required.

Is this a reasonably efficient way of providing medical care for the majority? What proportion of the population does it reach? And how well does referral work *in practice*?

Pattern of coverage

The few surveys undertaken in underdeveloped countries in the 1960s–1970s indicated that most patients who visited health care facilities came from the immediate vicinity (see Figure 4.4). This pattern is still dominant today and is remarkably uniform across the underdeveloped world. So, for example:

- In Kenya, 40% of outpatients attending a health centre lived within 8 km (5 miles); 30% lived 8–16 km (5–10 miles) away; and 30% lived more than 16 km (10 miles) away (Fendall, 1965).
- In Tanzania, two separate studies showed that 80% of attending outpatients came from within 15 km (9.3 miles) of rural health centres (Gish, 1973).
- An Indian study revealed that for every additional half-mile (0.8 km) between the community and a dispensary, the number of people attending decreased by 50% (Frederiksen, 1964).
- Another study showed that over 60% of patients came from within a mile (1.6 km) of the primary health centre (Roemer, 1972).

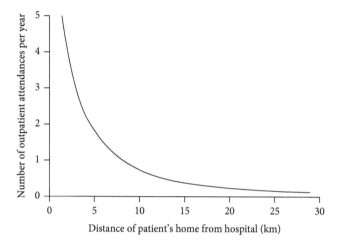

Fig. 4.4 Average number of outpatient attendances per year versus distance from home, Tanzania.

Source: King. (1975).

The decline in inpatient use of health facilities was less sharp than for outpatient care, but still dramatic. In Uganda, for example, outpatient attendances halved for every 3.2 km (2 miles), while the use of inpatient facilities halved for every 8 km (5 miles). A survey in Ghana showed that 80% of the inpatients at the five major hospitals came from surrounding urban districts (Saakwa-Mante, cited in Sharpston, 1972).

These and other studies clearly show that so-called referral hospitals often served as very expensive district hospitals for their local communities, who were often the elite who needed the facilities the least.

Health care workforce

A hospital-based system inevitably requires doctors and so the skewed distribution of facilities that is concentrated in urban areas is accompanied by the maldistribution of medical personnel.

The considerable disparities between the developed and underdeveloped countries in resources available for medical care were clear enough from the health budgets that we discussed in the section 'Health financing'. These disparities are equally obvious in the case of medical personnel. Since 1980, these disparities have worsened. In 2013, the global health care workforce was over 43 million, with an estimated global **needs-based shortage** of 17.4 million. The largest shortage was in South-East Asia (6.9 million) and Africa (4.2 million) (WHO, 2016a). By 2018, the global shortage of nurses alone was 5.9 million, and almost 90% of the deficit was in low- and lower-middle-income countries (WHO, 2016b). By 2030, the WHO (2020) estimates that 18 million more health workers will be needed in low- and lower-middle-income countries.

GLOSSARY

Needs-based shortage: the number of health care workers needed to meet population health needs exceeds the available supply of health workers (WHO, 2016a).

Figure 4.5 shows how Africa and South-East Asia, the regions that face the highest burden of disease, have the lowest health workforce densities.

But again, statistics like these understate the case because they do not take into account the great variation in the distribution of health workers within regions and countries. Doctors especially are concentrated in urban areas—particularly in the capital cities. For example, in 2001 in India, of all health workers, 59.2% were in urban areas, where 27.8% of the population resides, and 40.8% were in rural areas, where 72.2% of the population resides (WHO, 2016b).

Morley's 'three-quarters rule' accurately describes the allocation of health care resources in underdeveloped countries in the colonial and post-colonial periods:

Although three-quarters of the population in most countries in the tropics and subtropics live in rural areas, three-quarters of the spending on medical care is in the urban areas, and also three-quarters of the doctors (and other health workers) live there. Three-quarters of the deaths are due to conditions that can be prevented at low cost, but three-quarters of the medical budget is spent on curative services, many of them provided at high cost (Morley, 1973.)

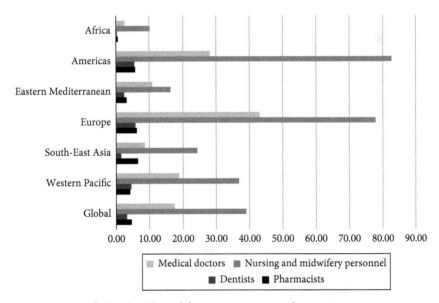

Fig. 4.5 Density of select health workforce per 10 000 population, 2013–2019.
Source: WHO. (2021).

In Chapter 3 we looked at the drain of resources in general from the poor to the richer sectors of underdeveloped countries and thence to the developed world. The situation with respect to medical personnel is much the same. Not only do health workers congregate in the major cities, but also a significant proportion actually leave their countries for Europe, North America and Australasia.

International migration: 'the brain drain'

The training of medical personnel in the colonies and ex-colonies made them suitable for employment in the developed world. The expansion of the health care system in developed countries in the 1950s and 1960s increased the need for the intensified recruitment of health personnel, including from former colonies. As Lord Cohen of Birkenhead in the UK House of Lords commented in 1961: "*The Health Service would have collapsed if it had not been for the enormous influx from junior doctors from such countries as India and Pakistan.*"

The push of poor working conditions in their own countries and the pull of higher salaries abroad drove thousands of health workers from underdeveloped countries to work in developed countries. By 1972, approximately 6% of the world's 140 000 physicians were in countries other than those of which they were nationals. Significantly, about 86% of all migrant physicians were working in just five countries—Australia, Canada, the Federal Republic of Germany, the UK and the USA (WHO, 1979).

The export of health personnel was not confined to physicians. It included vast numbers of nurses, midwives and unskilled hospital workers. A survey in the late 1960s showed that four out of every seven newly trained West Indian midwives were working in Britain, while only three remained in the Caribbean (Gish, 1971). South Korea had an official programme for 'exporting' nurses and nursing aides to Austria, West Germany, Japan and Switzerland. The Philippines had similar programmes in Europe and North America (Gish & Godfrey, 1977).

By the 1990s, as we saw in Chapter 3, the WTO had formalised the trade in health services and health workers between countries, through GATS. GATS has enabled the ongoing drain of skilled health care resources from underdeveloped to developed countries that generally only benefits the industrialised world, known as the 'brain drain'. It has resulted in an immense loss of human capital and financial resources and is in effect another mechanism to transfer resources from the poor to the rich, from the underdeveloped to the developed world.

In 2015, for example, there were 13 584 African-trained health care professionals practising in the USA, with 86% of them having been trained in Egypt, Ghana, Nigeria and South Africa (Mo Ibrahim Foundation, 2018). At that time, it cost approximately US$21 000–59 000 to train a doctor—the cost of which is not paid by the recruiting country. In other words, the importing country saves training costs and the home country loses what it has invested in educating its health care professionals. This is essentially a transfer of wealth from underdeveloped to developed countries.

According to the Mo Ibrahim Foundation (2018):

One in ten doctors working in the UK comes from Africa, allowing the UK to save on average $2.7 billion on training costs. Similarly, the US, Australia and Canada save respectively about $846 million, $621 million and $384 million in training cost from African *physicians they recruit. It is estimated that Africa has lost $4.6 billion in training cost for home-trained doctors, recruited by these four-top destination countries.*

In July 2020, in an attempt to strengthen its own health care system in the midst of the COVID-19 pandemic, the UK government relaxed its migration requirements to recruit health workers from around the world. Not only do recruitment drives like these leave already weak and overburdened health care systems in underdeveloped countries with enormous health workforce shortages, but also they have a dire impact on other life-saving health programmes. As an example, Zimbabwe has one of the largest HIV and TB burdens globally, and nurses play a key role in the response to these two diseases. However, with the steady flow of health workers out of Zimbabwe to developed countries, there is a serious risk of losing gains made to date in the HIV and TB programmes (Dzinamarira & Musuka, 2021).

The brain drain has left underdeveloped countries with health workforce shortages and generally weakened and overburdened public health care systems. It has impacted health and health equity, further disadvantaging the poorest and most vulnerable social groups. The brain drain is likely to continue to the developed world long after the shock of the COVID-19 pandemic has passed.

Auxiliaries (mid-level health providers)

We saw in previous chapters that the pattern of disease in underdeveloped countries during colonisation and into the post-colonial period was one of nutritional and communicable diseases. This meant that the number of conditions seen and the major causes of death—particularly among children—were limited. Therefore, the number of interventions needed to prevent or cure most of these diseases was relatively small and they were simple and yet effective to implement. It was unnecessary for health workers to have a sophisticated and extensive knowledge of modern medical methods.

These were some of the important factors behind the development of the category 'auxiliary' workers. They were traditionally considered as health workers with less education and less-developed skills than professionals, doing part of the work of professionals and under their direction. They were, and still are, an integral part of the health team, which was conceived of being made up of different categories of health workers whose collective efforts covered the medical need. The composition of the team varied in different countries and different contexts, but the primary health worker—the person who had *first* direct contact with the recipient of health care—was most important. In underdeveloped countries, auxiliaries were developed to fill the role of primary health workers.

Late in the nineteenth century, *single-purpose* auxiliaries were trained to combat single diseases—especially as smallpox vaccinators. After 1920, they were trained to treat yaws, yellow fever, sleeping sickness, leprosy, TB and venereal disease; and more recently they have been used in health care campaigns such as in the eradication of malaria.

The need to improve quality and coverage of health services prompted the training of *multipurpose auxiliaries*, the earliest of these being the dispensary auxiliary or wound dresser. But most categories of auxiliaries were developed to correspond to categories of professional and paramedical personnel: nursing, midwifery, health visiting, environmental health, laboratory, technology, pharmacy, radiography and entomology, and in some places medical care (Bryant, 1969).

Because of the population structure and distribution in most underdeveloped countries, health problems affecting pregnant and nursing mothers and small children constituted a significant proportion of health needs—which is still the case. For this reason, one category of auxiliary—the auxiliary worker for maternal and child-care or auxiliary nurse midwife (ANM)—became almost universal. These workers, usually women, had around two years' training both in preventive and in curative care. They operated from 'under-five clinics' with the aim of extending low-cost curative and preventive care to as large a proportion of the population as possible (Morley, 1975).

An obvious financial advantage in the use of auxiliaries over doctors was the low cost of both their training and employment. While originally candidates for auxiliary training were illiterate, gradually the educational requirements increased, so that by the 1960s there existed many different categories of auxiliaries, requiring different educational levels—from an ill-defined apprenticeship through to two years of formal training.

NOTE: Auxiliaries are a different cadre of workers to community health workers (CHW), which will be described in more detail in Chapter 7.

Today, most auxiliaries—referred to as mid-level health providers (MLPs)—have a formal certificate and accreditation from a higher education institution. They are able to diagnose, manage and treat illness, disease and impairments, and undertake preventive and promotive health care, either independently or under the supervision of a professional. Their role has progressively expanded, particularly in low- and middle-income countries, to help overcome the growing shortage of health workers and to improve people's access to essential health services. Examples occur in Tanzania, Mozambique and Malawi where such mid-level workers are trained for specific functions, such as caesarean section and provision of anaesthesia (Doylo, 2004).

In summary, colonial countries exploited the colonies and left their populations in poverty and in a state of underdevelopment. Sufficient progress in addressing structural inequalities and systemic underdevelopment has not occurred in the post-colonial era, and there has been a failure to develop resilient health care systems (Shoman et al., 2017). The case study below illustrates the failure of weak health systems in underdeveloped contexts to manage severe epidemics—in this instance, Ebola.

CASE STUDY: Failure of weak health systems to manage epidemics like Ebola

Ebola virus disease (EVD) is so called because the first outbreak in 1976 occurred simultaneously in a village close to the Ebola River in the Democratic Republic of

Congo (DRC) and in South Sudan (WHO, 2021b). The virus continued to spread, with the 2014–2016 outbreak in West Africa being the largest, with more cases and deaths than in all other outbreaks combined.

By 2014, civil wars in Guinea, Liberia and Sierra Leone had left the health systems of these countries in total collapse, with limited health infrastructure, significant shortages of health care workers and limited financial resources. Their health systems were simply unprepared and ill-equipped to manage and control an Ebola outbreak. The Ebola outbreak itself further weakened these countries' already fragile health care systems in a reinforcing negative cycle.

Those health care workers who had direct contact with symptomatic Ebola patients were at high risk of infection and death (Shoman et al., 2017) (see Figure 4.6). This placed added strain on the remaining health care workers, who had to prioritise managing the Ebola outbreak at the expense of providing adequate health care for other diseases and conditions. This led to additional outbreaks. Health workers working with Ebola were stigmatised and isolated by communities and patients with other conditions, who refused to seek treatment from them, fearing that the health workers themselves would infect them with Ebola (Shoman et al., 2017). This affected the health outcomes of these patients. The weak health care system enabled Ebola to thrive and cause devastation.

From 2014, the WHO led the Ebola response, adopting a classic 'outbreak control' strategy called STEPP—Stop the outbreak; Treat the infected; Ensure essential

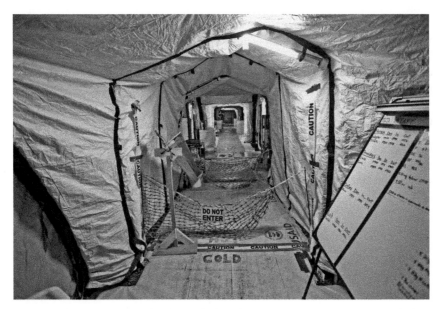

Fig. 4.6 The Monrovia Medical Unit for health workers who contracted the Ebola virus in the line of duty, 2015.
Source: Neil Brandvold, USAID. (2015).

services; Preserve stability; and Prevent further outbreaks. Although STEPP had worked in previous Ebola outbreaks, these had been limited in size and geographic spread. However, this outbreak spiralled out of control.

> *While some postulate a change in the distribution of animal vectors for the emergence of this current EVD epidemic, the escalation is driven by other factors . . . such large outbreaks almost invariably occur where there is severe poverty and health systems are compromised . . . All three countries had pre-existing challenges in their health systems with inadequate infrastructure, severe shortages of trained health workers, shortages of basic medicines and very weak health information and disease surveillance systems* (Scott et al., 2016).

Health services in the developed world

As discussed in Chapter 3, the decrease in deaths from infectious diseases in the British population from the mid-nineteenth century onwards occurred mainly because of improvements in social and economic conditions and public health interventions rather than due to advances in medical science.

Changes in the population structure and disease pattern emerged in the developed world and among the privileged groups living in the developed sectors of the underdeveloped world. In Britain, for instance, a country in the late phase of **demographic transition**, the proportion of old people in the population has been increasing rapidly since the 1900s: in the 25 years between 1949 and 1974, the number of people over 75 years increased by 55%; and in the following 40 years (up to 2014), the proportion of those aged 65 or over increased from 13.8% of the UK population to 17.7% (Office for National Statistics (ONS), 2017).

GLOSSARY

Demographic transition: the change from high death rates matched by high birth rates; to low death rates with still high birth rates; then finally to low death rates with low birth rates.

Certain conditions have supplanted the diseases of undernutrition and poor hygiene as the major causes of illness and death—heart disease, cancer, stroke, chronic lower respiratory diseases, influenza, pneumonia and Alzheimer's disease, among others.

However, differences in living and working conditions in different sections of the population are still reflected in marked differences in health. For example, while the

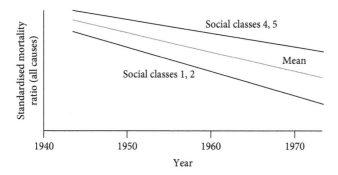

Fig. 4.7 Standardised mortality ratio (all causes), Britain.
Source: Registrar General's Occupational Mortality Tables, 1940s–1970s.

overall health of the British population improved from the 1950s onwards, the health gap between social classes has actually *increased* (see Figure 4.7).

We know that factors like industrial disease and accidents, poor living environments, inadequate housing, stress and cigarette smoking, disproportionately affect the working class. But what about the allocation of health services? Did the medical contribution counteract this imbalance in health-promoting resources in the developed world?

Health care facilities

It was not investment in health care that improved levels of health in the developed world. Greater investment in health care does not necessarily have much impact on the statistics of disease and death. However, health services are indispensable not so much for the small number of 'cures' they effect, but for the care they provide for the seriously ill and many others with disabling and uncomfortable conditions. Personal social services are also important in providing help and care for the especially vulnerable members of society—older people, children, people living with a mental health condition, and those living with mental and physical challenges.

We use the UK as the exemplar of a national health service in the developed world from its inception in 1948 until about 2000 because it is well documented and, although unique, it does have many similarities to health services in other developed countries. It has also played an important role in shaping health services in former British colonies.

NOTE: The landscape of the British National Health Service changed in the 1980s when the Thatcher government introduced a market-based system. We will discuss the reforms designed to increase competition and privatisation in Chapter 6.

CASE STUDY: The British National Health Service (NHS)

Introducing a national health service

Prior to 1948, British health care was a patchwork of voluntary, private and public provision, and millions of people still had little or no reliable health care. Popular opinion was that the provision of health care was a right that the State was responsible for providing, based on need rather than payment of fees or insurance.

In 1948, the ruling Labour Party's health minister, Nye Bevan, established the British National Health Service (NHS). The main aims were to provide universal health coverage, and the comprehensive provision and services free at the point of use—funded by public taxes. It had ambitions of equity of access to high-quality health services and to place service before profit (Gorsky, 2015). As Bevan explained, "*The essence of a satisfactory health service is that the rich and the poor are treated alike, that poverty is not a disability, and wealth is not advantaged*" (Nuffield Trust, 2020). The Conservative Party and the doctor's professional body, the British Medical Association (BMA), strongly opposed the establishment of the NHS, fearing that doctors would lose their independence and their right to buy or sell their services.

There were three main strands of the NHS, which were financed centrally:

- All hospitals were nationalised and managed by Regional Hospital Boards.
- General Practitioners (GPs) or family doctors remained independent but became consultants to the NHS and were responsible for primary care (first level of care).
- Local authorities were responsible for home nursing, public and environmental health and health prevention/promotion.

Over time, this division of functions together with the division of the medical profession into NHS salaried employees (hospital specialists and hospital doctors in training) and independent contractors (GPs) made it difficult to provide comprehensive and coordinated services. NHS hospital consultants could work part-time for the NHS and part-time in the private sector. This too had an impact on health care services, at times creating "*a battlefield for power and control*" (Greengross et al., 1999).

Spending on health care services (as a percentage of GDP) increased from the late 1940s until the 1980s—by 2% in 1947; about 3.5% in 1951; 4% in 1970; and 5% in 1980 (UK Public Spending, 2022) (see Figure 4.8). However, from the mid-1970s until the late 1980s, spending on personal social services (e.g. social care and social work services) began to fall dramatically, with only 0.38% of the total health care budget being devoted to preventive work, and the health education budget of the NHS only accounting for 0.01% of the total (Evans & Simpson, 1976).

In each decade between the 1950s and the 1980s, hospital services consumed the greatest percentage of the inadequate health care budget, with acute hospitals claiming nearly half of the total expenditure (see Table 4.1). Teaching hospitals, which catered for a disproportionately high number of middle- and upper-class patients, consumed more than a quarter of the total NHS capital budget, and this added to the recurrent budget too.

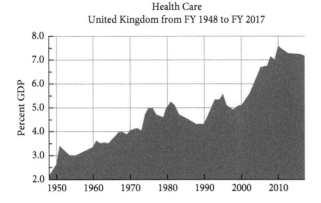

Health Care
United Kingdom from FY 1948 to FY 2017

Fig. 4.8 UK public health care spending as a percentage of GDP.

Source: UK Public Spending. (2022).
www.ukpublicspending.co.uk.

Distribution of facilities by sector and region

A brief examination of one of the most important sectors of the NHS—care of older people—reveals its inappropriate development. From the 1970s and into the 1980s, because of the small number of geriatric day hospitals in Britain, older people accounted for around 30% of admissions to acute wards of general hospitals (National Co-ordinating Committee Against the Cuts, n.d.).

It was not just by sector but also by geographical region that NHS facilities were unfairly distributed. Figure 4.9 shows the percentage four regions spent on their hospitals in terms of the national average in the 1970s, with London spending above the national average and the others spending below (Heller & Jenkins, 1976).

This unevenness occurred not just between regions but also within regions. For example, in the 'rich' metropolitan London region there were gross local discrepancies. Many teaching hospitals in London inflated their budgets and gave the impression that the region was overprovided in services. East London, for example, was an area of particular need, with an infant mortality rate 20% above the national average and hospital admissions nearly 30% higher than the national figure. Yet,

Table 4.1 Percentages of NHS gross expenditure

Year	Hospital services	GP services	Community health
1951	55.7	9.5	8.5
1961	57.0	9.6	9.3
1971	66.6	8.3	7.1
1980	62.7	6.2	6.2

Source: Taylor, D. (1981). *Health Research in England: a topic for debate*. Office of Health Economics: London.

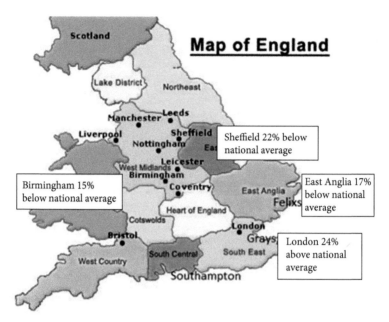

Fig. 4.9 Spending on hospitals in terms of national average, 1970s.
Source: Heller & Jenkins. (1976).

as part of a 'rationalisation of services', 21 hospitals in that area were closed and six partially closed.

Prior to the COVID-19 pandemic, the NHS was already in crisis as it had failed to keep pace with the increasing need for health care services. By late 2019, there were over 100 000 staff vacancies, including vacancies for 40 000 nurses. The NHS also lacked the equipment it needed to meet population needs. For the first time on record, the NHS was missing key targets, including patient waiting times for Accident and Emergency (A&E) care, cancer care and non-urgent operations (*The Lowdown*, 2020).

In 2020, millions of patients had their treatment put on hold as the NHS battled COVID-19. As mentioned previously, in July 2020, the UK government relaxed its visa requirements to attract health care workers from around the world to fill the gaps in the NHS. And, in August 2020, it was reported that the NHS would need to buy health care services over the next four years from the private sector, worth up to £10 billion, to bridge the gap in NHS capacity (*The Lowdown*, 2020).

Health care workforce

As in the rest of the world, urban areas are more attractive to health workers because they offer higher salaries and more social, cultural and professional opportunities. Furthermore, the geographical distribution of doctors—and other health workers— followed the same distribution of other resources, resulting in the same unequal access

Table 4.2 Career preferences of medical students: first choices (as percentages of total)

Career choice	Royal Commission	Manchester and Sheffield Enquiry	
	1968	1971	1972
Medicine	26.5	24.0	23.8
Surgery	17.8	19.9	13.5
Obstetrics and gynaecology	12.4	5.5	4.0
General practice	23.5	32.2	46.8
Psychiatry	5.2	1.4	2.4
Community medicine	1.6	2.0	1.6
Pathology	2.1	3.4	4.7
Anaesthetics	2.0	8.2	3.2
Radiology	0.8	0.8	–
Other	8.1	2.7	–

Hospital medical specialities (e.g. cardiology, chest medicine, clinical pharmacology, gastroenterology, general [internal] medicine, nephrology, neurology, occupational medicine)

Source: quoted in Heller, T. (1978). *Restructuring the Health Service*. Croom Helm: London, p. 39.

to health care services, particularly in rural areas and in socio-economically disadvantaged urban regions (Ono et al., 2014).

Medical education concentrates on the super-technological specialists. Medical students aspire to become specialists in those areas which are most prestigious and which also attract the lion's share of health service resources. The emphasis on technological specialisation is reflected in the career preferences of medical students in surveys undertaken in 1968, 1971 and 1972 (see Table 4.2).

Health team

In the underdeveloped world, primary health workers—auxiliaries—are seen as part of the health team. There is no exact equivalent of the auxiliary in the British health service, but the concept of a 'health team' does exist.

People in developed societies often need advice and care and not a super-technological intervention or the attention of a doctor. This has been acknowledged by the development of various workers whose operations are part of local authority health and social care services. They include health visitors, district nurses and home helps. Their functions include simple curative care, ante- and post-natal care and occasional home deliveries, rehabilitation, preventive measures and a certain amount of health education and domestic help for people who are ill or for older adults.

In summary, even in developed countries only a small proportion of the ill-health present in the community comes to the attention of the health and social care services. The most deprived are generally in areas with predominantly working-class populations.

The medical contribution in the developed world is effectively summed by the 'Inverse Care Law': "*The availability of good medical care tends to vary inversely with the need of the population served*" (Hart, 1971). In other words, those who need care most have the least access.

As far back as the 1960s it was clear that to cater for the health needs of people in both underdeveloped and developed regions of the world, a different approach to health care across all levels of care was needed.

The need for a different approach to health services

Foundations of the Primary Health Care approach

The first international policy-making conference that looked at a different approach to health care took place in Uganda in the mid-1960s. The conference proceedings were documented in the book *Medical Care in Developing Countries: A Symposium from Makerere* (1966), edited by Maurice King (1975). This book essentially explored the organisation and administration of health services in underdeveloped countries, focusing attention on the peripheral facility—the rural health centre—around which health services *should* be organised, with hospitals above and satellite clinics below. This came to be known as the 'basic health services approach' and fed into the development of the Primary Health Care (PHC) approach.

The King book was followed in 1975 by *Alternative Approaches to Meeting Basic Health Needs in Developing Countries: A Joint UNICEF/WHO Study*, edited by V. Djukanovic and E.P. Mach. This text articulated the official policy position of the WHO on a basic health system, again with a focus on health centres.

In addition to these publications and policies, there was the work of social epidemiologists, such as McKeown in England (see Chapters 2 and 3) and McKinley in America, that demonstrated the importance of socio-economic and environmental factors in the cause of disease and death. This understanding too fed into the development of the PHC approach.

In 1975, the WHO published *Health by the People*, edited by Professor Kenneth W. Newell. It documented several country studies of innovative ways of delivering PHC, mainly in the rural areas of countries like Bangladesh, Guatemala, Niger and Tanzania, and demonstrated the important role played by community-based workers in improving the health of communities, particularly child and maternal health.

Newell described several large-scale programmes and country experiences of PHC, significantly that of China following its liberation in 1949, through the 1950s, 1960s and into the 1970s. The health sector had been radically reorganised during the Chinese Cultural Revolution (1966–1976). Mobile health teams travelled all over the countryside to bring health care to rural areas. These teams trained peasants on farms, who could provide environmental sanitation, health education, preventive medicine, first aid and primary medical care while continuing their farm work. These were the 'barefoot doctors'—so-called because in the rural areas around Shanghai, much of the farm work is done barefoot in rice paddies. (This will be discussed in more detail in Chapter 7.)

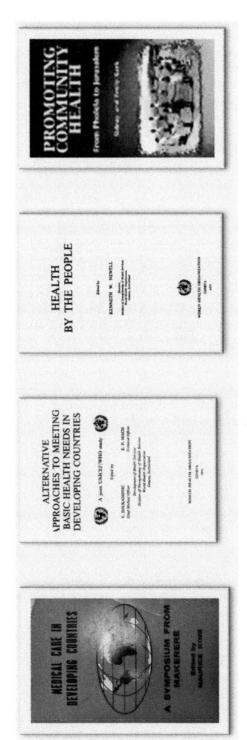

Fig. 4.10 The foundations of the Primary Health Care approach.
Source: King. (1966); UNICEF/WHO. (1975); WHO. (1975); Kark & Kark. (2000).

Newell compared China's experience with that of India. India had achieved independence from British rule in 1947 only two years before China had achieved liberation, and both countries had started off with high levels of infant, child and maternal mortality, many communicable diseases and a high incidence of violent injury. However, where China had achieved a dramatic drop in these health conditions, using barefoot doctors, India's health gains were much lower.

An experience that Newell did *not* describe, but which many argue was one of the main roots of the PHC approach, was the work done in South Africa in the 1940s by doctors Sydney and Emily Kark. They worked in a health centre in Pholela, a rural area in what is today KwaZulu-Natal, impoverished by the migrant labour system.

The Pholela health centre was inundated with cases of sexually transmitted diseases (STDs), which the Karks traced to the mining industry—men went to work in the mines, contracted an STD, returned home and transmitted the STD to their wives. The Karks understood that the health problems they were dealing with had their source in the living and working conditions in which people found themselves, and that these conditions were themselves a product of social, economic and political processes. The Karks introduced a highly integrated curative, preventive and promotive approach called Community Oriented Primary Care (COPC). The 'primary' part of it was the basic care within the clinic, as well as the use of trained community-based health assistants who "*combined treatment of the sick with household health education*" (Sanders & Reynolds, 2019). In addition, the community-based health assistants undertook community diagnosis to identify the causes of ill-health and to institute community-wide and **intersectoral** action to address these causes. Some root causes could be alleviated, but they could not address the underlying determinant—the migrant labour policy (Sanders & Reynolds, 2019).

GLOSSARY

Intersectoral: collaboration between health and other government sectors to jointly improve the health of populations; there may also be partnerships with government, private sector and non-profit groups.

All these interventions, policies and publications were the foundation upon which the PHC approach, which was discussed at the Alma-Ata Conference in 1978, was built (see Figure 4.10).

Primary Health Care (PHC)

A potential breakthrough in global health took place at the historic International Conference on Primary Health Care held in 1978 in Alma-Ata, which was then the

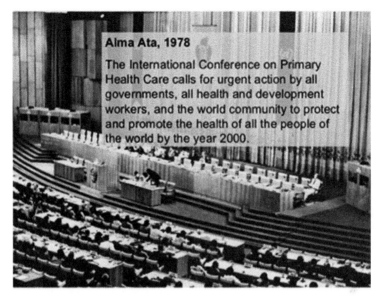

Fig. 4.11 The International Conference on Primary Health Care in Alma-Ata, Kazakhstan, Soviet Union, 1978.
Source: WHO. (1978). Alma-Ata Declaration.

capital of Kazakhstan, Soviet Union. The Conference was sponsored by WHO and UNICEF and was attended by ministers of health from 134 countries. Virtually all the nations there subscribed to the ambitious goal of achieving '*Health for All* by the Year 2000', calling for a more inclusive approach to health across all levels of care, with an emphasis on the primary and community levels. They further affirmed WHO's broad definition of health as "*a state of complete physical, mental, and social well-being*." These ideals were articulated in the Conference's final document—the Alma-Ata Declaration (see Figure 4.11).

To achieve the ambitious goal of *Health for All* and to reduce the gap between the health of people in underdeveloped and developed countries, the Alma-Ata Declaration called for economic and social development of countries, based on a **New International Economic Order** (NIEO). This call had been taken up by the group of **non-aligned countries** and by the United Nations (UN) General Assembly in 1974. It was:

... based on equity, sovereign equality, interdependence, common interest and cooperation among all States, irrespective of their economic and social systems, which shall correct inequalities and redress existing injustices, make it possible to eliminate the widening gap between the developed and the developing countries and ensure steadily accelerating economic and social development and peace and justice for present and future generations (UN, 1974).

GLOSSARY

New International Economic Order (NIEO): after the devastating effects of the global oil crisis in 1973 on underdeveloped countries, there was a call by non-aligned countries for a review of the existing Bretton Woods international economic system and a proposal for a new system that would empower underdeveloped countries to have more control over economic independence and political sovereignty (Gebremariam, 2017).

Some of the key elements of a NIEO included:

- Rights of states and peoples under 'colonial domination' to restitution and full compensation for their exploitation and that of their resources.
- Regulation of transnational corporations.
- Preferential treatment for underdeveloped countries in all areas of international economic cooperation.
- Transfer of new technologies.
- End the waste of natural resources.

Non-aligned countries: a group of countries that do not want to be officially aligned with or against any major power bloc.

The world's nations, together with WHO, UNICEF and major funding agencies, also pledged to work towards meeting people's basic needs through a comprehensive and remarkably progressive approach called Primary Health Care (PHC). Many of the principles of PHC were garnered from China and from the diverse experiences of small, struggling, non-governmental community-based health programmes (CBHPs) in the Philippines, Latin America and elsewhere.

What is Primary Health Care?

The concept of PHC as envisioned in the Alma-Ata Declaration has strong socio-political implications. It explicitly outlines a strategy that would respond more equitably, appropriately and effectively to basic health care needs; and would *also* address the underlying social, economic and political causes or determinants of ill-health.

The five main principles that underpin the PHC approach are as follows:

- **Equitable provision of services**: universal accessibility and coverage on the basis of need rather than privilege or power—supporting the principle of **health equity**.
- **Comprehensive health care**: with an emphasis on disease prevention and health promotion, but also including treatment and rehabilitation.
- **Intersectoral action for health**: collaboration between sectors to address the underlying social determinants of ill-health so as to improve the living and working conditions in which people find themselves.

- **Community and individual involvement and self-reliance**: a close link between the health and development of people living in poverty, and the need for active individual and community participation in planning, delivering and maintaining health services.
- **Appropriate technology and cost-effectiveness**: using appropriate low-cost technology and locally available and appropriate resources.

GLOSSARY

Health equity: those who have greater need get more services; the absence of systematic differences in health between different social groups in society; allowing all people to access the social, economic and political conditions they need to realise their fundamental human rights, including their right to health. The concept is built on the principles of social justice and fairness.

The principles of the PHC approach are embodied in what were identified as the essential elements or programmes:

1. Promotion of proper nutrition and adequate supply of safe water and basic sanitation (social determinants).
2. Maternal and childcare, including family planning.
3. Immunisation against the major infectious diseases.
4. Prevention and control of locally endemic diseases.
5. Health education concerning prevailing health problems, and methods of prevention and control.
6. Appropriate treatment of common diseases and injuries.
7. Mental health (included at a later stage).

PHC is a global approach, not only for low- and middle-income countries. Yet, as Sanders and Reynolds (2019) point out, the neglect of NCDs in the above list, which was dominant in developed countries at that time, but only beginning to be recognised in underdeveloped countries, suggests that this was in reality seen as an approach primarily for poor countries.

What is Comprehensive Primary Health Care (CPHC)?

The term Comprehensive PHC—which is used in the Alma-Ata Declaration—means providing PHC that "*addresses the main health problems in the community, providing promotive, preventative, curative and rehabilitative services accordingly*" (WHO, 1978, Alma-Ata Declaration).

Primary medical or clinical care that involves individually focused treatment and rehabilitation is part of CPHC, but not the whole of it. CPHC also engages with the social determinants of health, via its prevention and **promotive** role, and is predominantly population-focused. Thus, CPHC is a combination of individually and population-focused interventions.

GLOSSARY

Promotive: addresses the social determinants of ill-health through advocacy and lobbying government and policy-makers, for example to ban smoking in public places, as well as intersectoral interventions directed at households or communities to improve water supply, sanitation, housing, etc., and interventions that occur at the policy level, e.g. interventions to regulate alcohol or the food system.

An example of a comprehensive response to the management of a common illness in children is shown in Table 4.3. Note that the table does not show all interventions or the process of community participation and intersectoral action.

Different countries have applied CPHC in different ways, with progress being greatest in underdeveloped countries. Past and current examples of CPHC are described in Chapter 7. However, on the whole, CPHC in its complete form has been difficult to implement; and often when implemented, it has been short-lived mainly as a result of unfavourable political contexts. Resistance to CPHC was not unexpected. In fact, the last sentence of this statement in the Alma-Ata Declaration turned out to be quite prophetic:

> *It can be seen that the proper application of primary health care will have far-reaching consequences, not only through the health sector but also for other social and economic sectors at community level. Moreover, it will greatly influence community organisation in general. **Resistance to such change is only to be expected*** (WHO, 1978, Alma-Ata Declaration).

Table 4.3 Comprehensive management of diarrhoea

Rehabilitative	Curative	Preventive	Promotive
• After attack of diarrhoea: nutrition rehabilitation for children who are undernourished or become undernourished	• Treatment of dehydration: Oral Rehydration Therapy • Nutrition support (especially continued breastfeeding for the infant)	• Education of caregiver for personal and food hygiene (to understand and prevent diarrhoea being transmitted) • Measles vaccination • Breastfeeding • Rotavirus vaccination	• Improve environment: water supply and clean water • Sanitation • Household food security

Resistance to Comprehensive Primary Health Care

UNICEF and WHO represent a diversity of world governments, and for this reason they had to dilute much of the language used in the Declaration so that governments could translate it as they saw fit. This undermined the essence and muffled the power of Alma-Ata's call for *Health for All* and the sweeping changes in power structures and economic systems that were required.

One of the major disagreements was around the definition of PHC itself—some saw it as an approach that would enable health care for all; others as a level of care, as in the primary or first point of medical care. These two understandings have persisted up until today and have led to different and often conflicting views and ways of working. PHC as a first line of medical care came to be seen as a cheap option mainly aimed at poor countries (Sanders & Reynolds, 2019).

The biggest assault on CPHC came from within the international public health establishment itself. As early as 1979, before the debt crisis and Structural Adjustment Programmes (SAPs) were used as arguments against it, Julia A. Walsh and Kenneth S. Warren of the Rockefeller Foundation argued that the 'comprehensive' version of PHC formulated in the Alma-Ata Declaration was too costly and unrealistic (Walsh & Warren, 1979). If health statistics were to be improved, they argued, high-risk groups must be 'targeted' with carefully selected, cost-effective interventions. This new, narrower approach became known as Selective Primary Health Care (SPHC).

We will continue to discuss SPHC in Chapter 5.

Conclusion

The health systems of underdeveloped countries were shaped by their colonial roots, so that today the majority of the inadequate health care budgets are still spent on predominantly urban-based curative hospital services. Too often people living in poverty have no or extremely limited access to health care services or are forced to deal with medical expenses that push them further into poverty and ill-health. The globalisation of health care has promoted the recruitment and migration of health care workers from underdeveloped to developed countries, exacerbating the health–human resources crisis in the underdeveloped world.

The medical contribution in the developed world is effectively summed up by the 'Inverse Care Law'. This phenomenon is stimulated by increasing provision of health care to those who can afford it, as even the most socialised health systems (as in the British NHS) are now giving way to private initiatives.

The Alma-Ata Declaration of 1978, with its goal of *Health for All*, urged governments, global health institutions and major funding agencies to work towards realising people's right to health through a comprehensive approach to PHC. However, CPHC was rapidly reinvented as SPHC, stripped of most of its essential principles and reduced to selected high-priority technological interventions, determined not by communities but by international health professionals and experts. However, CPHC as envisaged under the Alma-Ata Declaration is still the most appropriate approach to achieve *Health for All*, and its components still need to be implemented in all settings.

References

Beck, A. (1970). A history of the British Medical Administration of East Africa, 1900–1950. Cited in Doyal, L. & Pennell, I. (1976). 'Pox Britannica'. Health, medicine and underdevelopment. *Race & Class*, 18(2):155–172.

Bryant, J. (1969). *Health and the Developing World*. Cornell University Press: Ithaca, p. 164.

Doyal, L. & Pennell, I. (1976). 'Pox Britannica'. Health, medicine and underdevelopment. *Race & Class*, 18(2):155–172.

Doylo, D. (2004). Using mid-level cadres as substitutes for internationally mobile health professionals in Africa. A desk review. *Human Resources for Health*, 2(1):7.

Dzinamarira, T. & Musuka, G. (2021). Brain drain: an ever-present; significant challenge to the Zimbabwean public health sector. *Public Health in Practice*, 2:100086.

Evans, J. & Simpson, L. (1976). The Radical Statistics Group. In: Yasukawa, K. & Black, S. (eds). Beyond Economic Interests. International Issues in Adult Education. SensePublishers: Rotterdam.

Fendall, N.R.E. (1965). Medical planning and the training of personnel in Kenya. *Journal of Tropical Medicine and Hygiene*, 68:12–20.

Frederiksen, H. (1964). Maintenance of Malaria Eradication, Duplicated Report, WHO/Mal/429. WHO: Geneva, pp. 2, 6.

Gebremariam, F.M. (2017). New International Economic Order (NIEO): origin, elements and criticisms. *International Journal of Multicultural and Multireligious Understanding*, 4(3).

Gish. O. (1971). *Doctor Migration and World Health. The impact of the international demand for doctors on health services in developing countries*. Bell: London.

Gish, O. (1973). Resource allocation, equality of access and health. *World Development*, 1(12):37–44.

Gish, O. & Godfrey, M. (1977). Why did the doctor cross the road? New Society, 17 March.

Gorsky, M. (2015). The NHS in Britain: any lesson from history for universal health coverage? In: Medcalf, A., Bhattacharya, S., Momen, H., et al. (eds). *Health for All: The Journey of Universal Health Coverage*. Orient Blackswan: Hyderabad, India, Chapter 7.

Greengross, P., Grant, K. & Collini, P. (1999). *The History and Development of the UK National Health Service 1948-1999*. DFID Health Systems Resource Centre: London.

Hart, J.T. (1971). The Inverse Care Law. *The Lancet*, 1(7696):405–412.

Heller, T. (1978). *Restructuring the Health Service*. Croom Helm.

Heller, T. & Jenkins, D. (1976). *Evidence for the Royal Commission on the National Health Service*. The William Temple Foundation.

Kark, S. & Kark, E. (1999). *Promoting Community Health: From Pholela to Jerusalem*. Witwatersrand University Press.

King, M. (1966). *Medical Care in Developing Countries: a Primer on the Medicine of Poverty and a Symposium from Makerere*. Based on a conference assisted by WHO/UNICEF and an experimental edition assisted by UNICEF. Oxford University Press: Oxford, pp. 2, 5.

Meredith, D. (1975). The British Government and colonial economic policy 1919–39. *Economic History Review*, 28(3):484–499.

Mo Ibrahim Foundation. (2018). Brain drain: a bane to Africa's potential. https://mo.ibrahim.foundation/news/2018/brain-drain-bane-africas-potential.

Morley, D. (1973). *Paediatric Priorities in the Developing World*. Butterworth: London.

Morley, D. (1975). The large teaching hospital—A disaster? In British Health Care Planning and Technology, British Hospitals Export Council Year Book, pp. 119–122.

National Co-ordinating Committee Against the Cuts. (n.d.). Publication No 1, p. 13.

Nuffield Trust. (2020). Health and social care explained. https://www.nuffieldtrust.org.uk/health-and-social-care-explained/nhs-reform-timeline/.

Ono, T., Schoenstein, M. & Buchan, J. (2014). *Geographic Imbalances in Doctor Supply and Policy Responses*. OECD Health Working Papers, No. 69. OECD Publishing: Paris.

ONS. (2017). People, population and community. https://www.ons.gov.uk/peoplepopulationandcommunity/populationandmigration/populationestimates/articles/overviewoftheukpopulation/july2017.

Pounds Sterling Live. (2022). Historical Reference Rates from Bank of England for 1975. Pounds Sterling Live. https://www.poundsterlinglive.com/bank-of-england-spot/historical-spot-exchange-rates/gbp/gbp-to-usd-1975.

Roemer, I.M. (1972). *Evaluation of Community Health Centres*. WHO: Geneva, p. 25.

Sanders, D. https://www.youtube.com/watch?v=EnHDnl7uFy0

Sanders, D. & Reynolds, L. (2019). *The Politics of Primary Health Care*. Global Public Health, in *Oxford Research Encyclopedias*. https://doi.org/10.1093/acrefore/9780190632366.013.50.

Scott, V., Crawford-Browne, S. & Sanders, D. (2016). Critiquing the response to the Ebola epidemic through a Primary Health Care approach. *BMC Public Health*, 16(410).

Sharpston, M.J. (1972). Uneven geographic distribution of medical care: a Ghanaian case study. *Journal of Development Studies*, 8(2):210.

Shoman, H., Karafillakis, E. & Rawaf, S. (2017). The link between the West African Ebola outbreak and health systems in Guinea, Liberia and Sierra Leone: a systematic review. *Globalization and Health*, 13(1). https://doi.org/10.1186/s12992-016-0224-2.

Taylor, D. (1981). *Health Research in England: a topic for debate*. Office of Health Economics: London.

The Lowdown. (2020). £10bn spend on private hospitals to bridge gap in NHS capacity, 24 August 2020. https://lowdownnhs.info/private-providers/10bn-spend-on-private-hospitals-to-bridge-gap-in-nhs-capacity/.

UN. (1974). Resolution adopted by the General Assembly. http://www.un-documents.net/s6r3201.htm.

UNICEF/WHO. (1975). *Alternative Approaches to Meeting Basic Health Needs in Developing Countries*. WHO: Geneva.

UK Public Spending. (2022). UK Public Spending Since 1900. Compiled by Christopher Chantrill. https://www.ukpublicspending.co.uk/past_spending.

WHO. (1975). *Health by the People*. WHO: Switzerland.

WHO. (1978). Alma-Ata Declaration.

WHO. (1979). Physician and nurse migration: analysis and policy implications, report on a WHO study, by Alfonso Mej'ia, Helena Pizurki, Erica Royston. World Health Organization. https://apps.who.int/iris/handle/10665/37260.

WHO. (2016a). Health workforce requirements for universal health coverage and the Sustainable Development Goals. *Human Resources for Health Observer*, Series No. 17.

WHO. (2016b). *The Health Workforce in India*. WHO: Geneva.

WHO. (2021a). The 2021 update. Global Health Workforce statistics database. https://www.who.int/data/gho/data/themes/topics/health-workforce.

WHO. (2021b). Ebola virus disease. Key facts. https://www.who.int/news-room/fact-sheets/detail/ebola-virus-disease.

World Bank. (1975). Health sector policy paper. https://documents.worldbank.org/en/publication/documents-reports/documentdetail/649631468138271858/health-sector-policy-paper.

World Bank. (2017). World development indicators: health systems. http://wdi.worldbank.org/table/2.12.

5

Health Policies and Health Care in the Context of Neoliberal Globalisation

The previous chapter explored the Primary Health Care (PHC) approach outlined in the Alma-Ata Declaration, ratified by 134 United Nations member states in 1978. The vision was of a more comprehensive and inclusive approach to *Health for All*, underpinned by the principles of health equity, social justice and fairness.

This chapter examines what has happened since the late 1970s in the struggle for accessible and affordable health care for all, within the context of neoliberal globalisation, and explores some of the forces that have led to and shaped the privatisation of health care.

From Comprehensive to Selective Primary Health Care

Within a few years of the Alma-Ata Declaration, the Rockefeller Foundation—an influential voice in global public health—argued against the implementation of Comprehensive Primary Health Care (CPHC) and in favour of a more selective approach targeting high-risk groups only with carefully chosen cost-effective interventions (Walsh & Warren, 1979). In this reinvention of PHC, many of the key concepts were removed, including:

- The emphasis on social and economic development.
- The inclusion of all other sectors that relate to health in the focus of PHC programmes.
- The keystone of involving communities in the planning, implementation and control of PHC.

This selective, politically sanitised (and thus unthreatening) version of PHC was reduced to a few high-priority technological interventions, determined not by communities but by international health professionals and experts (see Table 5.1). Selective Primary Health Care (SPHC) was quickly embraced by national governments, ministries of health and many of the larger, mainstream international organisations.

As discussed in Chapter 3, by the early 1980s the world was in the midst of a major economic recession, which was accompanied by a conservative shift in domestic and foreign policies of the most powerful industrialised countries, especially the USA and the UK. The new policies—dubbed neoliberal because they 'liberalised' or freed major markets from government regulation or interference, rolling back the role and power of the public sector—systematically put the growth of national economies before

The Struggle for Health. David Sanders with Wim De Ceukelaire and Barbara Hutton, Oxford University Press.
© Oxford University Press 2023. DOI: 10.1093/oso/9780192858450.003.0005

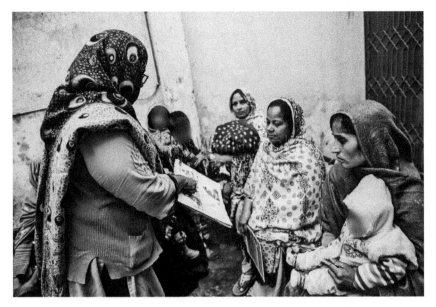

Fig. 5.1 Rural health in Pakistan. A Lady Health Worker (LHW) conducts a health session for her community in Nazampur Dhaka, Sheikhupura district.

Source: WHO/Asad Zaidi. (2018).

https://whohqphotos.lightrocketmedia.com/search/results?sort_by=date_created_s&s%5Bkeywords%5D=health+promotion+Punjab&s%5Bclass%5D=.

the basic needs and rights of people living in poverty. Social programmes, including health programmes to assist people living in poverty, such as the health session shown in Figure 5.1, were cut back or dismantled, both in the developed and underdeveloped world. More information about the neoliberal agenda can be found in Chapter 3.

Table 5.1 Comprehensive versus Selective PHC

	CPHC	SPHC
View of health	*"A state of complete physical, mental, and social well-being"* (WHO, 1946)	Absence of disease
Locus of control over health	Individuals and communities affected	Health professionals and experts
Major focus	Health services, as well as addressing the underlying social, economic and political causes of poor health	Medical and technological interventions
Health care providers	Multidisciplinary teams	Medical personnel
Strategies for health	Multisectoral collaboration	Medical interventions

Source: Adapted from Vuori (1986).

A new strategy: 'Child Survival and Development Revolution'

Confronted by these escalating obstacles to the goal of *Health for All*, the United Nations International Children's Emergency Fund (UNICEF) began backing away from its advocacy of a comprehensive, equity-oriented approach to primary health care. In 1983 it announced that it was adopting a new strategy designed to achieve a *"revolution in child survival and development"* (UNICEF, 1982a), at a cost that poor countries could afford. Falling clearly within the paradigm of SPHC, UNICEF presented the Child Survival Revolution as a streamlined, cheaper, more feasible version of PHC, designed to shelter children from the impact of deteriorating economic conditions. Its goal was to halve the U5MR in the underdeveloped world by the year 2000. To this end, it prioritised four important health interventions, together bearing the acronym GOBI:

- Growth monitoring
- Oral Rehydration Therapy (ORT)
- Breastfeeding
- Immunisation.

In response to concerns that GOBI might be too narrow, in 1984 UNICEF recommended an expanded version, GOBI–FFF, adding Family planning, Food supplements and Female education (UNICEF, 1982b).

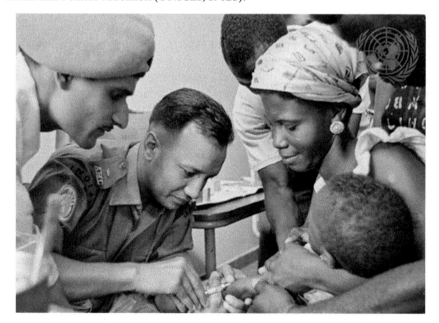

Fig. 5.2 First Bacillus Calmette–Guérin (BCG) vaccination centre opened in the Congo, 1962.

Source: United Nations. (1962).

https://dam.media.un.org/package/2am9lot_4.

Although the response to the limited version of GOBI had been enthusiastic, this expanded version made little headway among health ministries and donors. In fact, in practice GOBI was often trimmed further. Many nations limited their major child survival campaigns to ORT and immunisation (e.g. measles, DPT [diphtheria, pertussis and tetanus] and polio vaccinations), which UNICEF called the 'twin engines' of the Child Survival Revolution. However, some countries put most of their resources into only one of these 'engines', while neglecting the others.

Figure 5.3 illustrates the main differences between CPHC and SPHC, using the example of diarrhoea in children. The comprehensive management of diarrhoea includes all the rehabilitative, curative, preventive and promotive actions and interventions depicted in the example, whereas the selective management of diarrhoea only includes those actions and interventions that are circled and ignores the others, especially the promotive interventions which address the social determinants of health.

UNICEF's argument for GOBI can be summed up as follows (Wisner, 1988):

- Financial and human resources for PHC in poor countries are scarce and growing scarcer due to the persisting international economic crisis.
- Simple, low-cost, widely accessible technologies for saving children's lives exist.
- A method for popularising these technologies at low cost (i.e. social marketing) exists.
- Therefore, GOBI should be implemented as a priority now.

If funding and government support are used as the determining indicators, the Child Survival Revolution was an almost instant success. Governments in both hemispheres that had shown little support for CPHC welcomed GOBI enthusiastically. Both USAID—the lead US government foreign funding agency—and the World Bank

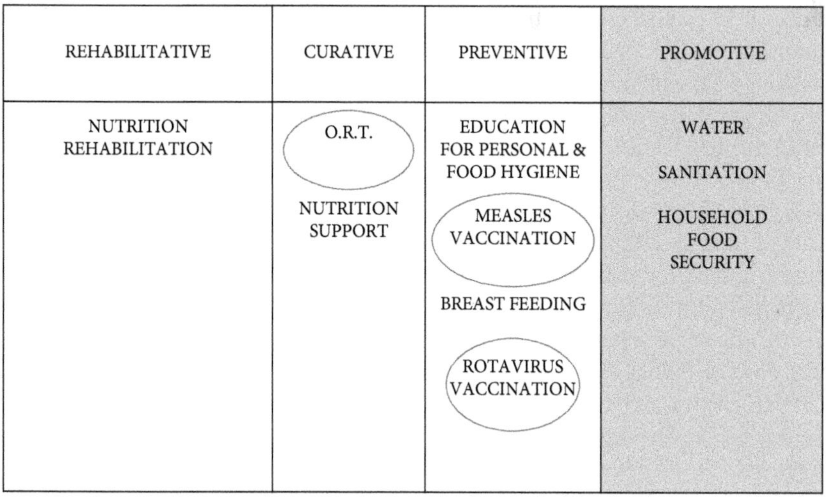

REHABILITATIVE	CURATIVE	PREVENTIVE	PROMOTIVE
NUTRITION REHABILITATION	O.R.T. NUTRITION SUPPORT	EDUCATION FOR PERSONAL & FOOD HYGIENE MEASLES VACCINATION BREAST FEEDING ROTAVIRUS VACCINATION	WATER SANITATION HOUSEHOLD FOOD SECURITY

Fig. 5.3 Example of the actions and interventions required to manage diarrhoea in children. CPHC includes all the interventions, while SPHC includes only those that are circled.

pledged major financial support. By the mid-1980s virtually every underdeveloped country had launched a campaign promoting some or all the GOBI interventions.

Indisputably, immunisation and ORT are effective, low-cost interventions that can help to save many children's lives, if sometimes only temporarily. However, the shift from CPHC to SPHC and GOBI was a way for governments and health professionals to avoid dealing with the social and political causes of ill-health and thus, in effect, was a way to preserve the inequities of the status quo.

The evolution from CPHC to SPHC fitted nicely into the general shift in high-level development planning:

- From social to technological solutions.
- From community participation and cooperatives to private enterprise.
- From a bottom-up to a top-down approach.
- From process to product.
- From problem-posing learning to pre-charted training techniques.
- From critical analysis or awareness raising to social marketing.
- From a comprehensive vision of *Health for All* to raising child survival rates.

Because it represents a compromise away from the potentially more empowering CPHC to a more limited and conservative SPHC, some critics have called the Child Survival Revolution *"the revolution that isn't"* (Schuftan, 1990). The health measures of the Child Survival Revolution did not adequately combat the underlying social causes that contributed to children's deaths. They were much less 'life-effective' than they would have been if implemented as part of a more comprehensive strategy.

Health as an investment

The rise of PHC coincided with the world recession and debt crisis and conservative macroeconomic policies. Throughout the late 1980s and early 1990s, the World Bank became increasingly influential in international health, both through lending money for health sector programmes and by including health policy reforms in the conditions for structural adjustment lending. The Bank's agenda for redirecting health policy and restructuring the health systems of underdeveloped countries was spelled out in its 1993 World Development Report *Investing in Health* (see Figure 5.4). This report had (and continues to have) a profound influence on health policy in underdeveloped countries. Countries willing to implement Bank-endorsed policies were regarded as appropriate candidates for aid and the World Bank encouraged other donor agencies to assist these compliant countries to finance the transitional costs of structural change in the health sector.

The powerful influence of the World Bank on the WHO was demonstrated in the 2003 WHO report by the Commission on Macroeconomics and Health (CMH), chaired by Jeffrey Sachs. *Investing in Health: a summary of the findings of the Commission on Macroeconomics and Health*, echoed the 1993 World Development Report. The WHO publication employed market principles, economic efficiency and a **cost-effectiveness analysis** to define priority health interventions, which were grouped into costed 'packages' of care. For example, hygiene promotion (especially handwashing) was promoted

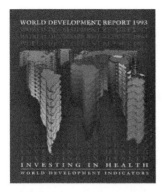 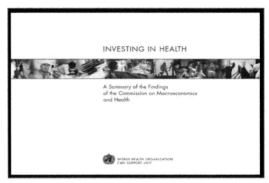

Fig. 5.4 The title of the Commission on Macroeconomics and Health's 2003 report echoes that of the 1993 World Bank report.

Sources: World Bank. (1993). *World Development Report 1993: Investing in Health*. New York: Oxford University Press. World Bank. https://openknowledge.worldbank.org/handle/10986/5976; WHO Commission on Macroeconomics and Health. (2003). *Investing in health: a summary of the findings of the Commission on Macroeconomics and Health*. World Health Organization. https://apps.who.int/iris/handle/10665/42709.

as a much more cost-effective means of reducing diarrhoea over improved water supply and sanitation (WHO, 2001). This reasoning obviously has its limitations, as it excluded the many indirect effects and benefits of improved water supply and sanitation that are difficult to calculate but impact positively on health, such as saving (mostly) women's time in water collection, improving household agriculture, improving household income and food security (Sanders et al., 2009).

GLOSSARY

Cost-effectiveness analysis: analysis focused only on certain easily measurable interventions and proposed limited 'packages' of mainly personal preventative and curative care—reminiscent of SPHC.

Health activists argued that the Commission had failed to examine the root causes of ill-health and that it had narrowly portrayed health as primarily a requirement for productivity and economic growth, as illustrated by this statement from the Commission:

> *Increased life expectancy and low infant mortality are linked to economic growth. Healthy people are more productive, healthy infants and children can develop better and become productive adults. And a healthy population can contribute to a country's economic growth* (WHO, 2001).

International donors were quick to adopt the cost-effectiveness analysis and the justification of top-down vertical health programmes advocated by the World Bank and reinforced by the WHO's Commission on Macroeconomics and Health. We will discuss the specific role of international donors in global health a later in the section, 'Global Health Initiatives (GHIs) (early 2000s)'.

The consequences of health sector reform

Initiated in the late 1980s, health sector reform that was promoted by the evolving global health governance structure, where the World Bank and new public–private entities became more prominent, accelerated the expansion of local private health care. Whereas before it was accepted that a strong public health system was the only viable option for underdeveloped countries to provide health care to their poor populations, a new paradigm gained ground: that the market should and could take care of the health of people living in poverty. The reasons for this were two-fold: on the one hand, as part of Structural Adjustment Programmes (SAPs), governments had to cut budgets for public health care and resort to hidden or outright privatisation of health care. On the other hand, there was the emergence and expansion of a local middle class with the appropriate purchasing power to make private health care profitable. The result was the **commercialisation of health care.**

GLOSSARY

Commercialisation of health care: the provision of health care goods and services to those who can afford it, to make a profit. It includes providing services through market relationships to those who can pay, an investment in those services to make a profit and a payment system based in individual payment or private insurance (Mackintosh, 2003).

Other multilateral organisations and donors also pressured governments of underdeveloped countries to commercialise health care. A key idea was that purchaser and provider functions had to be separated to create a 'market' for health care services. This means that the State alone could not both provide health care services and pay for them.

Concrete policy prescriptions included various combinations of decentralisation, liberalisation, user fees and cost-recovery in public health services, contracting out of services, corporatisation of government hospitals and encouraging competition among insurers and health care providers (Mackintosh & Koivusalo, 2005).

Reducing public funding for health care services

According to the World Bank's 1993 *Investing in Health* report:

> *The case for government financing of discretionary clinical health care—services outside the essential package—is far less compelling. In fact, governments can promote both efficiency and equity by reducing—or when possible eliminating—public funding for these services.*

Governments were encouraged to transfer all 'non-essential' public health services to private providers. This doctrine was introduced in underdeveloped countries where the local population was considered to have the necessary means to purchase health services, such as in parts of Asia and Latin America. As a result of this policy, public health systems tended to focus on disease control programmes, while curative health care, for which there was sufficient demand, was transferred to the private for-profit sector (Unger et al., 2008).

In certain cases, international institutions, most notably the IMF, wanted to suppress government spending even further, using the so-called public sector wage bill ceilings, i.e. capping the amount of money used to pay the wages of public sector employees. Such wage bill ceilings have hindered governments' ability to educate, hire and retain enough doctors, nurses and health workers. In Kenya, for example, this policy led to several thousands of professionally trained nurses remaining unemployed over many years (Rowden, 2008).

Cost-recovery, user fees

The public sector was required to not only cut costs but also recover costs and enhance revenues. To this end, international institutions recommended that governments impose user fees for health services. According to Whitehead and colleagues (2001) the arguments they put forward were as follows:

- Free services were incompatible with quality care.
- Being paid a fee would offer financial possibilities to health providers to provide quality services.
- Privatisation would increase the public's appreciation of health services and prevent overuse.

User fees in public health care did enhance the income of the public system. More importantly, it made private for-profit health care more competitive and stimulated the expansion of the private sector, but without a free alternative. The consequences of this policy were dramatic. As an example, in 1987, the WHO/UNICEF Bamako Initiative was adopted by African health ministers in Bamako, Mali. The aim was for PHC services to become more self-sustaining in Sub-Saharan African, "*by generating funds in communities through the sales of drugs at a price considerably higher than cost*" (Hardon, 1990). Although measures were meant to be implemented to exempt the poorest patients (particularly aimed at women and children), these were not applied. The approach was widely criticised by development workers because of the equity impacts on the most vulnerable communities and due to concerns about efficiency and sustainability (Gilson, 1997).

According to Whitehead et al. (2001), the negative social effects of direct user fees for health care are greater than most other fees, because these expenses are unexpected and the total cost is often unknown until after treatment. The greater the commercialisation of health care, the greater the exclusion of children from treatment when ill and the greater the inequality in rates of immunisation. Of all the types of commercialisation studied, fee-for-service provision in conditions of generalised poverty had the strongest association with low-quality care, exclusion and neglect (Mackintosh, 2003).

> *Commercialisation—sometimes, discreditably, 'sold' as a policy for increasing equity—has generally acted to embed inequality in new forms . . . commercialization has to be at least partially blocked if socially inclusive development is to be possible . . .* (Mackintosh, 2003).

Critics of the narrowly focused SPHC approach and of the later health sector reforms believe that the move from equity and comprehensiveness to technical efficiency and selectiveness has led to:

- A return to vertical programmes.
- Fragmentation of health services.
- Neglect of the social determinants of health.
- Erosion of intersectoral work and community health infrastructures and "*at best delayed, and at worst undermined the implementation of the comprehensive strategy codified at Alma-Ata*" (Sanders et al., 2008).

The shifting global funding architecture

International and foreign donors enthusiastically embraced the cost-effectiveness analysis and the justification of top-down selective, technocratic, vertical approaches and fragmented health systems advocated by the World Bank and reinforced by the WHO's Commission of Macroeconomics and Health.

Project support or aid (1970s–1990s)

Up until the early 1990s (with SAPs in operations), the bulk of donor funding for health in underdeveloped countries was either channelled from international organisations, like the World Bank, in the form of loans and credits, or from earmarked **project** and **programme** aid through **bilateral** and **multilateral** donors, such as USAID, the World Bank and UN agencies like UNICEF.

GLOSSARY

Project: an individual development intervention designed to achieve specific objectives within specified resources and implementation schedules; it often is part of a broader programme.

Programme: a time-bound intervention involving multiple activities that may cut across sectors, themes and/or geographic areas, e.g. funding for the health sector.

Bilateral aid: aid given by one government directly to another.

Multilateral aid: aid given through the intermediary of an international organisation, such as the World Bank, which collects donations from several governments and then distributes them to recipients.

Project and programme aid allowed donors to have direct control over their money, to hire technical staff from their own countries and to take the lead in the implementation of their projects (Mosley & Eeckhout, 2000). However, the sustainability of such projects was problematic for several reasons:

- The proportion of public funds for health care in many underdeveloped countries such as Zimbabwe, was (and still is) low in comparison to the contributions from donors.
- Recipient governments did not have ownership of the projects.
- It was difficult to coordinate the different autonomous and separately managed donor projects.
- At times, these donor projects were implemented or administered by institutions that did not have the capacity to manage them (Buse & Walt, 2000).

The Sector Wide Approach (SWAp) (1990s)

To address the ongoing problems of project support or aid, in the late 1990s the Sector Wide Approach (SWAp) emerged as a financing or organisational mechanism. Donors began to shift from earmarked funding for specific diseases, sectors or themes to supporting the health sector as a whole, in a more coordinated way.

SWAps included five key elements (Walford, 2003):

1. All significant funding agencies supported one shared, sector-wide policy and strategy.
2. There was a medium-term budget to support this policy.
3. There was a partnership between government and the funding agencies.
4. There were shared processes for implementing and managing the sector strategy and work programme.
5. There was a commitment to move to greater reliance on government financial management, policy development, coordinated planning and accountability systems.

The goals were to minimise duplication and competition and to encourage more coherent country-led policy development and health system strengthening (Buse & Walt, 2000). However, there were several challenges, including the weak institutional capacity of recipient governments to coordinate and manage different and competing donors. Thus, some donors started to shift funds out of SWAps to the general budget in the finance ministries of underdeveloped countries, allowing governments the freedom to decide their own priorities.

Global Health Initiatives (GHIs) (early 2000s)

The term, 'Global Health Initiative' refers to entities that mount a selective response to specific aspects of the global public health agenda (WHO, 2008b).

By the early 2000s, more than 80 Global Health Initiatives (GHIs) had emerged as new global funding mechanisms for development assistance in the fight against specific diseases (such as HIV/AIDS) in low- and middle-income countries (Brugha, 2008). Their funding came partly from governments of developed countries and partly from philanthropic organisations like the Bill and Melinda Gates Foundation (BMGF). They were *"a blueprint for financing, resourcing, coordinating, and/or implementing disease control across at least several countries in more than one region of the world"* (Brugha, 2008).

GHIs earmarked funds for focal diseases, independent of country context, for example the Global Fund to Fight AIDS, TB and Malaria (GFATM), Roll Back Malaria (RBM), the World Bank's Multi-Country HIV/AIDS Program (MAP), and the US President's Emergency Plan for AIDS Relief (**PEPFAR**), which was established during President G.W. Bush's term to channel US bilateral funds specifically for HIV/AIDS programmes.

A NOTE ABOUT PEPFAR

PEPFAR is the US government's agency that is committed to addressing the global HIV/AIDS epidemic. It is implemented by seven other US government departments and agencies including the US Agency for International Development (USAID), the US Department of Health and Human Services and its agencies, including the Centers for Disease Control and Prevention (CDC), Health Resources and Service Administration, and the National Institutes of Health (NIH), the US Department of Defence, the Peace Corps, the US Department of Labour, the US Department of Commerce and the US Department of the Treasury.

According to Buse and Walt (2000), the main GHIs were formed around three key categories:

- Product/commodity (drug or vaccine) development, such as the Global Alliance for Vaccines and Immunization (GAVI).
- Improving access to health products, such as the Mectizan Donation Program—a drug donation programme established by the multinational pharmaceutical company Merck & Co., for neglected tropical diseases, river blindness and elephantiasis in particular.
- Global coordination mechanisms, including funding vehicles such as the GFATM.

Most GHIs were established between 1998 and 2003, resulting in, among other effects, a dramatic increase in funding for HIV/AIDS (see Figure 5.5).

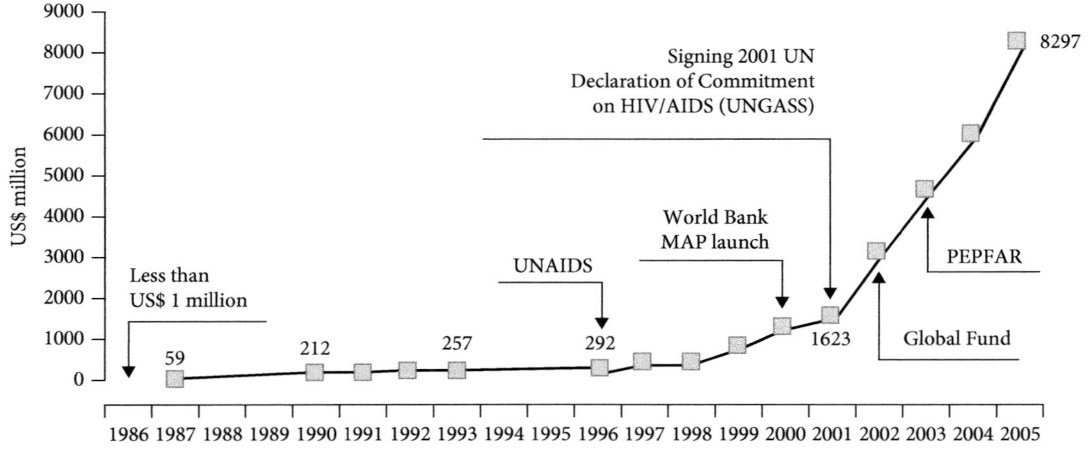

US$ million
9000
8000
7000
6000
5000
4000
3000
2000
1000
0
Signing 2001 UN
Declaration of Commitment
on HIV/AIDS (UNGASS)
8297
World Bank
MAP launch
UNAIDS
PEPFAR
Less than
US$ 1 million
Global Fund
59
212
257
292
1623
1986 1987 1988 1989 1990 1991 1992 1993 1994 1995 1996 1997 1998 1999 2000 2001 2002 2003 2004 2005

Notes: [1] 1986–2000 figures are for international funds only
[2] Domestic funds are included from 2001 onwards

[i] *1996–2005 data: Extracted from 2006 Report on the AIDS epidemic (UNAIDS 2006)*
[ii] *1986–1993 data: AIDS in the World II. Edited by janathan Mann and Daniel J.M. Tarantola (1996)*

Fig. 5.5 Total annual resources available for AIDs, 1986–2005.

Source: World Bank (1993). World Development Report 1993: Investing in Health. New York: Oxford University Press. World Bank.

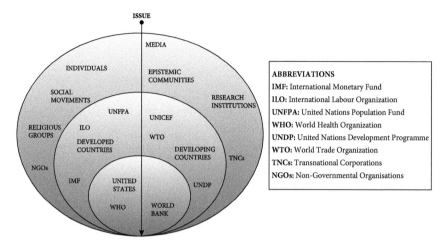

Fig. 5.6 Global health governance mapped.
Source: Dodgson et al. (2002).

Each GHI works with recipient countries in different ways. With some GHIs, recipient countries are expected to submit specific proposals for aid. For example, in the case of GAVI, country applications have to specify levels of immunisation coverage and how they would increase these with new-generation vaccines. The performance of the country is assessed against the country's stated goals. Grants are disbursed only in partial payment and once results are demonstrated.

By 2002, although the key actors in **global health governance** were the WHO (with its health expertise) and the World Bank (with its development finance expertise), both organisations were linked to other global actors which had political or economic influence. Several 'non-state' actors (e.g. private companies, non-governmental organisations [NGOs], research institutions, charitable foundations, faith-based and social movements) were becoming more visible in health and in their efforts to influence policy-making and global health governance (see Figure 5.6).

GLOSSARY

Global health governance: includes political collaboration of different actors, across different levels (local, national, global), to develop and institute health policies and to resolve health problems. It uses an infrastructure of global agreements and institutions. This 'global policy space' can be used to set regulatory rules and to limit or promote different agendas.

In this complex arena of actors, the issue of leadership and authority is a difficult one … the absence of a single institution, with the authority and capacity to act decisively, to address health issues of global concern in another (Dodgson et al., 2002).

Several important new **global private–public partnerships** (GPPPs) began to emerge, including, for example, between the WHO and other UN agencies, governments, the corporate sector and GHIs (see Figure 5.7). These organisations were increasingly recognised as the new system of global health governance (Buse & Walt, 2000). Since then, developments in global health governance have to a large extent been shaped by the evolution of contemporary globalisation and the processes used to promote its agenda.

GLOSSARY

Global private–public partnerships (GPPPs): a collaborative relationship between at least three parties, including one in the private for-profit sector and an intergovernmental organisation and perhaps a recipient government—which transcends national boundaries (Buse & Walt, 2000).

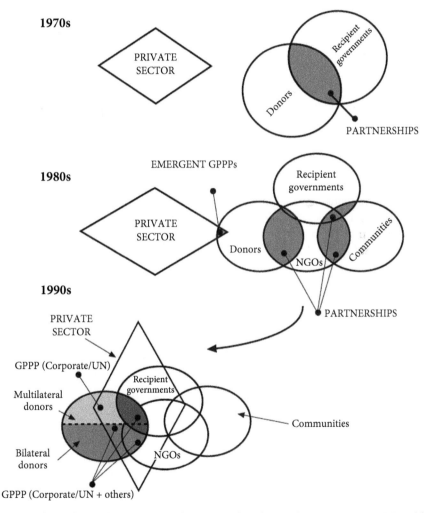

Fig. 5.7 The shift to global private-public partnerships (GPPPs) over time. UNDP/World Bank/WHO Special Program for Research and Training in Tropical Diseases.
Source: Data from Buse & Walt. (2000).

Philanthrocapitalism

Some GHIs (although not all of them) include, or are often partially funded by, philanthrocapitalist foundations. These are private initiatives (that use the private capital of an individual rather than donors) that operate on a business model, harnessing the power of the market to achieve social outcomes or to pursue a philanthropic goal. They invest in socially responsible programmes that will bring about both a financial return and a social good.

Since the late 1990s, the philanthropic sector has grown enormously in number, size of annual giving and scope of activities. It has the power to harness new resources and significant amounts of money, partners, technical capacity and political commitment. In 2017, *Global Health Watch 5* (GHW 5) estimated that there were approximately 200 000 philanthrocapitalist foundations globally—86 000 in the USA, 85 000 in Western Europe and 35 000 in Eastern Europe. Estimates of how much money is given range from US$7 billion to more than US$10 billion per year. The largest and most influential organisation is the BMGF (The Gates Foundation), with an estimated US$2.9 billion per year allocated for health (People's Health Movement, 2017).

The main concerns with GHIs and philanthrocapitalist foundations

In 2003, the OECD published the findings of a Needs Assessment Survey commissioned in 11 countries representing different geographic regions and levels of development. The Survey asked two main questions:

- How can donors improve development assistance in ways that support country-owned and -led development strategies?
- Which donor practices are most undermining of the effectiveness of these strategies?

It was found that the five highest burdens on donor practices for low- and middle-income countries were:

1. Donor-driven priorities and systems, rather than supporting national needs and priorities.
2. Difficulties with different donor procedures, systems and policies.
3. Uncoordinated donor practices resulting in difficulties in fulfilling the multiple, diverse requirements of different donors.
4. Excessive demands on government time.
5. Delays in disbursements (OECD, 2003).

As an example, in 2000, Tanzania was preparing 2400 quarterly reports on separate aid-funded projects and hosted 1000 donor visit meetings a year (Kenny, 2006).

The fragmentation created by funding by separate agencies and GHIs is illustrated in the 'Spaghetti Complex Diagram' in Figure 5.8, which focuses on only one component of the health system, namely supplies and logistics in the pharmaceutical sector in Kenya. Multiple partners play different roles in supplying a variety of commodity types, with little coordination between them. Funds are sourced from multiple donors, including government, the World Bank, bilateral donors, multilateral donors and private and NGO sectors.

The complexity in medicines supply arrangements was mainly centred on the sources of financing and the procuring entity (i.e. 'who pays for what' and 'who buys what'). Once the medicines were procured, however, warehousing and distribution were mainly handled by Government and NGO/faith-based organizations. But there was often no logistical support provided for this purpose. The delivery of supplies to the point of warehousing was uncoordinated and the warehousing and distribution capacity were severely constrained, resulting in clogging of the distribution system. This situation was particularly acute for KEMSA, which handled the majority of supplies from the numerous procurement agents. Consequently, in spite of holding large stocks in the warehouses, the country still experienced frequent stock-outs in health facilities and sometimes expiries of essential medicines at the central level (WHO, 2010).

There are major concerns about the increasing influence of these multiple donors on global health governance and decision-making, including the power to preserve the status quo and as a way for those people who are mega-rich to achieve their own agendas and shape social outcomes, which are not always in the best interests of those on the receiving end or supportive of national needs and priorities.

Given current priorities identified by leading philanthropic organisations, an over reliance on such funding risks a singularly technology-driven, biomedically-centred approach, rather than one that simultaneously supports policies and new knowledge that more effectively deals with equity and the social determinants of health (Labonte & Schrecker, 2007).

Most philanthropic foundations operate on the same principles promoted by US steel tycoon Andrew Carnegie over a century ago. He suggested that:

[Philanthropy would enable the] problem of rich and poor to be solved. The laws of accumulation will be left free, the laws of distribution free. Individualism will continue, but the millionaire will be but a trustee of the poor, entrusted for a season with a great part of the increased wealth of the community, but administering it for the community far better than it could or would have done for itself (McGoey, 2016, cited in People's Health Movement, 2017).

Health care, it is argued, is a public good and should be provided by the public sector, funded through money generated through taxes. In other words, tax should be the instrument we use to achieve equity. However, the philanthrocapitalist model *"exacerbates growing inequality rather than mitigates it, by depriving treasuries of*

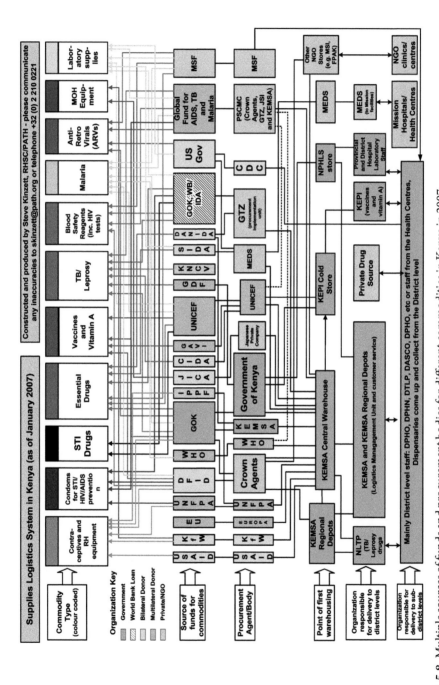

Fig. 5.8 Multiple sources of funds and procurement bodies for different commodities in Kenya in 2007.

Source: Constructed and produced by Steve Kinzett.

tax revenues that could be spent on redistributive welfare policies" (People's Health Movement, 2017).

Money channelled into philanthropic foundations may be accumulated in many different ways, including by not paying taxes commensurate with profits earned and by investing money offshore to maximise returns and reduce taxes owed in the home nation. In addition, in some countries, like the USA, some of the funding supplied by philanthropic foundations or as part of the 'corporate social responsibility' of a company or corporation are exempt from taxes, and private individuals who donate to these foundations can get a tax deduction. This means that some of this funding in fact consists of a public subsidy, i.e. money foregone by the State due to tax exemptions (McCoy et al., 2009).

With reference to The Gates Foundation, the following concerns have been articulated:

- *They apply a business model to measure results*: they focus on selective, short-term projects with demonstrable donor-driven and defined results, for example disseminating insecticide-treated bed nets in malaria areas, rather than also tackling the social determinants of the problem.
- *They rely on technical solutions to complex global health problems*: they provide vaccines only, for example, as an 'elegant technology', rather than also treating the underlying causes of various communicable diseases, such as the lack of sanitation, safe drinking water and better nutrition.
- *They influence policy-making and agenda setting*: The Gates Foundation, "*through its practice of providing matching funds and active advocacy, influences priority setting in the World Health Organization (WHO) and promotes an emphasis on vertical, disease specific programmes*" (People's Health Movement, 2017).
- *They lack transparency and accountability mechanisms*: they are governed by and only accountable to their own boards or trustees and secretariats, rather than to any government, international organisation or community, even though they wield enormous power over the policies and priorities of countries and organisations like the UN, WHO and World Bank.
- *They foster privatisation, fragmentation and weakening of global governance*: when working with governments, a precondition set by The Gates Foundation is the involvement of the private sector and public–private partnerships, often devaluing the role of governments (People's Health Movement, 2017).

The problem of domination of national health systems by international donors and policies is compounded by neoliberal policies at national level, weak governance and accountability systems and corruption in several low- and medium-income countries. The latter refers to financial kickbacks to local companies for government contracts.

CASE STUDY: Cases of corruption in South Africa

- According to Tayler and Dickinson (2006), from the early 2000s, evidence of corruption in South Africa impeded efforts for prevention and treatment of HIV and AIDS. Such corruption included, for example, materials never being purchased; false claims of treatment; procurement and distribution; the sale of antiretroviral drugs; theft; and government corruption.
- The Judicial Commission of Inquiry into Allegations of State Capture (the Zondo Commission) was established in 2018 purely to probe such examples of state capture, fraud and other allegations in the public sector.
- More recently, in 2021, in a second special report on the financial management of COVID-19 initiatives, the Auditor-General has said that contracts for the supply of personal protective equipment (PPE) are the biggest target in COVID-19-related corruption (Ndenze, 2021).

Recent global policies to address the crisis of development

After a decade of UN conferences and summits focused on addressing extreme poverty, hunger and disease worldwide, in September 2000, 189 UN member nations committed to achieving eight measurable and time-bound goals by 2015. These became known as the Millennium Development Goals (MDGs)—goals that were based on a commitment to a human rights-based development approach. Before examining the MDGs in more detail, it is important to consider what the right to health means and how it intersects with other human rights.

The human right to health

The increasing prevalence of human rights discourse, particularly since the early 1990s, has led to a new emphasis on the right to the *highest attainable standard of physical and mental health*, to use the wording of the International Covenant on Economic, Social and Cultural Rights, one of the key human rights instruments. This echoes similar wording in the Constitution of the WHO. It is important to note that the reference is to health, not health care, and that this is understood to mean that the right to health intersects with many other human rights, particularly those in the social and economic sphere. This intersection may be both positive and negative. For instance, failure to adequately protect human rights may have adverse health consequences by the damage that it causes, for example through physical violence and abuse. Secondly, there may be circumstances where measures to protect health may themselves violate human rights, for example by coercive treatments or violations of a patient's privacy and dignity. More positively, realisation of the right to health can contribute to other rights, such as access to education or political participation, and the protection and fulfilment of a range of human rights contribute to health—including adequate food, sanitation, housing and employment (Marks & Clapham, 2005). So, even in the abstract, the right to health cannot easily be separated from the whole range of human rights.

The UN International Covenant on Economic, Social and Cultural Rights (ICESCR) defined the right to health as:

> *an inclusive right extending not only to timely and appropriate health care but also to the underlying determinants of health, such as access to safe and potable water and adequate sanitation, an adequate supply of safe food, nutrition and housing, healthy occupational and environmental conditions, and access to health-related education and information, including on sexual and reproductive health* (UN, 2000).

An additional element of the right to health, and one of primary importance, is the principle of non-discrimination. According to the late Jonathan Mann, one of the leading authorities on health and human rights, *"inadvertent discrimination is so prevalent that all public health policies and programmes should be considered discriminatory until proven otherwise"* (Marks & Clapham, 2005).

The centrality of non-discrimination is one of the ways in which a human rights approach can be said to add value to the struggle for health. Another 'value-added' element is that by framing health as a universal entitlement, both individuals and groups may be able to challenge government policies and the actions of private companies using tactics such as litigation. There have been clear examples of this from South Africa, among many other countries, where courts have ruled against pharmaceutical transnationals on the question of availability of antiretroviral (ARV) drugs and against the government itself for the neglect of the issue of mother-to-child transmission of HIV in the rollout of ARVs.

Millennium Development Goals and human rights

The Millennium Declaration, which was adopted by world leaders in 2000, recognised the importance of human rights as being fundamental to achieving the MDGs. Each of the eight MDGs is underpinned or related to a specific human right, as shown in Table 5.2.

In 2010, the MDG Summit concluded with member nations recommitting to achieving the MDGs and adopting a global action plan specifically aimed at accelerating the progress of women and children's health.

However, by 2014, as the deadline approached, the achievement of the MDGs was limited and uneven across regions, especially across Africa where the challenges were enormous, including, among others, unacceptably high poverty rates and child and maternal mortality, the devastating effects of rapid climate change, mass migration and recurring wars.

Table 5.2 MDG and related human rights

MDG	Related human rights
Goal 1: Eradicate extreme poverty and hunger	Right to adequate standard of living; right to work; right to food
Goal 2: Achieve universal primary education	Right to education
Goal 3: Promote gender equality and empower women	Women's right to equality
Goal 4: Reduce child mortality	Right to life
Goal 5: Improve maternal health	Women's right to life and health
Goal 6: Combat HIV/AIDs, malaria and other diseases	Right to health
Goal 7: Ensure environmental sustainability	Right to environmental health; right to water and sanitation; right to adequate housing
Goal 8: Develop a global partnership for development	Right to development; economic, social and cultural rights; right to health

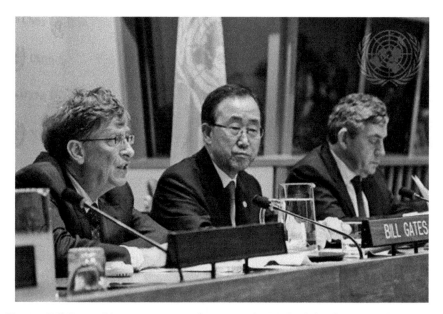

Fig. 5.9 Bill Gates addresses a press conference on the UN high-level event on the MDGs. Also participating are Secretary-General Ban Ki-moon (centre) and Gordon Brown, Prime Minister of the United Kingdom of Great Britain and Northern Ireland.
Source: United Nations. (2008).
https://dam.media.un.org/package/2am9lot_4#/searchresult&vbid=2am94sgd3q62&pn=7&ws=search results; UN7644103.

The MDG framework itself is seen by various authors as problematic on several levels. A review undertaken by Fehling and colleagues (2013) identifies the following important concerns (among others):

- The process used to develop and formulate the MDG goals and targets was driven by the USA, Europe and Japan and co-sponsored by the World Bank, IMF and OECD, with little input from developing countries and civil society organisations (see Figure 5.9).
- The MDGs were too simplistic, unachievable, focusing on 'quick fix' selective interventions only and failing to address the social determinants of health. For example:

Langford (2010) writes that the MDGs of 'gender equality and the empowerment of women' were narrowed down to gender equality in education, and the target for 'affordable water' was dropped from the MDG list in order to allow for privatisation in the sector (Fehling et al., 2013).

- The focus on halving the proportion of people suffering from hunger and poverty rather than on halving the absolute numbers of people suffering was seen as a major limitation, as was the failure to sufficiently address inequity and inequalities (which were said to often be used interchangeably).
- Progress towards the MDGs was measured in mostly national averages or aggregated data, which do not provide a detailed understanding of progress in each region and within-country inequalities.

Vandemoortele (2011) even calls it a 'tyranny of averages' where issues of inclusive and equitable progress are ignored within the framework due to 'abstractions and over-generalization' (Fehling et al., 2013).

The problem with using national and global averages to plan health interventions and make decisions about resource allocation is that they tend to mask the reality of what is happening at the local level—where interventions are most needed. UNICEF (2021), for example, notes that while there have been dramatic decreases in the under-five mortality rate globally, from 12.5 million in 1990 to 5.2 million in 2019, when the data are analysed at the local level a different picture emerges, "*some countries showing a national reduction in child mortality rates over the past decade also show an increase in child mortality rates in certain areas*" (UNICEF, 2021). In Nigeria, for example, the under-five mortality rate was 117 deaths per 1000 live births in 2019. However, at a more local level in 2019, the under-five mortality rate ranged from 58 to 261 per 1000 live births (UNICEF, 2021).

Despite these concerns, however, the targets of child mortality reduction by 50% and maternal mortality by 75% by 2015 did act as a spur to national action, and marked improvements did occur in some countries, although falling short of these targets and not decreasing inequities (UN, 2015).

Sustainable Development Goals

This set the scene for the UN to launch a new agenda to build on and finish what the MDGs did not achieve. In September 2015, *Transforming Our World: The 2030 Agenda for Sustainable Development* was launched and included 17 Sustainable Development Goals (SDGs) and 169 targets to be met by 2030, with a pledge that *"no one will be left behind"* (Preamble to Transforming Our World: The 2030 Agenda for Sustainable Development).

> *The Sustainable Development Goals (SDGs), otherwise known as the Global Goals, are a universal call to action to end poverty, protect the planet and ensure that all people enjoy peace and prosperity. These 17 Goals build on the successes of the Millennium Development Goals, while including new areas such as climate change, economic inequality, innovation, sustainable consumption, peace and justice, among other priorities* (UNDP, 2019).

According to Ekram and Bradford (2018), the estimated annual price tag to deliver the SDGs was US$3.5 trillion, jointly funded by governments, private donors and philanthropic foundations. Since January 2016, philanthropic foundations have contributed more than US$50 billion. Most of the funding has been invested in SDG 4: Ensuring inclusive and equitable quality education for all, and SDG 3: Ensuring good health and well-being—each receiving more than US$18 billion. In addition, foundations have contributed to combatting various health emergencies, such as avian influenza, Zika virus, Ebola virus and Middle East respiratory syndrome (MERS), as well as public health emergencies caused by natural/human-made disasters like wars, cyclones and earthquakes.

Critics have argued that the SDGs are yet another top-down UN process and that failure to implement previous agendas has eroded the confidence of organisations in the practicality of achieving goals such as these. They have also cautioned that there is a risk that because the SDGs are so extensive and ambitious, sectors will become even more siloed and will not be able to provide an integrated and comprehensive approach to achieving health outcomes, including addressing the social determinants of health.

CASE STUDY: COVID-19 and the SDGs

The COVID-19 pandemic has impeded progress towards reaching the SDGs. It has hindered progress in slowing the rate of global poverty, hunger and food insecurity and global ill-health. The pandemic has highlighted the fragility and weaknesses in health care services throughout the world and how unprepared they are to respond to a global pandemic.

For example, access to child immunisation was negatively affected. Maternal mortality increased directly due to COVID-19 pneumonia deaths in pregnant women and indirectly due to the indirect effects of COVID-19 causing disruption of regular maternity services. Sexual and reproductive services for contraception and termination of pregnancy have been particularly affected, causing a reversal of gains in reproductive choices for women.

The little progress that had been made in gender equality has been slowed down (with gender-based violence increasing in many countries as a consequence of lockdowns), as has been the provision of clean water and sanitation and access to electricity and other forms of energy.

COVID-19 school closures have impacted on gains made in universal primary school enrolment. It has impacted economic growth and employment opportunities. There has been a considerable decline in remittances—money transfers sent home by workers living and working abroad—which were trending upwards before the pandemic. There has been an unexpected decline in transport and travel worldwide.

Overall, all countries exhibit inequality—with the gap between people who are rich and people who are poor growing even wider within and across countries. Worldwide, there has been a crisis in leadership with governments. Climate change threatens to further undermine progress in almost every area of human development (Pirlea et al., 2020). As temperatures increase, scientists are warning that there may be an increase in vector-borne and zoonotic diseases.

Universal Health Coverage (UHC)

Central to SDG 3 and contributing to other SDGs is Universal Health Coverage (UHC) with its focus on:

- **Equity in access to health services**: those who need the services should get them, not only those who can pay for them.
- **Access to quality health care services**: services should be good enough to improve the health of those receiving them.
- **Access to safe, effective, quality and affordable essential medicines and vaccines**: all who need them should get them.
- **Achieving financial-risk protection**: the cost of using care should not put people at risk of financial hardship.

Of all components of SDG 3, the UHC target should be the one that potentially tracks the right to *Health for All* most closely, especially as it is firmly based on the principle of equity. However, there are some major concerns, not least of which are the different understandings of UHC which impact on how it is operationalised. In 2013, Oxfam warned:

Universal health coverage (UHC) has the potential to transform the lives of millions of people by bringing life-saving health care to those who need it most. UHC means that all people get the treatment they need without fear of falling into poverty. **Unfortunately, in the name of UHC, some donors and developing country governments are promoting health insurance schemes that exclude the majority of people and leave the poor behind** (Oxfam, 2013).

Initial indicators to measure UHC included health services *coverage* and financial protection *coverage*. The use of the term 'coverage' rather than 'universal health care' suggests either a limited scope of care or enrolment in a government-funded or a for-profit private health insurance scheme, aggravating health inequities (Sanders et al., 2019).

A recent publication by Brazilian senior health policymakers warns that 'emphasis on coverage in UHC may undermine the comprehensive, integrated approach of PHC and limit the population's access to the first level of care or to the supply of basic packages based on persons' ability to pay ...' (Giovanella et al., 2019, p. 3). Additionally, a recent report of a PAHO High-Level Commission expresses concern that '... reform agendas exclusively focused on the health sector, centered on medical care services and the expansion of insurance coverage, has displaced public health and the processes of social determination of health ...' (Pan American Health Organization, 2019, p. 6) (Sanders et al., 2019).

By 2016, with the increasing focus on finances and the acceptance of austerity measures, the global health conference in Bangkok on Priority Setting for UHC concluded with a statement about the importance of deciding which services and policies to prioritise, based on 'cost-effectiveness with respect to health outcomes' (Prince Mahidol Award Conference, 2016). The health emphasis embodied in this statement further waters down the policy of *Health for All* through the implementation of CPHC, as enshrined in the 1978 Alma-Ata Declaration. As stated by Wong et al.:

The current global emphasis is clearly narrowed down to health care financing followed by clinic health services. This is not surprising given that the implementation of UHC is not independent of the health system it is in. In an era of privatization, private health care services have increasingly replaced public services as the main provider of health care to population and predictably, its emphasis has been in financing, and biomedical interventions and research (Wong et al., 2016).

What of the Alma-Ata Declaration and its PHC agenda? What has happened alongside the development agenda, and where is PHC now?

Primary Health Care 40 years on

Five years after the MDGs were adopted, the UN *The Millennium Development Goals Report 2005* highlighted the following:

- Poverty rates were falling mainly in Asia, but that 1 billion people still lived in extreme poverty (subsisting on less than US$1 a day); more than 800 million people had too little to eat; and more than a quarter of children under five years old in underdeveloped countries were malnourished.

- Death rates in children under five years were dropping, but 11 million children a year still died from preventable or treatable causes.
- Some progress had been made in reducing maternal deaths in underdeveloped regions, but more than half a million women still died each year during pregnancy or childbirth in the countries where giving birth was most risky.
- More people had access to safe drinking water, but half the underdeveloped world still lacked toilets or other forms of basic sanitation.

Commission on the Social Determinants of Health (CSDH)

It was within this context that the WHO established the Commission on the Social Determinants of Health (CSDH) in 2005, to identify the underlying root causes of persisting and widening health inequities within and between countries and to formulate recommendations on how to reduce these.

The launch of the Commission brought renewed hope that there would be a return to the principles and ideals envisioned in the Alma-Ata Declaration—of health as a fundamental human right with intrinsic value, and of the importance of tackling the chain of social, economic and political determinants which contribute to ill-health and health inequities.

Policy-makers, donor agencies, international organisations and others gave input to the Commission. An important submission was made by the People's Health Movement (PHM) in which it called for the revitalisation of the promises of the Alma-Ata Declaration (including PHC) and for the underlying causes of inequity to be addressed:

> We strongly believe that the ultimate goal, is not merely to look for health policies that favour the poor. Rather we seek significant policies that directly address the social determinants of the inequitable distribution of resources at a global, national and subnational level... The Commission has a historic opportunity to advocate for equity and for the structural changes that will do away with the social, economic and political determinants of health (People's Health Movement, 2007).

You can read more about the PHM, a large global civil society movement comprised of health activists supportive of the WHO policy of *Health for All*, in Chapter 7.

The *Civil Society Report on the Social Determinants of Health* (2007), in which the PHM played a major role and which was submitted to the Commission, examined why the global vision of the Declaration of Alma-Ata had *not* been achieved and why PHC as envisioned in the Declaration had been virtually abandoned. It cited the following key reasons:

- The tendency to confuse PHC with health care delivery at the 'primary' level of the health care system, which was often seen as "*cheap, low-technology care for poor people in poor countries*" (WHO, 2007).
- The economic crisis that started in the 1970s which made it virtually impossible for underdeveloped countries to provide the resources needed to sustain their health care systems.
- The health sector reforms—underpinned by neoliberal economic policies— imposed on poorer countries by the IMF and World Bank, which systematically weakened the public health system and promoted private and commercial health care, promoting cost-effective packages that ignored the underlying causes of ill-health.
- SPHC which was largely biomedical in orientation and delivered by separate programmes, each targeting a specific health problem. Many of these programmes relied on donor funding and were driven, controlled and implemented by international donor agencies.

In introducing the final WHO Commission Report in 2008—*Closing the Gap in a Generation*—the chair, epidemiologist Sir Michael Marmot, stated that the:

> *inequalities in health, avoidable health inequalities, arise because of the circumstances in which people grow, live, work and age, and the systems put in place to deal with illness. The conditions in which people live and die are, in turn, shaped by political, social and economic forces ... Reducing health inequities is for the Commission on Social Determinants of Health, an ethical imperative. Social injustice is killing people on a grand scale* (WHO, 2008a).

Based on the interrelated values of social justice and health equity, health as a human right and the empowerment of people, the report highlighted the relationship between access to the social determinants of health and the social production and distribution of health/ill-health across different social groups. It called for a broader approach to addressing the unfair and avoidable differences in health and survival through intersectoral action, community participation and the empowerment of those who are most vulnerable to health risks and threats, within and across countries. The health status of people, it argued, was the responsibility of all policy-makers and not only those in the health sector. We need not only good health policies, but also health in all policies. Four sets of reforms were identified:

- Universal coverage reforms to improve health equity, social justice and access.
- Health service delivery reforms to make health systems more relevant and responsive to people's needs and expectations.

- Healthy public policies reforms that promote and protect the health of communities.
- Leadership reforms to ensure that health authorities take responsibility for the health care of their people.

Alma-Ata to Astana: from PHC to UHC
Astana Global Conference on PHC, 2018

On 25–26 October 2018—40 years after the Alma-Ata Declaration was endorsed—1200 global health leaders gathered in Kazakhstan, this time in the capital city of Astana, at the Global Conference on Primary Health Care. The Declaration of Astana (2018) (see Figure 5.10) states:

*We acknowledge that in spite of remarkable progress over the last 40 years, **people in all parts of the world still have unaddressed health needs. Remaining healthy is challenging for many people, particularly the poor and people in vulnerable situations.** We find it ethically, politically, socially and economically unacceptable that inequity in health and disparities in health outcomes persist* (WHO & UNICEF, 2018).

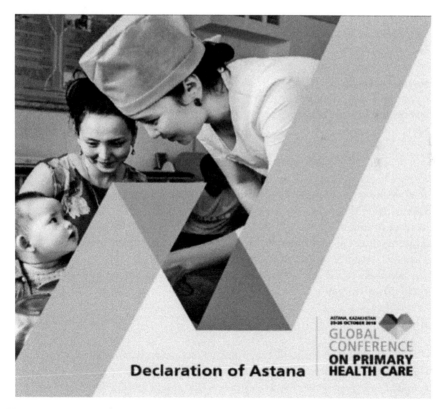

Fig. 5.10 Astana Declaration on PHC.
Source: WHO & UNICEF. (2018).

The aim of the conference was to endorse a declaration renewing the commitment of the member states of the WHO to Primary Health Care as a way of achieving universal health coverage and the health-related SDGs.

> We are convinced that **strengthening primary health care (PHC)** is the most inclusive, effective and efficient approach to enhance people's physical and mental health, as well as social well-being, and that **PHC is a cornerstone of a sustainable health system for universal health coverage (UHC) and health-related Sustainable Development Goals** (WHO & UNICEF, 2018).

The call was summed up in the WHO's call for a *'triple billion target'* by 2023:

> 1 billion more people with universal health coverage; 1 billion better protected from health emergencies, and 1 billion enjoying better health and well-being (WHO, 2020).

Discussion centred on domestic mobilisation of the estimated cost of US$350 billion annually for a package of 'essential cost-effective PHC-based interventions'.

> There were also constant reminders that foreign investment can be attracted for primary care by linking it to pre-existing global commitments. Virtually all Member States have signed up to the Sustainable Development Goals which includes a commitment to Universal Health Coverage (UHC)—the tripartite aspiration of delivering universal access to comprehensive health services with adequate financial protection—strongly boosted by Gates, the World Bank, and WHO. Dr Tedros, WHO Director General, repeatedly stressed that primary care (PHC) is the best (and cheapest) platform for improving access and increasing services; 'no UHC without PHC' (Allen, 2018).

People's Health Assembly 4, 2018

A few weeks after the Astana Global Conference on PHC, the People's Health Movement (PHM) held its fourth People's Health Assembly (PHA4), also returning to its place of origin—Savar, Bangladesh (see Figure 5.11). Delegates reaffirmed their commitment to PHC to achieve health equity and their commitment to the principles and agenda presented in the Alma-Ata Declaration of 1978.

The preamble to the *Alternative Civil Society Astana Statement on Primary Health Care* (PHM, 2018) states:

> We envision:
>
> - Societies and environments that prioritize, protect and promote people's health;
> - Health care that is accessible, affordable and acceptable for everyone, everywhere;
> - Health care of good quality that treats people with respect and dignity;
> - Health systems over which communities are able to exert control.

> Although these objectives are shared in the official Astana Declaration it is concerning that the latter frames PHC primarily as a 'cornerstone', i.e. a foundation of Universal

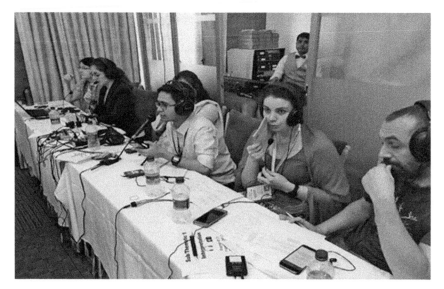

Fig. 5.11 PHA (16–19 November 2018) BRAC University, Savar, Dhaka, Bangladesh.

Health Coverage (UHC). PHC is broader and indeed subsumes UHC, which is, in many countries, being implemented by private health insurance companies and aggravating health inequities. While the official declaration recognises that it is 'ethically, politically, socially and economically unacceptable that inequity in health and disparities in health outcomes persist' it does not acknowledge that health gains in some places are being reversed. The declaration also recognises the risk factors for NCD's as well as premature deaths 'because of wars, violence, epidemics, natural disasters, the health impacts of climate change and extreme weather events and other environmental factors', yet nowhere are the fundamental economic and political causes responsible for this as well as for widening inequalities worldwide explicitly stated (People's Health Movement, 2018).

CASE STUDY: Health gains being reversed in the USA

According to the National Center for Health Statistics, in 2015, for the first time since 1999, the overall death rate in the USA rose by 1.2% for White men, Black men and White women. Heart disease and cancer accounted for nearly half of all deaths. Much of the increase in mortality can be explained by obesity, although poverty and its associated struggles like stress, depression and poor nutrition also play a role.

'We might be seeing the drag that decades of stagnant wages, growing inequality, and the associated behavioral (e.g. smoking, diet, activity) and psychosocial (e.g. chronic stress, depression) factors have on eventual mortality', said Michael Kramer, a professor of epidemiology at Emory University, via e-mail. Americans are hit harder

than other rich countries are by these forces, he posits, both because of our skimpy preventive health care and because 'the U.S. has higher income inequality and less comprehensive social safety net, so the ill-effects of poverty may take an undue toll' (Khazan, 2016).

Table 5.3 outlines the main concerns the PHA had with statements in the Astana Declaration. The PHA4 urged civil society organisations, health professionals and students, to challenge the inequitable macroeconomic regime and inappropriate policies, through evidence-based advocacy and social mobilisation.

Table 5.3 Alternative Civil Society response to Astana Statement on PHC

Astana statement on PHC	Alternative Civil Society responses
PHC is a means to achieving UHC.	It is the reverse: UHC is a means to achieving PHC.
*We will continue to address the **growing burden of noncommunicable diseases**, which lead to poor health and **premature deaths due to tobacco use, the harmful use of alcohol, unhealthy lifestyles and behaviours**, and insufficient physical activity and unhealthy diets.* *Unless we act immediately, we will continue to lose lives prematurely because of **wars, violence, epidemics, natural disasters, the health impacts of climate change** and extreme weather events and other environmental factors.*	No mention is made of addressing the structural determinants of the 'commercial' drivers of NCDs and climate change. The focus needs to be on prioritising and promoting working and living conditions that promote healthy lives; and a healthy and protected natural environment.
*We call on **all stakeholders—health professionals, academia, patients, civil society, local and international partners, agencies and funds, the private sector, faith-based organisations and others**—to align with national policies, strategies and plans across all sectors, including through people-centred, gender-sensitive approaches, and to **take joint actions to build stronger and sustainable PHC towards achieving UHC.***	It is not in the interests of the private sector—driven by the profit motive—to reduce the commercial determinants of health. How will conflicts of interest be managed?
It is *ethically, politically, socially and economically unacceptable that inequity in health and disparities in health outcomes persist.*	In contrast to the Alma-Ata Declaration, no reference is made to the need for a 'New International Economic Order' to address global wealth inequities and for mitigating the destructive impact that neoliberalism has had on global poverty, inequality and inequity, and on the health of people and the natural environment.
The Astana agenda achieves *health for some, not health for all* (Dr Tedros, WHO Director General, cited in Allen, 2018).	No mention is made of *Health for All* as a basic human right; and on quality health care that is accessible, affordable and acceptable to everyone, everywhere.

The struggle is not merely a struggle about a methodology or level of health care. It is a struggle about fundamental human rights to health, to accessible and affordable health care, and a struggle for *"equitable economic and social development [which] will require rejection of the currently dominant neo-liberal paradigm and establishment of a sustainable and equitable economic order globally and nationally"* (People's Health Movement, 2018).

Conclusion

SPHC matched the general shift in high-level development planning to technical solutions and privatisation of public services, and from the comprehensive vision of *Health for All* to survival rates. The health care reform that was then promoted by the evolving global health governance structure, as a subset of conservative neoliberal economic policies, gave rise to the privatisation and commercialisation of health care—from *Health for All* to health care that people could afford. There was a concomitant reduction in government health spending in many low- and middle-income countries with increasing dependence on multiple international donors and the reduced ability of countries to determine their own health agendas.

While there has been some progress in some health outcomes in some countries, others have been left behind, particularly the least developed regions of the world, where extreme inequalities have been worsened by neoliberal globalisation. In October 2018, world leaders met in Astana, Kazakhstan to renew a commitment to PHC as a 'cornerstone' to achieving UHC. An alternative statement to the Astana Declaration was put forward by health activists, reaffirming civil society's commitment to CPHC in pursuit of health and well-being for all, and to achieve equity in health outcomes globally and nationally.

References

Allen, L. (2018). After Astana: the post-conference agenda for global primary health care. *PLoS Global Health blog*, 30 October 2018.

Brugha, R. (2008). Global health initiative and public health policy. In: Quah, S.R. & Heggenhougen, K. (eds). *International Encyclopaedia of Public Health*, Volume 3:72–81. Academic Press/Elsevier: Amsterdam.

Buse, K. & Walt, G. (2000). Global public–private partnerships: part 1—a new development in health? *Bulletin of World Health Organisation*, 78(5):699–709.

Dodgson, R., Lee, K. & Drager, N. (2002). *Global Health Governance: A Conceptual Review*. Centre on Global Change and Health, London School of Hygiene and Tropical Medicine: London, and WHO: Geneva.

Ekram, A. & Bradford, L. (2018). Foundations have invested $50 billion in the SDGs, but who's counting? Foundation SDG Funders. http://sdgfunders.org/sdgs/dataset/historical/.

Fehling, M., Nelson, B. & Venkatapuram, S. (2013). Limitations of the Millennium Development Goals: a literature review. *Global Public Health*, 8(10):1109–1122.

Gilson, L. (1997). The lessons of user fee experience in Africa. *Health Policy Plan*, 12(4):273–285.

Giovanella, L., Mendonça, M.H.M., Buss, P.M., Fleury, S., Gadelha, C.A.G., Galvão, L.A.C. &, Santos, R.F.D. (2019). *From Alma-Ata to Astana. Primary health care and universal health systems: an inseparable commitment and a fundamental human right.* Cad Saude Publica, 25;35(3):e00012219. English, Portuguese. doi: 10.1590/0102-311X00012219. PMID: 30916174.

Hardon, A. (1990). Ten best readings in ... the Bamako Initiative. *Health Policy and Planning,* 5(2):186–189.

Kenny, C. (2006). What is effective aid? How would donors allocate it? World Bank Policy Research Working Paper 4005, September 2006.

Khazan, O. (2016). Why are so many Americans dying young? *The Atlantic.* https://www. theatlantic.com/health/archive/2016/12/why-are-so-many-americans-dying-young/ 510455/).

Labonte, R. & Schrecker, T. (2007). Globalization and social determinants of health: promoting health equity in global governance (part 3 of 3). *Globalization and Health,* 2007(3):7.

Mackintosh, M. (2003). Health care commercialisation and the embedding of inequality, RUIC/UNRISK Health Project Synthesis Paper. United Nations Research Institute for Social Development (UNRISD): Geneva.

Mackintosh, M. & Koivusalo, M. (2005). Health systems and commercialization: in search of good sense. In: Mackintosh, M. & Koivusalo, M. (eds). *Commercialization of Health Care. Social Policy in a Development Context.* Palgrave Macmillan: London. https://doi.org/ 10.1057/9780230523616_1.

Marks, S. & Clapham, A. (2005). *International Human Rights Lexicon.* OUP: Oxford.

McCoy, D., Chand, S. & Sridhar, D. (2009). Global health funding: how much, where it comes from and where it goes. *Health Policy and Planning,* 24(6):407–417.

Mosley, P. & Eeckhout, M.J. (2000). From project aid to programme assistance. In: Tarp, F. & Hjertholm, P. (eds). *Foreign Aid and Development.* Routledge: New York.

Ndenze, B. (2021). COVID-19: AG Maluleke says procurement of PPEs saw the biggest corruption. *Eyewitness News.* https://ewn.co.za/2021/02/19/covid-19-ag-maluleke-says-procurem ent-of-ppes-saw-the-biggest-corruption.

OECD. (2003). DAC Guidelines and Reference Series. Harmonising donor practices for effective aid delivery. https://www.oecd-ilibrary.org/docserver/9789264199835-en.pdf?expires=1565683135&id=id&accname=guest&checksum=2a21f7ffdf29f165f 44d64ce631c50b2.

Oxfam. (2013). Why health insurance schemes are leaving the poor behind. https://policy-pract ice.oxfam.org/resources/universal-health-coverage-why-health-insurance-schemes-are-leaving-the-poor-beh-302973/.

Pan American Health Organization. (2019). Universal health in the 21st century: 40 years of Alma-Ata. Report of the High-Level Commission. Washington, D.C: Pan American Health Organization. http://iris.paho.org/xmlui/bitstream/handle/123456789/50742/ 9789275120682_eng.pdf?sequence=16 (accessed June 28, 2019).

People's Health Movement, Medact, Third World Network, Health Poverty Action, Medico International and ALAMES. (2017). *Global Health Watch 5: An Alternative World Health Report.* Zed Books: London.

People's Health Movement. (2018). Alternative civil society Astana statement on primary health care. https://phmovement.org/alternative-civil-society-astana-declaration-on-primary-hea lth-care/.

Pirlea, A.F., Serajuddin, U., Wadhwa, D., Welch, M. & Whitby, A. (eds). (2020). *Atlas of the Sustainable Development Goals 2020: From World Development Indicators.* World Bank: Washington, DC.

Prince Mahidol Award Conference (PMAC). (2016). Report on the 2016 Conference on Priority Setting for Universal Health Coverage, 26–31 January 2016, Bangkok, Thailand.

Rowden, R. (2008). *Changing IMF Policies to Get More Doctors, Nurses and Teachers Hired in Developing Countries*. Actionaid: London.

Sanders, D., Baum, F., Benos, A. & Legge, D. (2011). Revitalising primary healthcare requires an equitable global economic system—now more than ever. *Epidemiology Community Health*, 65(8):661–665.

Sanders, D., Nandi, S., Labonte, R., Vance, C. & Van Damme, W. (2019). Alma Ata to Astana: From Primary Health Care to Universal Health Coverage–One Step Forward and Two Steps Back. *The Lancet*. 394(10199):619–21. doi: https://doi.org/10.1016/S0140-6736(19)31831-8.

Sanders, D., Schaay, N. & Mohamed, S. (2009). Primary Health Care. In: Carrin, G., Buse, K., Heggenhougen, K. & Quah, S.R. (eds). *Health Systems Policy, Finance and Organization*, Chapter 2:284–295. Elsevier: Amsterdam.

Schuftan, C. (1990). The child survival revolution: a critique. *Family Practice*, 7(4):329.

Tayler, L. & Dickinson, C. (2006). The link between corruption and HIV/AIDS. *IAPAC Monthly*, 12(2):37–39.

Unger, J.P., De Paepe, P., Buitrón, R. & Soors, W. (2008). Costa Rica: achievements of a heterodox health policy. *American Journal of Public Health*, 98(4):636–643.

United Nations (UN) Human Rights Office of the High Commissioner (2000). Millennium Declaration. https://www.ohchr.org/en/instruments-mechanisms/instruments/united-nations-millennium-declaration.

UN. (2000). ICESCR General Comment 14, 11 August 2000, E/C.12/2000/4. UN: Geneva.

UN. (2005). UN Millennium Development Goals report. https://unstats.un.org/unsd/mi/pdf/mdg%20book.pdf.

United Nations. (2008). https://dam.media.un.org/package/2am9lot_4#/searchresult&vbid=2am94sgd3q62&pn=7&ws=searchresults; UN7644103.

UNDP. (2019). *Transforming Our World: The 2030 Agenda for Sustainable Development*. United Nations Development Programme: New York.

UNICEF. (1982a). *The State of the World's Children 1982–83*. Oxford University Press: New York.

UNICEF. (1982b). *The State of the World's Children 1984*. Oxford University Press: Oxford.

UNICEF. (2021). *Subnational Under-Five Mortality Estimates, 1990–2019: Estimates Developed by the United Nations Inter-Agency Group for Child Mortality Estimation*. UNICEF: New York.

Vuori, H. (1986). Health for all, primary health care and the general practitioners. *J R Coll Gen Pract*. 36(290):398–402.

Walford, V. (2003). *Defining and Evaluation SWAps: A Paper for the Inter-Agency Group on SWAps and Development Cooperation*. Institute for Health Sector Development (UK): London.

Walsh, J.A. & Warren, K.S. (1979). Selective Primary Health Care: an interim strategy for disease control in developing countries. *New England Journal of Medicine*, 301(18):967–974.

Whitehead, M., Dahlgren, G. & Evans, T. (2001). Equity and health sector reforms: can low income countries escape the medical poverty trap? *The Lancet*, 358:833–836.

WHO. (1946). Constitution of the World Health Organization. https://apps.who.int/gb/bd/pdf_files/BD_49th-en.pdf#page=6.

WHO Commission on Macroeconomics and Health. (2003). *Investing in health: a summary of the findings of the Commission on Macroeconomics and Health*. WHO: Geneva.

WHO. (2007). Civil society report. Commission on Social Determinants of Health. https://www.ghwatch.org/sites/www.ghwatch.org/files/Civil%20Society%20Alternative%20Report%20SDH.pdf.

WHO. (2008a). *Closing the Gap in a Generation: Health Equity Through Action on the Social Determinants of Health—Final Report of the Commission on the Social Determinants of Health*. WHO: Geneva.

WHO. (2008b). WHO and World Bank join forces for better results from global health investments. https://www.who.int/news/item/05-08-2008-who-and-world-bank-join-forces-for-better-results-from-global-health-investments.

WHO. (2010). Experience with supporting pharmaceutical policies and systems in Kenya. Progress, lessons and the role of WHO. https://www.who.int/medicines/publications/who_emp_mpc_2010_2.pdf?ua=1.

WHO. (2020). Thirteenth General Programme of Work (GPW13): methods for impact measurement. https://www.who.int/publications/m/item/thirteenth-general-programme-of-work-(gpw13)-methods-for-impact-measurement.

WHO & UNICEF. (2018). Declaration of Astana. Global Conference on Primary Health Care, Astana, Kazakhstan, 25–26 October 2018. https://www.who.int/docs/default-source/primary-health/declaration/gcphc-declaration.pdf.

Wisner, B. (1988). Gobi versus PHC? Some dangers of selective primary health care. *Science Direct. Social Science & Medicine*, 26(9):963–969.

Wong, Y.S., Allotey, P. & Redipath, D.D. (2016). Sustainable development goals, universal health coverage and equity in health systems: the Orang Asli commons approach. *Global Health, Epidemiology and Genomics*, 1:e12.

World Bank. (1993). *World Development Report 1993. Investing in Health*. World Bank: Washington, DC, and Oxford University Press: Oxford.

6

The Commercialisation of Health Care
Medicine, Business and the State

Chapter 3 looked at the reasons for the widening inequality between people who are rich and those who are poor, between and within both the underdeveloped and developed world, and the resulting inequitable distribution of the resources necessary to promote health. Chapter 4 showed that the medical contribution does little to change the effects of the social conditions on the health of most people. Chapter 5 explored how in the latter part of the twentieth century, in the context of neoliberal globalisation, health care became increasingly privatised and commercialised, as well as civil society's struggle against this (see Figure 6.1). This shift was accompanied by changes in the global funding architecture, which saw the rise of a plethora of global public–private partnerships (including philanthropic private foundations), all of which channelled aid—and influence—into underdeveloped countries. This raises certain questions in relation to the commercial determinants of health which we will unpack in this chapter:

- Why are health services inappropriate in nature and inequitably distributed?
- What role have the health professions played in creating and maintaining this set-up?
- What role have big business and the State played in producing and maintaining such health inequities?

The role played by the health professions

Many of the fundamental characteristics of today's medical profession in developed and underdeveloped countries can be traced to the period of the Industrial Revolution in Britain, when the capitalist system became dominant and created an impoverished and urbanised working class. For this reason, it is once again important to discuss how this history laid the foundations upon which the medical profession developed, especially in those countries with a colonial link.

History: status, craft and trade

The medical profession in Britain originated as one of the 'status occupations' of the leisured gentry. Physicians (or doctors) possessed no specialised knowledge or skills, but derived their position from title and tradition, supported by inherited wealth

The Struggle for Health. David Sanders with Wim De Ceukelaire and Barbara Hutton, Oxford University Press.
© Oxford University Press 2023. DOI: 10.1093/oso/9780192858450.003.0006

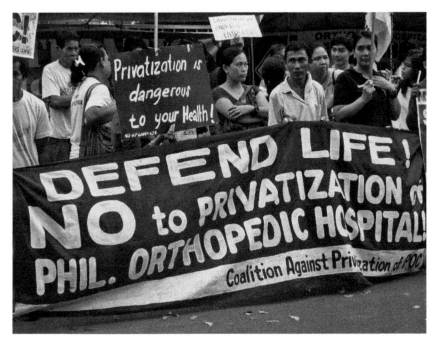

Fig. 6.1 Viva Salud (formerly Third World Health Aid [TWHA]) protest against privatisation of health care, the Philippines.
Source: Wim De Ceukelaire—Viva Salud.

(Robson, n.d.). Their theoretical training was restricted largely to the works of the ancient Roman physician Galen. Doctors were not taught practical experimentation and they rarely saw patients. When confronted with a sick person, physicians resorted largely to superstition and quasi-religious rituals (Ehrenreich & English, n.d.). In 1518, the Crown recognised the first professional body—the Royal College of Physicians.

Surgeons, on the other hand, were condemned by the Church because of their blood-spilling, and in 1540 they formed an alliance with barbers in a barber-surgeon's guild. For centuries, barbers were seen as both grooming and medical specialists. They handled sharp instruments like scissors and razors and were allowed to practise minor surgeries like tooth extraction and bloodletting—the withdrawal of blood from patients was thought to cure or prevent illness and disease. From the sixteenth to the eighteenth century, it was barber-surgeons, and not doctors who were responsible for conducting surgical operations and even amputations. It was not until 1880 that the Crown recognised the Royal College of Surgeons.

Apothecaries (who sold medicines and potions) were considered by both physicians and surgeons to have a much lower social status. Up until 1815, they were not allowed to charge for their medical advice or their potions.

Thus, the medical profession that emerged under capitalism in the twentieth century grew out of three groupings: the physicians from the 'status occupations'; the surgeons from the craftsmen; and the apothecaries from the tradesmen.

The history of women in health care

Up until the eighteenth century, most practising physicians, surgeons and apothecaries were men. In 1859, the first woman graduated with a degree in medicine and was placed on the *Medical Register*; in 1865, the first woman was licensed as an apothecary; and in 1886, the first woman surgeon was approved and placed on the *Medical Register*.

Women had been involved in health care from early times, but mainly assumed the role of midwives, nurses and lay healers. In contrast to doctors, they practised especially among the peasant classes. They discovered and administered herbal remedies that are still important today, such as ergot for labour pains, belladonna to inhibit uterine contractions during threatened miscarriage, and digitalis for treating heart ailments (Ehrenreich & English, n.d.).

These 'wise women' as they were called by the people they served believed in trial and error and cause and effect. They relied on their intuition rather than doctrine or faith. Their methods and results consequently posed a great threat to the Church and to the emerging medical profession, which early on ensured their exclusion from the universities. Up until the eighteenth century, they were legally barred from surgical practice and from using surgical instruments. Despite this, the great majority of female healers remained in practice.

In the seventeenth and eighteenth centuries, the non-professional barber-surgeons led the assault on the last sphere of activity reserved for female healing—midwifery. The barber-surgeons claimed to be technically superior to midwives based on their use of obstetrical forceps during delivery—classed as a surgical instrument (see Figure 6.2). So began the rapid transformation of the neighbourly midwifery tradition into lucrative obstetrics, a business that physicians or doctors began to enter from the eighteenth century onwards.

In the middle of the nineteenth century, nursing was the only remaining occupation for women in health care. Prior to this, nursing was generally undertaken in the Church or in patients' homes. Most nurses did not have any formal training but were women who happened to be nursing someone—usually a sick relative (Ehrenreich & English, n.d.).

In 1834, the UK Poor Law was enacted to reduce the government's cost of looking after people living in poverty by placing them in workhouses (poorhouses) where they could live and work. Infirmaries were set up in the workhouses to provide care for older people, and sick and dying people who were poor. Conditions in these institutions were generally harsh, unclean and squalid and it was estimated that 10% of those admitted to the workhouse died afterwards (see Figure 6.3). By 1866, there were 53 nurses employed in 11 such workhouses in different urban areas.

To be acceptable to doctors and women of 'good character', nursing had to be reformed. Florence Nightingale, with her team of sober, disciplined, middle-aged Victorian women in the battle-front hospitals of the Crimean War, led the movement (see Figure 6.4). She was followed by Dorothea Dix in the USA in the military hospitals set up during the American Civil War (1861–1865). This nursing pursuit was thought to be 'natural' and acceptable for women of their (upper) class.

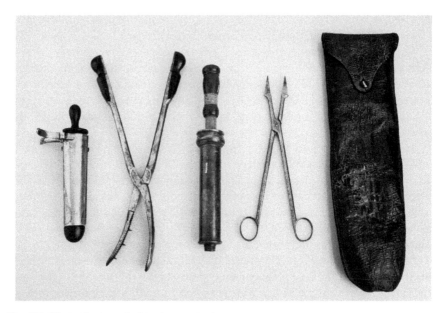

Fig. 6.2 Obstetrical surgical instrument set.
Source: Science Museum, London. Wellcome Collection.
https://wellcomecollection.org/works/rrcnb8da.

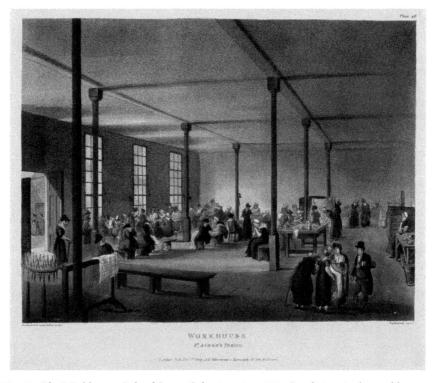

Fig. 6.3 The Workhouse, Poland Street, Soho: interior, 1809. Conditions in the workhouses were deliberately harsh, with some people describing them as 'prisons for the poor'.
Source: T. Sunderland after A.C. Pugin and T. Rowlandson, 1809. Credit: Wellcome Collection.

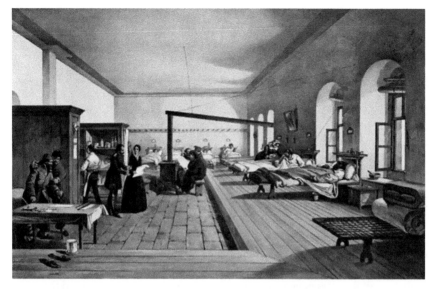

Fig. 6.4 Florence Nightingale assessing a ward at the military hospital in Scutari, *c*. 1856.
Source: E. Walker after W. Simpson. Wellcome Library, London. The National Archives.
https://www.nationalarchives.gov.uk/education/resources/florence-nightingale/source-1/.

Overall, in the mid- to late nineteenth century, nursing was largely low-paid, heavy-duty housework and began attracting fewer upper-class women. However, until recently, the teaching of upper-class graces was integral to nursing training. Nightingale further reinforced the prevailing attitudes in society towards women in general, and the position of nurses in particular, and confirmed the dominance of the male medical profession by reinforcing women's subservient role.

When some English nurses proposed that nursing be modelled on the medical profession with examinations and licensing, *Nightingale* responded that "*nurses cannot be registered and examined any more than mothers.*" She also said of the few female doctors of her time: "*They have only tried to be men, and they have succeeded only in being third-rate men*" (Ehrenreich & English, n.d.). Indeed, in the late nineteenth century, as the number of nursing students rose, the number of female medical students started to decline. Women had been prescribed their role in the health care system!

The evolution of the modern doctor

Many of the fundamental characteristics of today's medical profession can be traced to the period of the Industrial Revolution when the capitalist system became dominant and created an impoverished and urbanised working and middle class. Those doctors who had no private or inherited wealth were now forced to seek payment for their services among these people.

Doctors also found it necessary to unify to preserve their privilege and status. In 1834 they formed a collective organisation called the British Medical Association

(BMA). Initially this body represented doctors who provided services to people who were poor, under the UK 1834 Poor Law. The BMA represented the profession's views of the Poor Law, complaining that what workhouse doctors were paid was "*as insulting and degrading to the character of the medical profession as [it was] unjust and injurious to the poor*" (People's History of the NHS, People's Encyclopedia, n.d.).

The BMA played a key role in drafting and passing the Medical Act of 1858, which unified the factional medical groups and is seen as marking the beginning of the modern period of the medical profession in the UK. The aim of this Act was to regulate the qualification and registration of doctors, and university examinations replaced personal patronage as the qualification for membership of the medical profession. The General Medical Council (GMC) was set up to oversee the supervision of all educational and licensing bodies. Members of the GMC were drawn from government, universities and the medical profession, and this formally linked medicine with the State (Robson, n.d.).

Through the BMA and GMC, a 'code of practice' was formulated and activities that might be detrimental to the profession as a whole were legislated against, such as advertising and 'patient snatching'. Despite these controls, doctors continued to minister largely to working class people and so remained poor themselves. Around the turn of the twentieth century, a character in Bernard Shaw's play, *The Doctor's Dilemma*, sums up the situation perfectly:

> *When you are so poor that you cannot refuse eighteen pence from a man who is too poor to pay you any more, it is useless to tell him that what he and his sick child needs is not medicine but more leisure, better food and a better drained and ventilated house. It is kinder to give him a bottle of something almost as cheap as water and tell him to come again with another eighteen pence if it does not cure him. When you have done this over and over again every day for a week, how much scientific conscience have you got left?*

Perhaps a better example than the protracted British Industrial Revolution (1760–1840) is the French Revolution of 1789, when all areas of society, including medical institutions, came under close scrutiny. Two important ideas were born during this period: first, that health care was a function of the State; and second, that social change could eradicate disease and return humanity to a state of original health (Robson, n.d.). For a while, Faculties of Medicine were closed and doctors' societies and associations abolished—all doctors were to be employed by the State. Sickness was to be dealt with at home with state-administered public assistance. In fact, the first task of the doctor was seen as a political one: the struggle against disease was to be a fight against bad government. In the words of one French revolutionary:

> *Who then should denounce tyrants to [human]kind if not the doctors who make [humans] their sole study and who each day in the homes of poor and rich, among ordinary citizens and among the highest in the land, in cottage and mansion, contemplates the human miseries that have no other origin but tyranny and slavery?* (Robson, n.d.).

However, these ideals—and many others—did not materialise. Throughout Europe the medical profession developed and strengthened—a profession that still today insists on the *separation* of 'medicine' and 'politics', and which in its practice and education promotes this belief. The main causes of this reversal did not lie solely in the area of medicine. All kinds of **libertarian** ideals thrown up in the popular struggles that swept Europe in this revolutionary period soon became dreams of the past, as the previous ruling class of feudal lords and monarchs was replaced by the capitalists.

The most important way in which the new system of capitalism differed from pre-capitalist societies was in the area of production. Because of the Industrial Revolution, all kinds of goods and commodities necessary for a reasonable standard of living could now be produced on a large and much more efficient scale in factories and on farms. However, the means whereby these commodities were produced were owned by a very few people. The competitive nature of capitalism further heightened this and eventually resulted in today's monopoly ownership. In practice, therefore, ideals like 'Liberty, Equality and Fraternity', born in the overthrow of the old feudal order, inevitably failed because of new class division and inequalities between the wealthy class who owned the **means of production** and the impoverished and urbanised working class whose only source of wealth was its labour.

GLOSSARY

Libertarian: a political philosophy and movement that upholds liberty, i.e. being free from control or oppressive restrictions imposed by authority, as a core principle.

Means of production: everything that is needed and used to produce goods and commodities, e.g. factories, equipment, materials.

Health care as a commodity

Doctors had already secured a privileged position by forming an alliance with the wealthy and powerful who had helped them in the early nineteenth century to defeat competition from healers, such as women nurses and midwives. But with the emergence of capitalism, status was no longer enough. To survive, it was necessary to possess a commodity that both satisfied a human need or want *and* could be exchanged for money. The new capitalists had their products and workers had their commodity—their capacity for labour. Doctors too needed a commodity.

By the nineteenth century, it was possible for doctors to gain a greater understanding of the body's structure and function—anatomy, physiology and pathology—through the observation of corpses and ill patients. The invention of the microscope, one of the most advanced pieces of nineteenth-century technology, gave birth to microbiology, which in turn gave rise to the **germ theory of disease** (Robson, n.d.). For the first time in history, a rational basis for disease prevention and cure was established (Ehrenreich & English, n.d.). These advances were timely, as they constituted for doctors a body of knowledge which they appropriated for themselves and which became the basis for their commodity—modern health care (Segall, 1976).

GLOSSARY

Germ theory of disease: the accepted scientific theory that micro-organisms or 'germs', which are too small to see without magnification, invade humans, other animals and other living hosts and can lead to disease.

Doctors, through the BMA, had already played an important role in ensuring the passage of the Medical Act of 1858, which drew a line between qualified and unqualified practitioners and which created the GMC for professional regulation. They now consolidated their monopoly ownership of the commodity of health care by establishing and controlling professional associations, colleges and hospitals. Doctors now determined the entry, training, numbers and employment of graduates. In short, they controlled the production of their commodity. Similarly, they increasingly controlled its character and distribution.

But why did health care become so inappropriate in character and inequitable in distribution? Is it because doctors—and other health workers whom they dominate—are innately insensitive?

. When capitalism spread internationally, the 'capturing' of most of the world's population was not because the imperialists were particularly inherently malicious, but because they were merely obeying a law of the capitalist economic system: the result was the brutal exploitation of the colonised. By the same token, although some doctors and other health workers are often insensitive, their actions can only be understood as a result of the commodity-nature of health care within the context of capitalism.

Why has health care become so inappropriate?

Under capitalism, all production is geared to the production of commodities to be sold for the highest price possible. The business owner is not concerned about the usefulness of the product, but rather about the financial gain to be realised from its sale. Many expensive commodities may have little social utility. This applies also to health care as presently practised globally, which is largely inappropriate to health needs and does not cope with the health problems of the vast majority.

The germ theory of disease and advances in medical science in the nineteenth and twentieth centuries created the basis for what is termed the '**biomedical approach**' to health and illness. This approach persists today, where a patient is regarded as a set of systems, one or more of which go wrong in illness, and which health workers attempt to put right with drugs and advanced technology. The biomedical approach has further entrenched health care as a commodity that can be sold in the market and that can become a profitable business.

However, we know that most disease and illness in the developed and underdeveloped world has its origins in social conditions. This information is widely available. Indeed, some of it is even taught—albeit in abstract ways—in medical schools. But even **social medicine** does not attempt to dissect the social roots of the physical and psychological 'illnesses' of current-day society.

GLOSSARY

Biomedical approach: assumes that the causes of disease and illness are wholly physical and biological in nature—that they occur when there is a deviation from the norm of measurable biological variables.

Social medicine: based on an understanding that human health and disease are affected by social and biological factors; also incorporates preventive medicine.

As an example, it is accepted that tobacco use is one of the leading causes of preventable and premature death worldwide, from different cancers and cardiovascular and lung disease (Cahn et al., 2018). However, few doctors question why smoking has become such a widespread habit with such a marked social-class distribution (see Figure 6.5).

According to the advocacy organisation Campaign for Tobacco-Free Kids (2020):

- Approximately 19.2% of adults (more than 1 billion) worldwide are tobacco users—32.7% males and 5.8% females. Approximately 24 million youth between 13 and 15 years old smoke and 13 million use smokeless tobacco products.
- More than 80% of the world's adult tobacco users live in low- and middle-income countries.
- While tobacco use is declining globally, there are slower declines in low- and middle-income countries—this is due to population growth and the tobacco industry specifically targeting these markets.

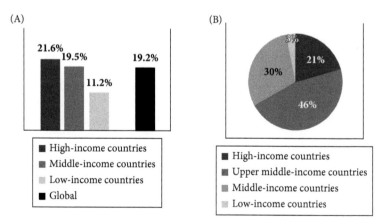

Fig. 6.5 A) Global adult smoking prevalence by country income level.
B) Global deaths from tobacco by country income level.
Source: Tobacco-Free Kids. (2020).

- In all countries, tobacco use is concentrated among the poor and less-educated groups, intensifying poverty by increasing health care costs and diverting family resources away from basic needs like food, shelter and education.
- Tobacco-related illnesses account for over 8 million global deaths annually. By 2030, it is estimated that 80% of these deaths will be in low- and middle-income countries (WHO, 2019a).

It is widely and increasingly acknowledged that living and working conditions and the social organisation of societies underlie such global 'epidemics' as tobacco use. However, this awareness is *in practice* negated by the concentration on a high-tech, individual-oriented, after-the-event curative medical approach. The half-understood lessons of social medicine and **epidemiology** are largely ignored.

GLOSSARY

Epidemiology: *"the study of how often diseases occur in different groups of people and why"* (Stewart, 2016).

The inappropriateness of this approach is even starker in underdeveloped countries where the social origins of disease are so obvious. This is because the fundamental causes of ill-health are out of the control of doctors. Indeed, any open recognition of the real causes would call into question the very system that allows doctors to own and market their commodity. In short, it is not in the interests of the medical profession to examine, and still less to confront, the fundamental social roots of illness.

It is not only this overwhelmingly important area of health promotion that is minimised and ignored. The medical contribution itself has been distorted in accordance with the demands of the market. Cure has become overdeveloped at the expense of care and prevention. Certain conditions susceptible to cure are highly researched and resourced. This is especially the case with those conditions that disproportionately affect people who are wealthy and powerful.

The anomalies inherent in this 'free market' system are particularly clear in the fields of acute medicine and surgery, especially in countries where the market is 'freeest'. For example, the disease pattern in various European countries and the USA is similar, yet the probability of a person in the USA undergoing surgery is much higher than in Europe. As an example: in a 12-year retrospective cohort study of primary care electronic records (2005–2016), it was found that tonsillectomy is the most common surgical procedure in children, with childhood tonsillectomy rates in Belgium, Finland and Norway being twice the UK rate; and the rates in the USA being three times higher than in the UK (Šumilo et al., 2018).

Heart disease is one of the top 10 causes of death in both developed and underdeveloped countries. Since the 1960s, intensive coronary care units (CCUs) have been developed in most hospitals to improve treatment of these cases. They are invariably expensively equipped and better staffed than other hospital facilities. The first critical assessment of the efficacy of this super-technological intervention was published in 1976. Although it found that patients kept at home had a slightly *higher* survival rate than those treated in intensive CCUs (Mather et al., 1976), the latter continue to be built!

At the same time, government spending on public services has been cut back. The caring services for older adults, people living with disabilities and those who are chronically sick are becoming increasingly inadequate. Waiting lists for many beneficial but not dramatically life-saving surgical operations, like hip replacement and gynaecological operations, have increased enormously. This has mainly affected working people who cannot afford to go 'privately'.

Victim blaming

The biomedical approach and the focus on the individual explains the obsession of modern medical science with 'lifestyle factors'. Those health care professionals who in the past advocated the most costly, sophisticated curative techniques are now advocating that if individuals take appropriate action, if they avoid unhealthy behaviour, then they may prevent most diseases produced by social conditions. Lifestyle and environmental factors are combined, and the message is that individuals are the primary agents in shaping or modifying the effects of their environment. It is implied that little can be done about the living and working conditions of modern industrial technological society, but we can do much for ourselves as individuals (Crawford, 1997). This is reminiscent of earlier attitudes to disease sufferers and all-too-prevalent attitudes towards people who are poor and ill in underdeveloped countries.

Attributing people's vulnerability to diseases to their failing to adopt healthy lifestyles is an example of 'victim blaming', because in reality people's vulnerability is determined to a large extent by their social class.

The hollowness of blaming people's vulnerability to diseases for failing to adopt healthy lifestyles is best demonstrated by a consideration of occupational disease. In the USA, in 2016, nearly 3.7 million workers across all industries had work-related injuries and illnesses. These figures are generally underreported and it is believed that the true estimate is two or three times higher. It is estimated that 50 000–60 000 workers die from occupational diseases each year and this does not include those who die from chronic occupational diseases that are not detected for years after workers are exposed to toxic chemicals (American Federation of Labor and Congress of Industrial Organizations [AFL-CIO], 2018). According to the ideology of adopting healthy lifestyles, these statistics are explained not by the hazards of the job, the speed of work required, the pollution of working environments, exposure to toxic chemicals or the danger of machinery, but by the lack of sufficient caution by the workers themselves, or even by their 'genetic susceptibilities'!

The unhealthy addictive habits of tobacco use and alcohol consumption are approached in a similar way. Health education attempts to persuade people to adopt healthier lifestyles. Yet neither the social stresses nor marketing and advertising pressures that induce the habits are effectively confronted.

The same 'victim blaming' argument is used in relation to the underdeveloped world's 'problems' of high population growth (solution: 'family planning') and undernutrition (solution: 'health education')—rather than tackling underdevelopment.

So, most people accept the proposition that illness caused by social conditions can and should be *individually* solved by *'professional'* medical interventions or *individual* preventive action. Consequently, any thoughts of a collective assault on the roots of illness—which are social—are undermined. This is one of the important ways in which the medical profession serves the interests of those in power and strengthens the status quo.

> *A strong ethos of **individualism** is likely to lead to victim blaming assumptions (Crawford, 1977). Such an attitude is obvious in the following comment by an Australian federal health minister, Tony Abbott (2005) on a television program on childhood obesity:*
>
> *'No-one is in charge of what goes into my mouth except me. No-one is in charge of what goes into kid's mouths except their parents. It is up to parents more than anyone else to take this matter in hand … if their parents are foolish enough to feed their kids on a diet of Coca Cola and lollies well they should lift their game and lift it urgently.' …)*
>
> *Tesh (1988) points out that the very research questions we ask are shaped by core values. Thus a focus on individualism would lead to questions about why individuals are overweight and explore their motivations, while a more collective ideology would explore questions about why it is that obesity levels in all high income countries have increased in the past decade and consider what features of the society have encouraged this (Baum, 2002).*

GLOSSARY

Individualism: to place the responsibility (and blame) for problems or conditions with the individual rather than with the structures that may influence or shape behaviour and experience.

Medicalisation and disease mongering

Modern medical science has not reduced the number of people who tend to get sick. To the contrary, there is little incentive to reduce the burden of disease, because more sick people means that the market for diagnostic and therapeutic interventions increases. In fact, the biomedical model with its focus on individual behaviour and its promotion of the role of medical professionals tends to **medicalise** common human problems, turning them into medical problems in an attempt to expand markets for treatment and new products. This is called **disease mongering**.

GLOSSARY

Medicalise: treating a natural human condition as if it were a medical condition that needs intervention.

Disease mongering: turning ordinary conditions into medical problems, seeing mild symptoms as serious, treating personal problems as medical and seeing risks as diseases, in order to expand markets for treatment and new products.

There's a lot of money to be made from telling healthy people they're sick. Some forms of medicalizing ordinary life may now be better described as disease mongering: widening the boundaries of treatable illness in order to expand markets for those who sell and deliver treatments. Pharmaceutical companies are actively involved in sponsoring the definition of diseases and promoting them to both prescribers and consumers. The social construction of illness is being replaced by the corporate construction of disease (Moynihan et al., 2002).

Doctors and pharmaceutical manufacturers, for example, have medicalised the natural process of menopause, which occurs in midlife and older women, claiming that it is a hormonal deficiency condition and that it places women at higher risk of heart disease, osteoporosis and Alzheimer's disease (Meyer, 2001). As a preventive measure they urge women going through menopause to take long-term hormonal replacement therapy, despite the associated increased risks of breast cancer and stroke. Another example is how the media have been used by doctors and the pharmaceutical industry to reframe irritable bowel syndrome—what for most people is a mild functional disorder—as a widespread and serious disease. Of course, there are many people with irritable bowel syndrome who are severely disabled by their symptoms, but the arrival of new drugs has seen manufacturers seek to change the way the world thinks about this ordinary condition. The effect is to shift the focus *"toward medical and technical solutions, neglecting necessary social, community, or political action"* (Clark, 2014).

Why has health care become so inequitably distributed?

Ever since products or commodities first began to be exchanged, there has had to be a common, socially acceptable measure of their value, something that establishes an equivalence between items with different uses and characteristics. This measure is roughly set by the amount of labour—mental and physical—that is spent producing the commodity. A manufactured product acquires its value from a combination of labour time needed to produce it and the previous labour time embodied in the capital goods that are used, such as machinery, equipment, tools, vehicles and other physical resources.

In the case of health care, this includes the labour expended by the student, the skilled labour performed by the teachers, and the labour embodied in the various commodities consumed in the process of training (Segall, 1976). When health care became a commodity, there was therefore an incentive for the producers and owners—the doctors—to obtain as long and as complex an education as possible to *raise the value of the commodity*.

Several years are spent on university training and compulsory internship, culminating in producing a 'jack of all trades'. But, before this highly educated graduate can actually provide even a primary care service proficiently, several further years of experience and often specialist training are needed. The effect of such an educational system is to increase the value of the doctors' commodity and allow them a wide choice of specialisation whereby their earning power can be further increased. However, the useful skills that doctors eventually acquire can be learned in a much shorter time and far less expensively.

The usual arguments for this 'professional' training cite the necessity of preserving 'standards of excellence' and 'equipping doctors with the education necessary to enable them to make the weighty decisions demanded of them'.

However, these assertions are unrealistic. Most doctors, because of their class backgrounds, will have had a different social experience from most of the population. Partly for this reason, but more importantly because of the inappropriate approach to health care already discussed, they may find it a challenge to approach health problems sensitively and realistically. Similarly, they are often unable to plan services that cater for the real health needs of most people. Doctors want to *market* their commodity profitably. Therefore, those in private practice in developed countries will work predominantly in those localities that house people who are rich and will perform the sort of care—mostly high-technology cure—that can be easily sold to buyers who can afford it. *In underdeveloped countries this means that doctors are concentrated in the towns and offer a service both inappropriate to and inaccessible to most people.*

Many doctors who work in the public sector tend to want to work in richer and more urban localities, in the most technologically sophisticated and advanced hospitals where prospects for private practice are greatest and in those specialities that provide the best possibilities for profits. Having said that, however, there are also many health care workers who understand 'service' but in public health care face a mix of gruelling hours and frontline danger, as we have seen for example, with COVID-19. They tend to become so overwhelmed by coping with overloaded services that they end up treating sickness rather than promoting health.

On the whole, however, *because doctors are so dominant in influencing the shape of the health sector, together with people who are wealthy and powerful whose diseases are most susceptible to high-technology individualised care, health services remain both inappropriate and inequitably distributed.*

In summary, doctors have not only appropriated health care as *their* commodity, but have also determined its value. They have achieved this by using various 'feudal-like' guilds. These have ensured the profession's near-monopoly of knowledge about health, allowing *it*—the profession—to pose the main questions about health in terms of *itself*. This prevents *people* learning about and acting confidently on their health problems—although most health care is in fact done by 'unqualified' people.

The other features of professionalism have resulted from the necessity for doctors to regulate the price of their commodity. This has been achieved by the guild mechanisms of controlling competition and monopoly price fixing. Rules about advertising, under-bidding and patient-snatching are examples of this within the profession.

To avoid competition from non-guild health workers, the profession strictly defines what a 'doctor' is and determines all the privileges that go with that. The work of other health workers is then defined in relation to that of doctors—to whom they are subordinated. The scope of their knowledge and skills is regulated and they are categorised as 'para-medical' or 'auxiliary'—to doctors.

These elitist set of norms and self-regulations have come to be accepted as 'natural' both by health workers and by the public. They ensure the continuation of the knowledge monopoly, regulate the supply of the commodity on the market, fix prices in private practice, and enable the medical profession to negotiate with government their terms in any nationalised health service. And this is done not only at a national level by licensing or registration bodies such as the GMC in Britain or the American Medical Association (AMA), but also on an international scale.

Still today, delegations from these registration bodies in developed countries visit medical schools in underdeveloped countries to assess the 'quality' of their medical education and to determine whether their graduates will be competent to practise in the developed world. In other words, the international value of doctors' health care—as with all other commodities—is regulated by the most powerful monopolies.

Speaking to a group of medical professionals at the Mayo Clinic in 1978, economist Milton Friedman argues for 'no licensure of physicians' [by government], because that would help to reduce and eliminate the monopoly power of the American Medical Association. That monopoly power is derived almost entirely from the fact that the practice of medicine is an activity which can be engaged in by only those who have licenses from government. And the control over that licensure procedure is what has enabled the AMA to exercise its monopoly power for these many decades (Worstall, 2017).

Reproduction of the profession

Another way in which the price of the health care commodity is indirectly regulated is through the *selection* of medical students and thus the control of the standard and supply of medical graduates. Most doctors still come from the upper social strata, whether in developed or underdeveloped countries, and thus the social gap between doctor and patient has actually widened.

In Britain, in 2016:

- 80% of students applying to enter medical school came from approximately 20% of schools which were typically selective or fee-paying.

- Only 17.6% of young entrants to medicine, dentistry or veterinary science were from the 'lower' socio-economic groups—the lowest percentage of any subject; and 4.7% of them were from the areas with the lowest levels of historical participation in higher education. Again, this was the lowest of any subject group (Social Mobility Commission, 2016).

This is not unique to developed countries. In underdeveloped countries, students from rural areas in particular are underrepresented in medical schools and face many challenges when compared to those whose parents are urban, wealthy and highly educated.

Once selected, medical students are effectively isolated from the community they will eventually serve, and even from other students, for entry to medical school means virtually exclusive contact with professionals. Consequently, many attitudes, often already present because of socio-economic class, are reinforced by the inappropriate approach to health care that is taught and those teaching it.

Having been socialised in the 'professional approach' to health and health care, medical students are taught a 'professional approach' to patients, who are regarded as passive objects of care. Most training is done in hospitals where patients are either so ill or too intimidated by the hospital environment to be anything but passive. 'Ideal patients' are those who are compliant, submissive, obedient and non-assertive, whereas those who ask too many questions about their illness are often seen as 'troublesome' (Parsons, 1972). An 'interesting' patient is one with a rare, complex and often fatal disease. The average patient living with a common degenerative disease or mental health condition may be disdained.

Given the social gap that we have referred to and the complex socialisation process, it is hardly surprising that class distinctions are seen here too. The interaction between doctor and patient is often described as being:

discriminatory, marginalising, abusive and mirrors social stratifications in society at large ... This experience of discrimination and poor quality care is even more marked for poorer, lower class, caste women and men and is also often mediated by other factors, including ethnicity, religion and language group ... (Govender & Penn-Kekana, 2007).

Gender too plays a specific role in shaping this interface, especially within the context of patriarchal societies, which we will look at in the next section.

In the past, when neither doctors nor patients possessed much knowledge about the causes of and cures for disease, practitioners relied on mystification to maintain their livelihood. However, with the knowledge of disease that is available today, most of which could be quite easily communicated to patients, mystification becomes quite unproductive. It prevents patients, that is all non-medical people, from learning about their own bodies and understanding and dealing with their illnesses, especially when people have no internet access to online medical information.

Doctors are reluctant to offer knowledge for fear of jeopardising their authority and threatening their monopoly hold over health care. Many find it difficult to talk to patients from quite different social backgrounds, who may speak a different language and who often have a different concept of the origin of illness. The problem is considerably magnified when doctors trained in developed countries work in underdeveloped countries.

Inequities in the health care workforce

Gender and the health profession

Global health is delivered by women and led by men (WHO, 2019b).

Chapter 3 showed how underdeveloped countries and even underdeveloped areas in developed countries provide labour for the more developed regions. But in all countries there is an ever-present potential reserve workforce. Women are drawn in and out of employment when needed, not only on a large-scale during times of boom and crisis, but also continually on a small-scale when labour is required for short intervals, such as harvesting or piece-work.

Like all other reserve workforces, because they are often temporary and therefore poorly organised and frequently unskilled, women are poorly paid for working long hours in bad conditions. Additionally, it is women who often face a double burden: working long shifts at work (albeit for low pay) and additional unpaid work in the home—cleaning and cooking, caring for children and nursing older people and sick family members. The common denominator of 'women's work' is low pay for less-skilled work. This is why the earnings of the vast majority of health workers, most of whom are women and immigrants, are so very low.

The composition of the health workforce reflects, in a concentrated form, the hierarchical arrangement of capitalist societies, with **gender** inequalities in the health care system being common in both developed and underdeveloped countries (Keynejad et al., 2018).

GLOSSARY

Gender: *"socially constructed norms that impose and determine roles, relationships and positional power for all people across their lifetime. Gender interacts with sex, the biological and physical characteristics that define women, men and those with intersex identities"* (Global Health 50/50).

According to Boniol et al. (2019), of the 234 million workers in the health and social sector globally in 2013, 70% are women (see Figure 6.6). They provide essential health

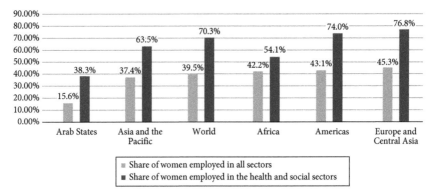

Fig. 6.6 Share of women employed in the health and social sectors compared to share of women employed in all sectors by International Labour Organization (ILO) region, 2013. *Source*: WHO. (2019).

services for approximately 5 billion people and contribute US$3 trillion annually to global health, with half of this being via unpaid care work.

In 2018, the WHO Global Health Workforce Network's Gender Equity Hub (GEH) identified four major gender inequity themes in the global health and social care workforce:

- **Gender pay gap**: on average, the differences in the average hourly wage between men and women across different health professions is 26%–28% higher than the average for other sectors. Several factors are said to account for this, such as different working hours for men and women, different occupations, women being underrepresented in senior positions, and having fewer opportunities for career advancement, and gender discrimination.

  While gender discrimination is more overt and visible in low-income settings where there is limited education and awareness, subtler forms exist at systemic levels in high-income settings (Keynejad et al., 2018). In the UK in 2018, for example, male doctors in the National Health Service (NHS) on average took home £67 788 a year in basic pay, compared to the £57 569 female doctors received—a gender pay gap of 15%. In 2019, the gender pay gap in the NHS had increased, with male doctors earning 17% more than their female peers and they continued to dominate the highest-paid consultants, like surgeons and urologists (*The Independent*, 2019).

- **Occupational gender segregation**: a large portion of the overall gender pay gap is driven by occupational segregation within the sector. In other words, although there are more women in the health sector, the sector is driven by gender norms and stereotypes which define 'men's' and 'women's' work (Boniol et al., 2019). 'Women's' work is typically assigned lower social value, status and pay. The majority of doctors, particularly in the high-tech specialties, are male, White and from the wealthy class, while many other health workers, especially unskilled workers, are female, Black, immigrants, and from the lower-middle or working class. Men are more likely to be employed in occupations in the private sector when there is a wage ceiling in the public sector. For example, 49.2% of men are more frequently employed as physicians or in other highly paid medical occupations in the private sector versus 39.2% of women. However, the opposite is true in the private sector for low-paid health care jobs, such as personal care workers, where 81.8% of women versus 53% of men are more frequently employed (Boniol et al., 2019).

- **Gender parity in leadership**: gender inequality is especially evident in the underrepresentation of women in management, leadership and governance roles in the health sector. In 2020, for example, only 5% of executives in global health organisations are women from low- and middle-income countries (Global Health 50/50) (see Figure 6.7).
- **Decent work free from bias, discrimination and harassment, including sexual harassment**: a large percentage of women in the health workforce, and especially frontline health care workers, face sexual harassment, violence and injury from male colleagues, male patients and members of the community.

Gender inequities remain a barrier to women advancing within the health care profession, despite greater gender awareness and social movements which are challenging gender power relations and policies around gender justice and equality.

The intersectionality of gender and race

GLOSSARY

Intersectionality: "*the interconnected nature of social categorisation such as race, class and gender, regarded as creating overlapping and interdependent systems of discrimination or disadvantage*" (Oxford English Dictionary, 2015).

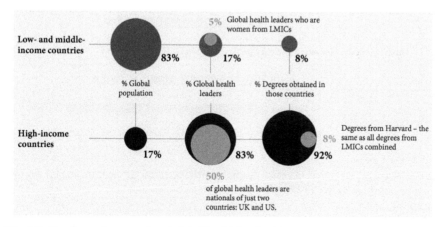

Fig. 6.7 Gender and geography of global health leadership.
Source: Global Health 50/50. (2020).

Class, gender, race, ethnicity, caste, disability, language, age and other identity factors, combined with poverty, determine our vulnerability to illness and disease and our access to health care (Yamin, 2020). The COVID-19 pandemic has exposed the multiple forms of inequalities and the specific health disparities that exist within and between countries, which are aggravated by weak health care systems, structural racism and a crisis of political leadership (Mendehnall, 2020). These factors intersect and put certain groups at high risk—people living in poverty, older adults, Black, Asian and minority ethnic (BAME) communities and key health care workers (the majority of whom we know are women) (*The Lancet*, 2020).

In the USA, for example, the Centers for Disease Control and Prevention (CDC) (Rossen et al., 2020) reported that the average percentage in excess deaths attributable to COVID-19 over an eight-month period (January–September 2020) were in adults aged 25–44 years, with Hispanic, Asian, other/unknown race or ethnicity, Black and American Indian or Alaska Native (AI/AN) being disproportionately affected (see Figure 6.8).

The same racial and ethnic determinants of health that impact disparities in COVID-19 in the general population play themselves out in the health care worker cohort globally. However, risk of infection is heightened among frontline health care workers (and their households)—many of whom are BAME women. An Amnesty International Report (2020) aptly entitled *Exposed, Silenced, Attacked: Failures to Protect Health and Essential Workers During the COVID-19 Pandemic* outlines how by June 2020, more than 230 000 health care workers globally had contracted COVID-19, and that in 79 countries, over 3000 were known to have died from the virus. However, these figures are likely to be a major underestimation because of the underreporting of cases.

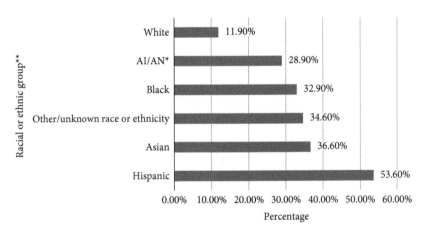

Fig. 6.8 Average percentage in excess deaths by racial or ethnic group from 26 January to 3 October attributable to COVID-19.

* AI/AN: American Indian or Alaska Native (AI/AN) persons.

** Total population: White 61.6%, Black or African American 12.4%, Asian 6%, American Indian and Alaska Native 1.1%, Native Hawaiian and Other Pacific Islander 0.2%, other 8.4%, two or more races 10.2% (2020 est.

Source: Rossen et al. (2020).

By September 2020, the WHO reported that health care workers accounted for one in seven COVID-19 cases globally—14% in most countries, but as high as 35% in some countries (Mellen & Taylor, 2020). Given that health care workers represent less than 3% of the population in most high-income countries and less than 2% in almost all low- and middle-income countries, these figures are disproportionate.

According to Public Health England (2020), 21% of health care workers employed by the NHS are BAME employees. However, they account for 63% of COVID-19-related deaths among the NHS workforce—a much higher proportion than expected. Of the 63%, 36% were Asian (compared to 10% of the workforce) and 27% were Black (compared to 6% of the workforce). More than a third of those who died were in nursing roles (Marsh & McIntyre, 2020).

There are three main causes of racial and ethnic disparities in infection and death during pandemics—disparities in exposure, susceptibility, and access to health care treatment.

- **Disparities in exposure**: this relates to the high-risk nature of the work of health care workers, combined with limited protections, for example, critical shortages of personal protective equipment (PPE). In a study undertaken among 2 135 190 people in the UK and USA, it was noted that frontline health care workers were at much higher risk (at least three times higher) of COVID-19 infection than the general community. This risk was much higher among BAME health care workers who reported that they had inadequate availability of PPE or who had to reuse PPE, and who were more likely to work in inpatient settings and nursing homes with greater exposure to COVID-19 patients (Nguyen et al., 2020).

  In the USA, structural racism in employment is partly a legacy of previous employment laws which protected White workers and disadvantaged racial and ethnic minorities. Although these laws ended in 1968, many racial and ethnic minorities still have limited access to paid sick leave or equal pay, *"forcing them to go to work even when they [are] sick and increasing disparities in their exposure to pandemic viruses, like COVID-19"* (Yearby and Mohapatra, 2020).

- **Disparities in susceptibility**: poor living conditions, housing challenges and other environmental factors (including overcrowded conditions, lack of hand-washing facilities and/or running water, and reliance on public transport), coupled with other pre-existing economic and social inequities, increase the risks associated with contracting an infectious disease. In the USA, for example, two-thirds of home care workers, who provide care to people living at home, are BAME persons. Twenty percent of these workers earn below the national minimum wage, live in substandard housing, do not get paid sick leave, do not have health insurance and work in close contact with patients who are ill or who are most vulnerable to infection (Yearby & Mohapatra, 2020; Rozenfeld et al., 2020).

[In the UK] individuals from BAME groups are more likely to work in occupations with a higher risk of COVID-19 exposure, this includes the health and social care workforce, as well as cleaners, public transport workers, and retail workers. The health and care workforce in England are significantly over-represented by people from BAME groups: 40% of doctors, 20% of nurses, and 17% of social care workforce

are from BAME groups ... Often, BAME workers are in lower paid roles within the NHS, which mean that these roles cannot be done remotely; this leads to greater exposure with other members of the community (Public Health England, 2020).

- **Disparities in treatment**: racial and ethnic disparities and discrimination permeate the health care system in many countries, placing both patients and health care workers at increased risk of illness. Public Health England (2020) reports that discrimination in the workplace based on race or ethnicity is a long-standing issue, and that because of this, during the initial stages of the COVID-19 pandemic in the UK, many BAME health care workers feared raising their concerns about the inadequate supply of PPE (or the supply of substandard PPE) to mitigate the risk of infection.

In summary, because of its narrow class background and its material interest in preserving the status quo, the medical profession retains an unquestioning belief in the values set by the ruling class and institutionalised by the State. Indeed, in the way it relates both to workers and to patients, it reinforces both sexist and racist assumptions. This 'medical consciousness' is transmitted first to other health professionals and then generalised to the population.

The medical profession believes itself to have a monopoly of the knowledge necessary for the health of the people. The two words 'health' and 'medicine' have become virtually interchangeable in the popular consciousness. Thus, people are actively discouraged from seeking non-medical causes—and therefore remedies—for their illnesses.

In short, one of the most important effects of the health care system is to support and reinforce the present arrangement of society. The health professions, under the dominance of doctors, have in large measure determined the nature of health care and the distribution of health care resources.

The role played by big business and the State

There is extensive evidence that the promotion of markets in healthcare leads to an increase in health inequities and inefficiencies. Despite such evidence, globally, privatisation of the health sector is being vigorously promoted. This policy push is a result of the strong influence the private sector wields on health policy-making. Private sector influence has risen exponentially with an increase in large private foundations and public–private partnerships (People's Health Movement et al., 2014).

In general, business interests and their representatives in government have resisted pressure to improve the living and working conditions of the majority and to provide more accessible, high-quality health care services. However, in some situations, business interests have recognised that it is in their interests to support certain reforms and social provisions. The best demonstration of this is the 1911 British National Health Insurance Act, which gave, for the first time, a measure of health care free at the time of use. However, it applied only to working males, while unproductive sectors of the population, such as wives, children and the unemployed were left to fend for themselves.

The Act reflected not just the demands of the people but also the needs of big business, which required a healthy working population for rapidly expanding industries, and also the needs of the State, which required a healthy fighting population for the wars of colonial expansion. It was only medical interests that remained opposed to the Act.

However, medical interests have not, for the most part, been in conflict with the State and business. Indeed, they have helped create the conditions for the continued operation of business interest and have even linked up with business in opposing the struggles of the people for health. *This alliance between medical, business and State interests has existed for a long time, but it has become increasingly prominent over the last few decades.*

As an example of this alliance, we will look at what came to be seen worldwide as a leading model for a public financed (from general taxes), public provided and managed and centrally planned universal health care—the National Health Service (NHS), England.

Privatisation of the public health sector: the British NHS

In Chapter 4, we presented a case study of the establishment of the British NHS in 1948, with its main aims being to ensure universal health coverage, comprehensive provision and health care services free at the point of use. From the late 1940s, spending on health care services (as a percentage of GDP) increased. However, from the mid-1970s until the late 1980s, the funding of social services and prevention and health education fell dramatically, and an unevenness in the financing of specific sectors and geographical regions began to emerge. In this section, we discuss how the British NHS began to change with the introduction of the neoliberal agenda and the increasing privatisation of health care. (See Chapter 4 for more details on the establishment of the NHS.)

Private health insurance schemes
In 1955, just over half a million people in the UK were covered by private health insurance; by 1978 this had grown to nearly 2.5 million people and by 1997 to 7 million. In 2015, approximately 10.5% of the UK population had private health insurance that covered services outside the NHS, as well as those freely available in the NHS (especially specialist services), but for which there are large waiting times for NHS patients.

The growth of private health insurance schemes has depended on tax relief and especially on their access to NHS facilities at low cost, and has created a corresponding increase in part-time private consultants to the NHS. The board members and directors of these schemes are business people and eminent doctors. Many of the latter, and most of the part-time private consultants to the NHS, receive **merit awards** and occupy influential positions in Royal Colleges and on the staff of teaching hospitals. Thus, the already inappropriate development of the health service has been further distorted by the influence of these powerful professionals who help decide siting of medical schools, plan medical training and in the many other ways help to 'socialise' medical students and doctors.

GLOSSARY

Merit award: a monetary award that can be given to a consultant for outstanding professional services. There are different levels, with each having a different monetary amount.

The marketisation and outsourcing of health care
The NHS landscape changed in the 1980s, with the government of Margaret Thatcher introducing a market-based system into health care.

> *The NHS became subject to a particular form of managerialism that in turn led to **marketization** and the introduction of a quasi-market and outsourcing in health-care centred around competition and 'choice'* (Hunter, 2008, cited in People's Health Movement et al., 2014).

GLOSSARY

Marketisation: the introduction of competition into the public sector in areas previously governed through direct public control.

One of the most controversial changes was the policy of outsourcing of services. Initially this was limited to subcontracting cleaning, catering and laundry services. By the 1990s, to open the NHS market forces, health authorities became the purchasers of health care from competing hospitals and other bodies, like ambulance and community health services. This split between 'purchasers' and 'providers', the latter becoming the first NHS trusts, is still in place today. NHS trusts also had to generate their own income so that they could buy services from private companies, such as for financial planning, information technology, for the design and building of hospitals and for their operation and management. By 2000, professional medical services were opened up to the market.

The Health and Social Care Act (HSCA) 2012 further extended these market-based approaches to health care, creating NHS England in 2013 as part of sweeping reforms designed to increase competition and keep the government out of the day-to-day running of the NHS. The number of contracts awarded to private providers increased substantially, making NHS England:

> *a sort of holding company 'franchising' health services out to various public and private providers. Thus, the NHS was to be the government-funded payer, but less and less*

the direct provider of health services. This model enables for-profit companies to siphon money directly from public coffers supposedly set aside for national healthcare (People's Health Movement et al., 2014).

As part of the HSCA, Clinical Commissioning Groups (CCGs), comprising groups of GPs, were established in 2013 to commission health care services for patients in their area, including, for example, mental health services, urgent and emergency care, elective hospital services and community care. They can buy services from different groups and organisations, including, for example, hospitals, community services, GPs and the private sector (such as dentistry, optical care and pharmacy). All the drugs, supplies and equipment used by the NHS are privately provided. NHS England generally commissions specialised health services, military and veteran health services, services for people in prisons and some public health services.

A 2019/2020 NHS Support Federation survey shows that, on average, approximately 15% of CCGs' costs go towards buying health services from non-NHS organisations, including from private companies, not-for-profit companies and charities (Davidson et al., 2020). This does not include their spending on GP surgeries, which are accounted for separately, and many of which are run by private providers. For example, in 2020/2021, a 10-year contract worth £1.06 billion was awarded to the Community Interest Company (CIC) Sirona by the Bristol, North Somerset and South Gloucestershire CCG. The contract covers both adult and children's community health care, as well as many of the public health services that are funded by the local councils.

NOTE ABOUT A COMMUNITY INTEREST COMPANY (CIC)

A CIC is a type of business or social enterprise that is meant to reinvest their profits in their business or in a community, rather than being driven by the need to maximise their profits for shareholders or owners. However, Davidson et al. (2020) report that in the past few years, Sirona has exhibited the same behaviour that "*private companies have been criticised for in the past—Sirona has both asked for more money for contracts and walked away due to a contract being financially unviable.*" It has also failed to assess vulnerable children in its area of work, saying that it needed extra money to do this.

Prior to the COVID-19 pandemic, the NHS was already in crisis as it had failed to keep pace with the increasing need for health care services. By late 2019, there were over 100 000 staff vacancies, including vacancies for 40 000 nurses. The NHS also lacked the equipment it needed to meet the needs of the population it served. For the first time on record, the NHS was missing key targets, including patient waiting times for Accident and Emergency (A&E), cancer care and non-urgent operations.

Then millions of patients had their treatment put on hold in 2020 as the NHS battled COVID-19. In August 2020, it was reported that the NHS would need to buy health care services over the next four years from the private sector, worth up to £10 billion, to bridge the gap in NHS capacity (*The Lowdown*, 2020). The fear is that "*without adequate scrutiny of the deal, the NHS could simply end up bailing out an ailing private sector—to the tune of billions of pounds*" (*The Lowdown*, 2020).

The increasing privatisation of the NHS in England is undermining the core values on which it was founded, i.e. to provide affordable universal health care to all regardless of income or geographical location. In purely economic terms, it is well established that the private sector is a parasite on the NHS. This parasitic nature can be seen in, for example, health worker training. The public sector trains health care workers at great expense for the private sector. The relationship between these sectors is analogous to that in the underdeveloped world between the developed sector of the economy, catering mostly for the external market, and the underdeveloped sector, where the majority lives.

Privatisation of health care globally

The neoliberal agenda and increasing privatisation of health care has impacted public health care systems globally. In India, for example, approximately 1% of GDP is allocated to public health; over 70% of all health care is private; and 84% of the population are not covered under any health scheme (Prasad & Sengupta, 2019). Disinvestment in public health care, ongoing neglect and the steady increase in privatisation through public–private partnerships (PPPs) and insurance models have perpetuated poverty and massive levels of health inequities.

The Indian government's proposed health scheme has two divisions:

- The creation of 150 000 health and wellness centres (HWCs), intended to improve primary health care in the public sector.
- A health insurance model called 'Modicare'—the National Health Protection Scheme (NHPS) which involves state financing and a choice of public or private provisioning.

The concern is that with the current weak public health system, the NHPS will lead to "*further privatization of an already privatized system; further medicalization of health with incumbent costs and further irrationalities in care considering the lack of regulation of the health sector*" (Prasad & Sengupta, 2019), the further inequitable distribution of health care resources and services, and that the basic health needs of the poorest would not be covered.

Indian health care is predicted to reach US$275 billion in the next 10 years. In other words, it is a massive potential industry, with the main 'products' being health care infrastructure, health insurance, medical tourism and drug trials—which the government is ill-equipped to provide or regulate (Prasad & Sengupta, 2019). The private sector is waiting in the wings.

According to the People's Health Movement et al. (2014), the problems with the privatisation of a public health system include:

- **Reduced accountability:** it undermines the state's responsibility for guaranteeing all citizens' access to affordable health care.
- **Fragmentation of services:** the public health system is no longer a comprehensive and universal system but is part of a broader system made up of private health care providers.
- **Increased costs:** the extra bureaucracy, administration, funding arrangements, management and coordination mean extra expenses.
- **Regressive financing:** in the era of austerity, public financing is reduced and more money must come from users themselves.
- **Decreased efficiency:** the private sector tends to increase efficiency by *"maximizing the gap between what they receive for their healthcare efforts [i.e. profit] and what they spend on them"* (People's Health Movement et al., 2014).
- **Decreased quality:** medical care may be compromised because of the conflict of interest between the profit motive of companies and the professional medical ethics of staff.
- **Increased inequity:** health equity is undermined because not all services are free at the point of use.
- **Weaker public health system:** the health care system is less able to provide preventive and promotive services and cannot address the social determinants of health.

Global neoliberal policies influence important policy decisions in ways that may perpetuate the suffering of the poorest sections of our societies. Nowhere is this more obvious than in the trade of and access to medicines.

Big Pharma (the 10 largest drug companies)

. . . under-medication remains an appalling problem in many parts of the world, while over-medication threatens others. Are these two world health crises related? In symbolic terms—like the contrast between obesity and emaciation from starvation—they clearly are. Beyond this, one may well conclude that excessive demand for medicines in richer countries perpetuates the growth of a global medicinal drug production system that by its nature neglects medical need where people cannot pay (People's Health Movement et al., 2014).

The trillion-dollar global pharmaceutical industry has had one of the greatest impacts on health services among business health interests throughout the world. Controlled by a small number of multinational corporations, which are among the most profitable in the world, this industry decides which drugs to research and develop, which to market and distribute and how to set drug prices.

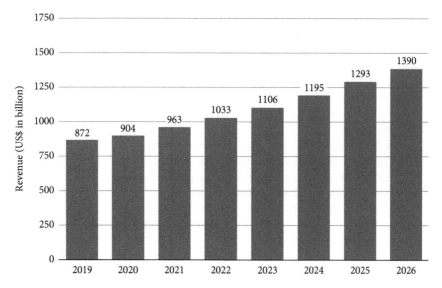

Fig. 6.9 Projected worldwide total prescription drug revenue, 2019–2026 (in US$ billion).
Source: Guttman. (2020). Statista.

Figure 6.9 shows the projected total global expenditure on prescription drugs from 2019 to 2026 (Guttmann, 2020). In 2020, global expenditure was expected to generate US$904 billion, increasing to US$1390 trillion in 2026. Table 6.1 shows the top 10 pharmaceutical companies (Big Pharma) in 2020 by total amount of revenue generated by the sale of goods.

Table 6.1 Top 10 global pharma companies, 2020, by revenue (US$ in billions)

Company	Revenue
Johnson & Johnson	82.6 billion
Roche	58.3
Novartis (Switzerland)	49.9
Merck	48
AbbVie (USA)	45.8
Bristol-Myers Squibb	42.5
Sanofi (France)	42.3
Pfizer (USA)	41.9
GlaxoSmithKline	34
AstaZeneca	26.6

Becker's Hospital Review. (2021).
https://www.beckershospitalreview.com/pharmacy/top-10-pharma-companies-by-revenue-in-2020.html.

The price of drugs: R&D or marketing?

Pharmaceutical companies claim that drug prices are so high because they need to recover the costs of research and development (R&D). However, most of these companies spend more of their budgets on marketing. On average, pharmaceutical companies spend approximately 17% of their revenue on R&D (Parrish, 2020). Ninety percent of the R&D budget is directed at pharmaceuticals for lucrative markets, for example, Viagra, anti-aging treatments, anti-depressants and tranquillisers (Lee & Collin, 2005). Investment in life-saving medications needed by underdeveloped countries is limited to the remaining 10% of their R&D budget (Kerry & Lee, 2007). However, even with major R&D spending, pharmaceutical companies remain highly profitable (Sherman, 2019). In addition, in countries like the USA, they can take advantage of federal and state R&D tax credits.

Interestingly, much of the R&D undertaken by pharmaceutical companies—including most R&D of the COVID-19 drugs and vaccines—have received significant amounts of public funding (Vieira & Moon, 2019; Dearden, 2020). Research into the development of 26 drugs or drug classes that were defined as **transformative** and granted approval by the US Food and Drug Administration (FDA) between 1984 and 2009 found that:

- Most of these drugs or drug classes were based on discoveries made by academic researchers supported by federal government funding.
- Others were jointly developed in both publicly funded and commercial institutions.
- A small number were developed exclusively in pharmaceutical industry R&D programmes.

That private companies are eventually reaping monopoly profits is a clear example of how medicine is used to transfer public resources towards private profit (Vieira & Moon, 2019).

GLOSSARY

Transformative drugs or drug classes: those that are innovative and have groundbreaking effects on patient care.

The marketing costs of pharmaceutical companies grew substantially from US$17.7 billion in 1997 (with US$17.1 billion on prescription drugs) to US$30 billion in 2016 (with US$26.9 billion on prescription drugs) (see Figure 6.10). In the same period, US spending on prescription drugs increased from US$116.4 billion in 1997 to US$329 billion in 2016 (Foley, 2019).

Of all the money spent advertising drugs, the majority went towards efforts to market to doctors. In 1997, the total spending on marketing to physicians was $15.6 billion. By 2016, it was $20.3 billion. Marketing to physicians includes sending paid representatives to doctors' offices to talk about a drug, free samples of it, or compensating physicians for speaking engagements about the drug (Foley, 2019).

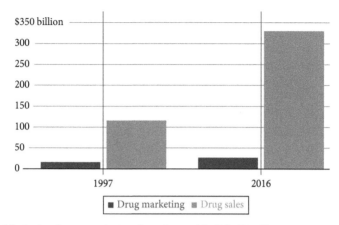

Fig. 6.10 Marketing for prescription drugs has paid off for Big Pharma.
Source: Schwartz & Woloshin. (2018).

'Regulation' of the global pharmaceutical trade

The World Trade Organization (WTO) regulates the global pharmaceutical trade through the Trade-Related Aspects of Intellectual Property Rights (TRIPS) Agreement, which was signed in 1995 (see Chapter 3). This Agreement deals with the granting of time-limited (20 years) monopoly intellectual property rights (IPRs) through a system of patents, copyright and trademarks, across countries. It also limits governments' control over their own domestic IPR and patent protection measures.

GLOSSARY

Essential medicines: medicines that satisfy the health care needs of the majority of the population. They should be available at all times in adequate amounts and in appropriate dosage forms, at an affordable price.

Most **essential medicines** are not subject to patent rights, except for new drugs. Sixty-nine percent of the total world population have access to essential drugs. However, this means that almost 2 billion people live *without* access to these medicines (WHO, 2017).

IPR and patents are a cornerstone of the global pharmaceutical trade. Without any competitors, a company can set any price on their products. And once a patent expires, the pharmaceutical company can make minor chemical modifications to the drug so that it is considered a new invention and is eligible for a new 20-year patent protection. This is called evergreening.

Patent law has been a battleground for access to medicines. Patent law helps influence what knowledge we produce, and who benefits from this knowledge. Patent law, in short, reflects what—and whom—society values (Section 27, n.d.).

Even though the stated purpose of the TRIPS Agreement is to ensure freedom of trade, the *effect* of the Agreement is to reduce competition and create a monopoly, increase the price of drugs (with no restrictions), stop countries from using the technology to produce cheaper, alternative drugs themselves, and ensure the outflow of foreign exchange from importing countries to exporting countries.

While modern medicine risks collapsing because of antibiotic resistance, these companies spend more resources inflating their stock price than developing new medicines. What useful medicines are produced depend on massive injections of cash from the public sector, which normally comes without any conditions constraining the prices these mega-corporations can charge for the final drugs produced (Dearden, 2020).

The overall health implications, in the short- to medium-term, are that drugs become unaffordable for the poor within and across countries, especially during public health crises. Those patients who need these medications most are denied the opportunity of receiving them. The long-term health implications of TRIPS are less predictable. If, for example, the TRIPS Agreement were absent, there would be little incentive for Big Pharma to invest in the R&D of new drugs or to improve existing drugs.

TRIPS flexibilities: grounds for overriding a patent

The TRIPS Agreement acknowledges that there are certain grounds for overriding a patent—called TRIPS flexibilities—especially where IPR conflicts with the right to health and with governments' responsibility to protect the public health of their citizens. In certain cases, a government has the right to important patented medicines produced elsewhere under **compulsory licensing** and **parallel importing**. Usually with a compulsory licence the patent holder receives a royalty either set by law or determined through arbitration.

GLOSSARY

Compulsory licence: the government forces a company that holds the patent to grant other companies a licence to manufacture their product (unlike a voluntary licence in which the patent holder chooses to negotiate with others or not).

Parallel importing: importing medicines from another country without the permission of the IP owner.

However, TRIPS flexibilities are extremely difficult to implement and are subject to a range of terms and conditions, most of which protect trade interests rather than public health. A significant obstacle is that each country must fight Big Pharma over each drug they need. Many countries that have hardly any local manufacturing capacity have come under pressure in trade negotiations not to use TRIPS flexibilities and to implement even tougher rules than those set out in TRIPS. High-income countries routinely use bilateral and regional trade agreements with some underdeveloped countries (called TRIPS-Plus) which impose stricter IP protection than under TRIPS.

The following case study illustrates the struggle of one country—South Africa—to bring TRIPS and the high cost of patented HIV medicines to the world's attention in 2001 and, in so doing, providing the opportunity for people who are poor in all countries to have greater access to life-saving medicines.

CASE STUDY: HIV/AIDS and access to antiretrovirals (ARVs)

In 1990, 8 million people worldwide were living with HIV/AIDS. Three years later, this figure had grown to a staggering 14 million. An estimated 9 million of those infected were living in Sub-Saharan Africa—a region that held 12% of the global population (WHO, 1995).

The first combination therapy to delay the onset of AIDS—Highly Active Antiretroviral Treatment (HAART)—became available in 1998, but it was so expensive (at US$10 000 a year per person) that only wealthy people, mainly in developed countries could afford it. Within four years, AIDS-related deaths in these countries had declined by between 60% and 80% (Avert, 2011). Only a handful of people in Sub-Saharan Africa had access to the treatment.

In an effort to fight the growing HIV/AIDS epidemic, in 1997 the South African government amended the Medicines Act. The aim was to reduce the price of drugs by allowing generic substitutions and parallel importation, making these medicines more accessible to all.

The South African Pharmaceutical Manufacturer's Association (PMA) (backed by the US government and European Union) and 40 multinational and national pharmaceutical companies sued the South African government, arguing that the amendment violated the terms of the TRIPS Agreement. What became known as the PMA case dragged on for three years, during which time the cost of HIV treatment remained prohibitively high.

Taking on goliath

It was against the backdrop of the ongoing PMA case that a civil society organisation, the Treatment Action Campaign (TAC), was established in 1998 to campaign for the rights of those living with HIV/AIDS, specifically the right to access affordable HIV treatment.

TAC, together with the AIDS Law Project (now called Section 27) and the international organisation Médecins Sans Frontières (MSF), used legal action, social mobilisation and public education to lead a global movement to take on Big Pharma.

They argued that patents and IPR allowed Big Pharma to price essential ARVs out of the reach of people living in poverty and were the main obstacles to the realisation of the right to health for people living with HIV. This violated a range of human rights that governments were tasked with protecting and promoting; and failure by governments to protect these rights was as much a barrier to the right to health as profiteering by Big Pharma.

In 2001, under mounting global pressure, the PMA case was dropped.

> *The PMA's withdrawal represented a remarkable victory for treatment activists. It provided proof that the world's most powerful multinational companies could be held accountable, and demonstrated the importance of treating health as a human right* (Section 27, n.d.).

The South African court case against Big Pharma spurred members of the WTO from the Global South to demand that the public health consequences of TRIPS be addressed at the Fourth WTO Ministerial Conference held in Doha, Qatar in 2001. This pressure led to the historic document, the *Doha Declaration on Public Health*, which confirmed the right of governments to protect public health by promoting access to existing and new medicines. Members had the ability to use the TRIPS flexibilities, including the right to use compulsory licensing and parallel importing. According to international medical activist Ellen t'Hoen, "*without the South African court case, we would not have had the Doha Declaration*" (Section 27, n.d.).

Today the use of these TRIPS flexibilities to increase access to drugs is seldom used, and, when used, is mostly limited to ARVs.

Fair trade?

> *Why do first-world ailments get cured faster than global health crises? Because Big Pharma doesn't serve sick people, it serves rich people …* (Hassoun, 2017).

Developing and producing pharmaceuticals is costly, and the expenses need to be covered by someone. So, what would fair trade in this industry look like? Is it fair, for example, that better-off middle-income countries like South Africa pay more for life-saving pharmaceuticals than low-income countries like Tanzania? Some would argue that it is not possible to achieve fair trade under the current market-driven system which is more concerned with servicing a market that can pay than with meeting the basic health needs of people who are poor. However, a number of proposals have been put forward to reform the existing system, so as to incentivise pharmaceuticals companies to invest money in the R&D of much-needed essential medicines, to delink R&D costs from drug prices, and to rather base the reward on innovation according to health care outcomes.

In the race to develop effective COVID-19 treatment and vaccines, Costa Rica has proposed a system that would allow researchers and countries to share technologies, collaborate with each other and produce patent-free medicines. Dearden says of this system:

> *The scheme is up and running, but its voluntary nature means that its impact will be limited. And while there are global programmes to support 'fair distribution' of medicines across the world, these schemes are all based on Big Pharma keeping its patents intact. The fact that rich countries are spending billions of dollars buying as many potential*

vaccines as possible suggests they do not have much faith in these schemes. They are, it seems, just for poor countries who have no better choice (Dearden, 2020).

The second case study discusses Big Pharma in relation to COVID-19 medicine and vaccine patents.

CASE STUDY 2: TRIPS and medical products for COVID-19

In October 2020, India and South Africa requested that the WTO consider a temporary waiver of TRIPS obligations related to COVID-19 medical products, such as diagnostics, medicines, vaccines, medical supplies and test data. Most underdeveloped countries supported the request, while most developed countries opposed it on the basis that TRIPS flexibilities cater for this purpose. They also pointed out that IPRs are not the only obstacle to accessing COVID-19 medical products, the inefficient health systems worldwide are another obstacle.

According to Labonte and Johri (2020), a few pharmaceutical companies have already given up their IP rights to a COVID-19 vaccine, promising once-off arrangements, for example:

- Moderna will not enforce its patent on a COVID-19 vaccine and will license its patent with other vaccine manufacturers, but will not share trade secrets.
- AstraZeneca will make its vaccine available on a cost basis until 31 July 2021.
- In an agreement with The Gates Foundation, Eli Lilly will give up its royalties for its COVID-19 antibody treatment for low- and middle-income countries.

A small group of high- and middle-income countries, representing about 13% of the world's population, secured deals with Big Pharma and their vaccine manufacturers to preorder more than 51% of the promised doses of the leading COVID-19 vaccines (Oxfam, 2020) (see Figure 6.11). The UK, for example, pre-ordered 40 million doses of the Pfizer/BioNTech vaccine—enough for 20 million people as it is a two-shot vaccine. On 2 December 2020 it was the first country to grant approval for the coronavirus vaccine and authorise the mass immunisation of the initial 800 000 doses.

In 2020, the fear was that the effect of these bilateral deals between governments and Big Pharma was that low-income or underdeveloped countries would be left behind. First, the underdeveloped world did not have the purchasing power of the wealthy countries and so risked being unable to get enough doses to vaccinate even their most vulnerable populations. Second, most of the world's vaccine production capacity would be tied up trying to meet the pre-orders, so that underdeveloped countries would have to wait up until 2024 for the vaccinations (Oxfam, 2020; Taylor, 2020). A third obstacle was related to logistics—most coronavirus vaccines must be stored at an unusually cold temperature. The Pfizer vaccine, for example, must be kept at $-94°F$ ($-70°C$), which was a great challenge to most countries, especially given the scale needed (Taylor, 2020).

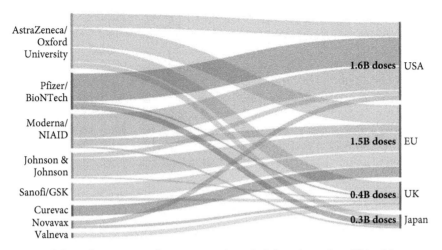

Note: Deals from other countries and economies not shown. Includes options to buy additional doses.
Sources: the companies; governments

Fig. 6.11 Rich countries that have pre-ordered the production of drug-makers.
Source: Data from Shah. (2020).

A NOTE ABOUT COVID-19 VACCINE GLOBAL ACCESS FACILITY (COVAX)

COVAX was an initiative of the Access to COVID-19 Tools (ACT) Accelerator, which was co-lead by the Coalition for Epidemic Preparedness Innovations (CEPI), Global Vaccine Alliance (GAVI), and the WHO. The main aim was to speed up the development and manufacture of COVID-19 vaccines in the quantities needed, secure the public funding to pay for them and organise effective systems to distribute them quickly, fairly and equitably to all countries of the world by the end of 2021. According to Médecins Sans Frontières (2021), "*the failure of the #COVAX facility to deliver equitable access to #COVID19 vaccines was a broken promise to the world*".

So far, we have examined the role played by Big Pharma in perpetuating the suffering of people who are poor within and across countries. Two further examples that we will consider are the breastmilk substitute industry (BSI) and the supply of medical equipment.

The breastmilk substitute industry

As in the developed world, the pharmaceutical industry has had the greatest impact among medical business interests on the health services of underdeveloped countries. However, it is the baby-foods industry that has probably attracted most attention. This has mainly been a result of the vigorous campaign over the past 40–50 years to expose the activities of the BSI.

Human breastmilk is nutritionally superior to artificial formulas and is nearly always available. It is important to the health of both the mother and the infant. It protects children against infection and contributes to their healthy growth and development. It can reduce childhood obesity, type 2 diabetes and leukaemia. It does not have any associations with allergic disorders such as asthma or with blood pressure or cholesterol issues. It reduces the nursing mother's risk of breast and ovarian cancer and diabetes. Breastfeeding acts as a contraceptive (although not fail-safe), both directly through its hormonal effects and often indirectly for cultural reasons. By 2025, the WHO's target global goal is a 50% increase in exclusive breastfeeding for the first six months of a baby's life for the following reasons (see Figure 6.12):

Not breastfeeding greatly increases child mortality. Infants who are not exclusively breastfed are 14 times more likely to die than those who are. Breastfeeding has been shown to protect against sudden infant death syndrome (WHO, 2020).

For the past 20 years, breastfeeding figures are as follows:

- 37% of infants younger than six months are exclusively breastfed in low- and middle-income countries and less than 20% in high-income countries, although there are important differences, ranging from less than 1% in the UK to less than 35% in Norway.
- Breastfeeding babies up to 12 months is highest in Sub-Saharan Africa, south Asia and parts of Latin America, but even in these regions still too few children are breastfed.
- In all countries, women who are poor tend to breastfeed longer than women who are wealthy (Victoria et al., 2016). Only 45% continue to be breastfed up until two years old (WHO, 2018).

Approximately 823 000 child deaths and 20 000 maternal deaths could be prevented each year in 75 high-mortality low- and middle-income countries if breastfeeding were scaled-up (Victoria et al., 2016).

Ingredients for the fatal cycle of undernutrition and bowel infection

A number of problems result from this decline in breastfeeding. Researchers have estimated that breastfeeding could prevent one in two cases of diarrhoeal disease and one in three respiratory infections in low- and middle-income countries (Victoria et al., 2016).

Although breastfed infants are not immune to bowel infections, they are considerably protected by the antiviral and antibacterial factors present in breastmilk. They are also spared exposure to infective organisms present on sometimes inadequately sterilised feeding bottles. Undernutrition can lead to more frequent and more severe diarrhoeal attacks and is aggravated if the powdered milk is overdiluted, which often happens.

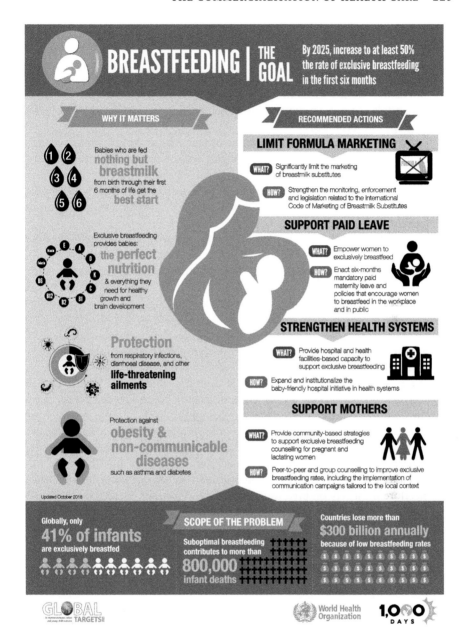

Fig. 6.12 WHO's target breastfeeding goal by 2025.
Source: WHO. (2020).

There are severe problems with breastmilk substitutes in underdeveloped regions, such as:

- Access to reasonable quantities of safe water is extremely limited in Africa, Asia and Latin America. In South Africa, for example, one in three households do not have drinking water on site, making bottle cleaning and preparing formula challenging (Lake et al., 2019).
- Few mothers can afford to carry out the instructions of the breastmilk substitute companies to wash their hands thoroughly with soap each time they prepare a meal for their baby (Muller, 1974).
- Although some products have accompanying instructions leaflets in the main languages of the countries of sale, many mothers in underdeveloped countries are illiterate.
- Breastmilk substitutes are unaffordable for the majority of poor families. In South Africa, for example, 37% of households live below the food poverty line (per capita income of less than US$34.78 per month) (Lake et al., 2019). Breastmilk substitutes can cost between US$22.60 and US$36.75 a month, depending on the brand. As a result, many families choose mixed feeding and/or dilute the formula to stretch it further.

Why is it then that breastfeeding has declined and been replaced by bottle feeding which is clearly so inappropriate and even dangerous in underdeveloped countries?
The impact of capitalism over the past decades has resulted in a large increase in the number of mothers in the labour force, whose working hours discourage or prevent the duration and frequency of breastfeeding. But to move from breastfeeding, it is necessary for an alternative form of infant feeding to exist. It is this 'alternative' that the breastmilk substitute industry (BSI) has vigorously promoted, to the extent of undermining efforts to protect and promote breastfeeding globally. The BSI justifies its operations by asserting that a large proportion of mothers are unable to breastfeed and therefore must rely on breastmilk substitutes. However, there is little scientific evidence to back this up, and failure to breastfeed for physical reasons is uncommon globally.

Promotional methods used by the BSI are strikingly similar to those used by Big Pharma, although the milk companies approach both health professionals and mothers directly. Doctors and maternity unit nurses are often already 'primed' by their training to accept the use of breastmilk substitutes. Many medical students receive no instruction about breastfeeding; and on maternity wards, often nursing staff see routine bottle feeding as 'convenient', which is likely to be viewed by both junior nurses and mothers as an endorsement of the practice. Health professionals are susceptible to the promotional activities of milk companies. They are visited by nurses and representatives who explain the 'benefits' of their products in much the same way as do the pharmaceutical representatives. Some companies create a relationship with the health profession through sponsoring and organising conferences on, for example, nutrition, using such occasions to promote their products. The professionals, now 'informed' about the 'advantages' of the breastmilk substitute, act, often unwittingly, as promotional agents.

In some underdeveloped countries, it is, ironically, at the 'well-baby' or under-five clinics that many mothers first encounter information about bottle feeding, usually in the form of milk company posters, which frequently decorate the buildings. The feeding bottle, which is part of the highly desirable overall image of the well-clothed, clean, chubby baby on the posters, becomes for many mothers an attainable symbol of hope and aspiration for their own babies.

But it was perhaps the operations of the 'milk nurses' in underdeveloped countries that were most unethical. In 1974, the publication '*The Baby Killer*' uncovered the following serious abuses by companies like Nestlé:

> *Medically unqualified sales-girls are hired and dressed in nurses' uniforms to give their sales pitch in the guide of nutrition advice. Mothers are encouraged to bottle feed their babies while they are breastfeeding them satisfactorily and before there is any need for supplements. 'Qualified' nurses are paid on a sales-related basis belying their educational role* (Muller, 1974).

That such promotional methods were effective was shown by Nigerian and Jamaican surveys. Mothers cited company nurses as an important reason for starting bottle feeding. Nine percent of the Nigerian mothers and a much larger proportion of the Jamaican mothers had received free samples of the formula either at a hospital or through nurses. Some companies even offered a free feeding bottle with their product. It could not be determined whether these were real or company 'nurses'. The proportion of illiterate mothers receiving samples was almost the same as educated mothers, showing that no attempt had been made to ensure that mothers were wealthy enough to be able to buy adequate quantities of the formula or sufficiently literate to mix it correctly. Small wonder that the feeding bottle has been termed 'the baby killer' (see Figure 6.13).

> *What unfolded was a tragedy: from mixing the baby water with unsafe water sources to not being able to afford the expensive baby formula and diluting it to make it last longer. The result was deaths of babies in the millions, malnourished babies with stunted growth condemned to a lifetime of physical and mental disability* (Ahthion, 2018).

'The Code'

In May 1981, the campaign against the BSI scored a major success when the WHO adopted a code of practice whereby the breastmilk substitute companies would stop advertising and start stressing the benefits of breastfeeding. The preamble to the *International Code of Marketing of Breastmilk Substitutes* (*the Code*) states that:

> *Inappropriate feeding practices lead to infant malnutrition, morbidity and mortality in all countries, and improper practices in the marketing of breastmilk substitutes and related products can contribute to these major public health problems.*

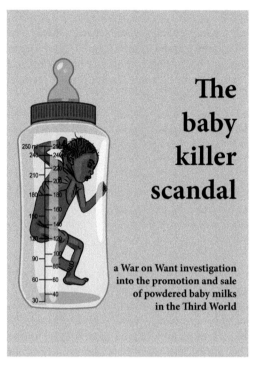

Fig. 6.13 War on Want was the first organisation to draw attention to the damage caused by baby milk companies with its groundbreaking 1974 publication *The Baby Killer*.
Source: War on Want & Muller. (1974).

One hundred and eighteen nations voted in favour of the Code, with only the USA voting against it. Since 1981, 136 out of 194 countries have adopted national legislation to give effect to the Code, to protect and support breastfeeding, regulate misleading and inappropriate marketing of breastmilk substitutes and remove commercial pressure from the baby-food landscape.

Although the Code is a step forward, there are still problems. For example, what constitutes advertising? Many breastmilk substitute companies reluctantly came round to supporting the Code because they realised that there was nothing to stop them sending promotional 'information' to the medical profession. As the Code is voluntary it is difficult to monitor and enforce, and so violations persist.

A voluntary code is all very well, but Nestlé, for example has an annual turnover larger than the gross national product of many African countries. In 2018, Nestlé spent US$7.3 billion on global advertising and marketing efforts (Guttmann, 2020)—more than the total budget of the WHO for 2018–2019 (US$4.4 billion), which is meant to police the Code (Moulds, 2020). In addition, in 2019, Nestlé reported total global sales of approximately US$93 billion and projections show that it expected its profit margin to continue to improve through to 2022 (Nestlé, 2020).

In 2018, the International Baby Food Action Network (IBFAN) Asia published a monitoring report in which they levelled serious accusations of Code violations by 28 breastmilk substitute companies, stating that:

> *37 years after the adoption of the International Code of Marketing of Breastmilk Substitutes, baby food companies continue to pay lip service and claim to be staunch breastfeeding supporters. But their actions prove otherwise as violations of the Code still happen frequently to undermine breastfeeding* (IBFAN, 2018).

Competing interests

> *There is only one reason for food companies to sponsor research—so they can use the results in their own interests. Sponsorship perverts science. Sponsored research is not about seeking truth or adding to public knowledge. It is about obtaining evidence to defend or sell the sponsor's product, to undermine research that might suggest that a product is unhealthy, to head off regulation, and to allow the product to be marketed with health claims* (Marion Nestle, 2013).

Very real concerns remain about the reach and influence of the BSI on, for example, academic research, sponsorship of conferences and national policy formulation and guidelines—all of which could be ultimately harmful to the health of mothers and their children. In 2018, for example, UK-based paediatric professor Chris van Tulleken raised concerns about whether the possible overdiagnosis of cow's milk protein allergy (CMPA) in infants could be *"acting as a Trojan horse for the US$50 billion (£40bn; €44bn) global formula industry to forge relationships with healthcare professionals in the UK and around the world"* (van Tulleken, 2018, cited in Lake et al., 2019).

Questioning the increase in prevalence of CMPA, van Tulleken, explains:

> *Between 2006 and 2016, prescriptions of specialist formula milks for infants with cow's milk protein allergy (CMPA) increased by nearly 500% from 105 029 to over 600 000 a year, while NHS spending on these products increased by nearly 700% from £8.1m to over £60m annually. Epidemiological data give no indication of such a large increase in true prevalence—and the extensive links between the formula industry and the research, guidelines, medical education, and public awareness efforts around CMPA have raised the question of industry driven overdiagnosis* (van Tulleken, 2018, cited in Lake et al., 2019).

While there is a place for breastmilk substitutes, there are very real concerns about the multilevel relationships that the BSI is capable of creating—from mother/child to the health care professionals, to the highest national level and through to global institutions.

The direct cost of the BSI falls on individual families rather than on countries' health budgets, although the treatment of childhood diarrhoea associated with bottle feeding or conditions that may be overdiagnosed, such as CMPA, certainly imposes a financial burden on the health sector. In both cases though, the costs in terms of human suffering are high partly as a result of blatantly unethical marketing practices—the very same kind of practices that happen in the pharmaceutical industry.

Medical equipment

A third example of capitalist medical technology is that of medical equipment. The operations of the medical equipment industry are not frankly 'unethical' and therefore do not attract investigation by the media—but they are important both in diverting health care resources and in influencing the shape of health care services. Although the 'market potential' in the underdeveloped world is necessarily limited by its lack of purchasing power, there are still some areas where such 'potential' exists and certain markets have presented themselves.

'The multibillion shilling medical equipment leasing plan'
In 2014, USAID announced that it had formed a partnership with the US multinational General Electric (GE), which would make up to US$10 million in credit available to Kenyan health facilities to buy GE medical equipment, such as ultrasound and magnetic resonance imaging (MRI) machines (Savchuk, 2014). It was expected that borrowers would be small and medium-sized health care facilities, faith-based or for-profit hospitals.

At the time, Monica Onyango, professor at Boston University's Centre for Global Health and Development, who had worked with the Kenyan Ministry of Health for many years, cautioned that these kinds of PPPs should rather respond to the priority needs of local communities before identifying what equipment to finance. "*The list should really come from the ground, not the donor*", she said.

However, in 2015 the Kenyan Ministry of Health launched 'the multibillion shilling medical equipment leasing plan', which would make specialised health care services and resources more accessible and affordable to its population. Under a Managed Equipment Supplies (MES) agreement, two hospitals in each county would be able to lease high-tech medical equipment from one of the following five multinational firms:

- GE from the USA: 98 hospitals would be equipped with digital X-ray, ultrasound and other imaging equipment.
- Philips Medical Systems from the Netherlands: 11 hospitals would be equipped with intensive care unit (ICU) facilities.
- Bellco SRL from Italy: renal and dialysis machines would be provided for each of the 47 counties and two national referral hospitals.
- Esteem Industries Inc from India: 96 hospitals would be equipped with sterilising equipment complete with surgical sets for all operations.
- Shenzhen Midray Bio-medical Ltd from China: 96 hospitals would be fully fitted with theatre equipment.

The total tender was worth about US$63 billion, with the condition that the suppliers train personnel on how to store, handle, operate, maintain and repair the machines. Although the hospitals received the medical equipment, in at least half of the counties it remained unused. This was in part due to the suppliers failing to fulfill their part of the agreement and partly because of the appalling conditions in some hospitals and the inadequate infrastructure needed to store and handle the equipment. However, one of the central problems was that the equipment did not address the most urgent public health needs in Kenya—HIV/AIDs, malaria, TB, improving family planning and maternal and child health—none of which necessarily required high-tech medical equipment.

How is this grotesque situation brought about?

Doctors in particular and health workers in general are, through their practice and training, oriented towards individual, curative medicine. They are therefore susceptible to sophisticated, expensive technology that may be inappropriate to the needs of most people. It is also the ruling elites who push for such medical services. They tend to live in the urban areas, suffer developed-country diseases and may have had treatment (often private) in the super-technological hospitals of London, Paris, New York and so on. They argue that it is scandalous that their country, now independent of the former colonial power, should still be dependent on medical services overseas.

Health sector aid

Another way in which the door is opened to the medical equipment business—and this is most relevant to concerned health workers who plan to work in underdeveloped countries—is through foreign 'experts' and expatriate health workers. Often unconscious of the negative aspects of their approach, these health workers bring with them not just their ideas about health and health care, but also their practical experience of using particular types of equipment. Hence, they may become the unwitting agents of big business. Undoubtedly, they are frequently seen as such by the companies concerned.

The form in which foreign aid is provided will help influence the approach taken by the recipient to health and health care. For example, foreign aid tied to technological inputs will reinforce the curative, technological approach to health care, as we have already seen in the example of managed medical equipment scheme in Kenya. But often the influence is more subtle, for example furthering political and/or economic interests.

Much of the foreign aid provided to underdeveloped countries is not only monetary, but also in the form of technical cooperation—providing essential skills and helping to train local people. While certain skills are always necessary, it is seriously questionable whether the ways in which many skills are applied are relevant to the majority in underdeveloped (and indeed in many developed) countries. For example, many physiotherapists in underdeveloped countries are trained to work only in well-equipped units in hospitals. Such skills are inappropriate to the needs of the vast majority. On the other hand, community and other health workers could be trained to perform certain basic physiotherapeutic techniques which have been developed to treat common local physical and disabling conditions. This would be an appropriate skill.

In the 1970s, the inappropriate contribution to health care by 'experts' is vividly illustrated in this account by a Bengali doctor. Fifty years later, the insight continues to be important:

> *Recently in Dacca airport I met an acquaintance who said to me in the course of our brief discussion that he had counted 72 experts in Dacca on that one day alone. And yourself, I asked. '73', he admitted.*
>
> *It will be an up-hill road overcoming this favourable bias towards the wisdom of the West. For a long time to come we will continue to credit foreign expertise unquestioningly with any knowledge they may lay claim to. Who are these experts that come from thousands of miles away with the perfect plan for a village they have never seen, and a culture they never lived?*
>
> *Our 'Western trained medical profession, sanitary inspectors originating in the British Empire, the malaria program established by the WHO, the Rural Health Centres devised by Western public health experts, and most recently, the family planning programs', all are forms of expatriate expertise that have left the health and family system of Bangladesh crippled, confused and utterly dependent . . .*
>
> *It is accepted that Bangladesh needs barefoot doctors, people trained in the village and able to meet the needs of the villagers, but the World Health Organisation experts proposed an elaborate 3-year programme to produce medical assistants. This training will take place in the towns, and most of the students will have a background of 12 years formal education. In one centre visited, 65 out of 80 enrolled had had 12 years or more educational background, and nearly all felt that the course itself should be 4 or more years if the programme was going to equip them to 'better serve the people'. Serve, no doubt in Dacca, or Libya, as experience attests. But the expert advisers of the WHO refuse to see any other way.*
>
> *These are the experts. They have been with us, as was noted earlier, for some time. Will we sell ourselves out to them unconditionally now? There are real experts however, and there is no such a thing as appropriate aid. Neither is it possible to discern the real from the 'invested aid'.*
>
> *Does it reach the real problems with realistic solutions? Does the plan provide for local responsibility in the foreseeable future? Is it honest in assessing its weaknesses as well as its strengths?* (Chowdhury, 1977).

Foreign aid of all kinds should in each case be critically evaluated, as it is by no means *always* disadvantageous or inappropriate to the recipient. There are many examples of foreign aid that tries to address important deficiencies, for example the Surgical Unit-based Safety Programme (SUSP) in African hospitals supported by the WHO and the Johns Hopkins Armstrong Institute for Patient Safety and Quality; programmes to promote safe pregnancy and delivery; and the global medical humanitarian organisation MSF which *"responds to the medical needs of people affected by conflict, disasters and epidemics and those excluded from healthcare"* (Doctors Without Borders [MSF], 2020).

Conclusion

As the capitalist economic and political system extended globally, capitalist medicine was introduced into underdeveloped countries. As in developed countries, many starkly inappropriate health services have been primarily a result of the transformation of health into a commodity. This has led to the neglect of health promotion, the stunting of preventive activities and the overinflation of the curative component of health care. In most post-colonial countries, both the health professions and the local elites have argued for western-style health care services. In many cases, they have sealed this by adopting the educational curricula and institutions of the former colonial power. In this way the international saleability of the professionals' skills is ensured and with it their frequent international migration. The transmission of this approach to health and health care to community and other health workers has created professional aspirations, upward migration and high drop-out rates.

This is further entrenched by medical business interests. The examples of the BSI, Big Pharma and the medical equipment industries show how the transfer of largely inappropriate technology aggravates the diversion of resources and the distortion of services in the interests of only a few. Frequently, foreign aid has similar effects, often benefiting the donor more than the recipient and often being dwarfed by health-sector trade, much of which is inappropriate to the needs of the majority of people.

The transfer of capitalist medicine to underdeveloped countries has had other important effects. The medical profession, as in the developed world, comes predominantly from the higher-income social classes and frequently allies with both local and international business interests, particularly in the medical field. Behind the apparently reasonable argument of 'professional freedom', doctors insists on the right to private practice, sophisticated and expensive facilities and equipment and unrestricted prescribing of expensive drugs. Their vested interests have led them to resist social change that would threaten the status quo nationally or globally.

From all that has been said, it becomes clear that the history of the medical contribution, like all history, is one of conflicts and relationships between certain social forces. In the case of health and health services, these forces are medical interests, business interests and the State, on the one hand, and the people, on the other.

References

AFL-CIO. (2018). Death on the job, the toll of neglect. Report, Workplace Health and Safety. https://aflcio.org/reports/death-job-toll-neglect-2018.

Ahthion, R.H. (2018). The sordid history of infant formula & the USA's attempt to bully, blackmail & threaten 3rd world countries. *Greanville Post*, 10 July 2018. https://www.greanvillepost.com/2018/07/10/the-sordid-history-of-infant-formula-the-usas-attempt-to-bully-blackmail-threaten-3rd-world-countries/.

Amnesty International. (2020). *Exposed, silenced, attacked: failures to protect health and essential workers during the COVID-19 pandemic.* Amnesty International: London.

AVERT (Averting HIV and AIDS). (2011). HIV and AIDS history. www.avert.org.hiv-aids-hist ory.htm.

Baum, F. (2002). Cracking the nut of health equity: top down and bottom up pressure for action on the social determinants of health. *Promotion & Education*, 2007;14(2):90–95.

Boniol, M., McIsaac, M., Xu, L., Wuliji, T., Diallo, K. & Campbell, J. (2019). Gender equity in the health workforce: analysis of 104 countries. Working paper 1. WHO: Geneva.

Cahn, Z., Drope, J., Hamill, S., et al. (2018). In: Drope, J. and Schluger, N. (eds). *The Tobacco Atlas*, 6th edn. American Cancer Society and Vital Strategies: Georgia.

Chowdhury, Z. (1977). Research: a method of colonisation. *Bangladesh Times*, 13–14 January 1977.

CIA The World Factbook. (2020). United States, People and Society. https://www.cia.gov/the-world-factbook/countries/united-states/#people-and-society.

Clark, J. (2014). Medicalization of global health 1: has the global health agenda become too medicalized? *Global Health Action*, 2014;7. https://www.ncbi.nlm.nih.gov/pmc/articles/pmc 4028930/.

Crawford, R. (1997). You are dangerous to your health—the ideology and politics of victim blaming. HMO Packet No. 3, p. 13. *International Journal of Health Services*, 1977;7(4):663–680.

Davidson, S., Evans, P. & Dawson, M. (2020). Revealed: NHS commissioners high spend on non-NHS care providers. *The Lowdown*, 14 September 2020. https://lowdownnhs.info/news/revealed-nhs-commissioners-high-spend-on-non-nhs-care-providers/.

Dearden, N. (2020). Big Pharma is not willing to help us defeat COVID-19. *AlJazeera*. https://www.aljazeera.com/opinions/2020/10/18/big-pharma-is-not-going-to-help-the-world-def eat-covid-19/.

Doctors Without Borders (MSF). (2020). About us. https://www.msf.org.za/about-us.

Ehrenrich, B. & English, D. (n.d.). *Witches Midwives and Nurses: A History of Women Healers, Glass Mountain Pamphlets*. Feminist Press at The City University of New York: New York.

Foley, E.K. (2019). HARD TO SWALLOW: Big Pharma spent an additional $9.8 billion on marketing in the past 20 years. It worked. *Quartz online*, 9 January 2019. https://qz.com/1517 909/big-pharma-spent-an-additional-9-8-billion-on-marketing-in-the-past-20-years-it-worked/.

Global Health 50/50. (2020). Towards gender equality in global health. https://globalhealth5 050.org/2020report/.

Govender, V. & Penn-Kekana, L. (2007). *Gender Biases and Discrimination: A Review of Health Care Interpersonal Interactions*. Women and Gender Equity Knowledge Network of the WHO Commission on Social Determinants of Health. WHO: Geneva.

Guttmann, A. (2020). Nestle: advertising spending worldwide 2015–2018. *Statista*. https://www.statista.com/statistics/286531/nestle-advertising-spending-worldwide/#:~:text=In%202018%2C%20the%20Swiss%20food,slightly%20more%20conservative%20market ing%20budget.

Hassoun, N. (2017). Fair trade pharma: a plan for more affordable prescription drugs. https://bigthink.com/videos/nicole-hassoun-how-to-incentivize-big-pharma-to-create-chea per-drugs.

IBFAN. (2018). Report on the Monitoring of the Code in 11 Countries of Asia: inappropriate marketing of baby foods and feeding bottles. https://www.ibfan-icdc.org/publications-for-free/.

Kerry, V. & Lee, K. (2007). TRIPS, the Doha Declaration and paragraph 6 decision: what are the remaining steps for protecting access to medicines? *BioMed Central, Globalization and Health*, 3:3.

Keynejad, R.C., Mekonnen, F.D., Qabile, A., et al. (2018). Gender equality in the global health workplace: learning from a Somaliland–UK paired institutional partnership. *BMJ Global Health*, 3(6):e001073.

Labonte, R. & Johri, M. (2020). COVID-19 drug and vaccine patents are putting profit before people. *The Conversation*, 5 November 2020. https://theconversation.com/covid-19-drug-and-vaccine-patents-are-putting-profit-before-people-149270.

Lake, L., Doherty, T., Sanders, D., et al. (2019). Child health, infant formula funding and South African health professionals: eliminating conflict of interest. *The South African Medical Journal*, 109(12):902–906.

Lee, K. & Collin, J. (2005). *Global Change and Health: Understanding public health*. McGraw-Hill Education.

Marsh, S. & McIntyre, N. (2020). Six in 10 UK health workers killed by COVID-19 are BAME. *The Guardian*. https://www.theguardian.com/world/2020/may/25/six-in-10-uk-health-workers-killed-by-covid-19-are-bame.

Mather, H.G., Morgan, D.C., Pearson, N.G., et al. (1976). Acute myocardial infarction: a comparison between home and hospital care for patients. *BMJ*, 1:925; quoted in Radical Statistics Home Group Pamphlet No. 2, p. 23.

Médecins Sans Frontières. (2021). COVAX: A broken promise to the world. Issue Brief, 21 December 2021. https://msfaccess.org/sites/default/files/2021-12/COVID19_IssueBrief_Covax_1708_ENG_21.12.2021.pdf.

Medenhall, E. (2020). The COVID-19 syndemic is not global: context matters. *The Lancet*, 396(10264):1731.

Mellen, R. & Taylor, A. (2020). Health-care workers make up 1 in 7 COVID-19 cases recorded globally, WHO says. *The Washington Post*, 17 September 2020. https://www.washingtonpost.com/world/2020/09/17/health-care-workers-make-up-one-seven-covid-19-cases-recorded-globally-who-says/.

Meyer, V.F. (2001). The medicalization of menopause: critique and consequences. *International Journal of Health Services*. https://journals.sagepub.com/doi/10.2190/m77d-yv2y-d5nu-fxnw.

Moulds, J. (2020). How is the World Health Organisation funded? The World Economic Forum COVID Action Platform. https://www.weforum.org/agenda/2020/04/who-funds-world-health-organization-un-coronavirus-pandemic-covid-trump/#:~:text=The%20who's%20total%20budget%20for,was%20approved%20at%20%244.4%20billion.

Moynihan, R., Heath, I. & Henry, D. (2002). Selling sickness: the pharmaceutical industry and disease mongering. *BMJ*, 324:886–891.

Muller, M. (1974). *The Baby Killer: A War on Want Investigation into the Promotion and Sale of Powdered Baby Milks in the Third World*. War on Want: London.

Nestle, M. (2013). Conflicts of interest and nutrition organizations. Dietitians for Professional Integrity. Nov 21, 2013. Online: https://integritydietitians.org/2013/11/21/conflicts-of-interest-and-nutrition-organizations/.

Nestle (2020). Nestle reports full-year results for 2019. https://www.nestle.com/media/pressreleases/allpressreleases/full-year-results-2019.

Nguyen, L.H., Drew, D.A., Graham, M.S., et al. (2020). Risk of COVID-19 among front-line health-care workers and the general community: a prospective cohort study. *The Lancet Public Health*, 5(9):E475–E483.

Oxfam. (2020). Small group of rich nations have bought up more than half the future supply of leading COVID-19 vaccine contenders. 17th September 2020. Online: https://www.oxfam.org/en/press-releases/small-group-rich-nations-have-bought-more-half-future-supply-leading-covid-19.

Parrish, M. (2020). Top 10 pharma companies by R&D spend. *Pharma Manufacturing*. https://www.pharmamanufacturing.com/articles/2020/top-10-pharma-companies-by-r-and-d-spend/.

Parsons, T. (1972). Definition of health and illness in the light of American values and social structure. In: Jaco, E.G. (ed.). *Patients, Physicians and Illness: A Source Book in Behavioral Science and Health*. Free Press: New York.

People's Health Movement, Medact, Medico International, Third World Network, Health Action International and ALAMES. (2014). *Global Health Watch 4: An Alternative World Health Report*. Zed Books: London.

People's History of the NHS, People's Encyclopedia. (n.d.). The British Medical Association. https://peopleshistorynhs.org/encyclopaedia/the-british-medical-association/. Accessed 4 December 2020.

Prasad, V. & Sengupta, A. (2019). Perpetuating health inequities in India: global ethics in policy and practice. *Journal of Global Ethics*, 15(1):67–75.

Public Health England. (2020*). Beyond the Data: Understanding the Impact of COVID-19 on BAME Groups*. PHE publications. https://assets.publishing.service.gov.uk/government/uploads/system/uploads/attachment_data/file/892376/covid_stakeholder_engagement_synthesis_beyond_the_data.pdf.

Robson. (n.d.). Quality, inequality and health care. *Medicine in Society, Special Edition*, 11.

Rossen, L.M., Branum, A.M., Ahmad, F.B., Sutton, P. & Anderson, R.N. (2020). Excess deaths associated with COVID-19, by age and race and ethnicity—United States, January 26–October 3, 2020. *MMWR Morbidity and Mortality Weekly Report*, 69:1522–1527. https://www.cdc.gov/mmwr/volumes/69/wr/mm6942e2.htm.

Rozenfeld, Y., Beam, J., Maier, H., et al. (2020). A model of disparities: risk factors associated with COVID-19 infection. *International Journal of Equity Health*, 19(126). https://doi.org/10.1186/s12939-020-01242-z.

Savchuk, K. (2014). USAIDS partnership with GE in Kenya will help health facilities buy high-tech equipment. *The World*, 23 March 2014. https://www.pri.org/stories/2014-03-23/usaids-partnership-ge-kenya-will-help-health-facilities-buy-high-tech-equipment.

Schwartz, L. & Woloshin, S. (2018). Medical Marketing in the United States, 1997–2016. *JAMA*, 321(1):80–96.

Section 27. (n.d.). Standing up for our lives: A history of the access to medicines movement in South Africa. https://standingupforourlives.section27.org.za/chapter-7/.

Segall, M. (1976). Health care as a commodity. *Medicine and Society*, 2(4).

Shah, S. (2020). In race to secure COVID-19 vaccines, world's poorest countries lag behind. *The Wall Street Journal*, 1 September 2020. https://www.wsj.com/articles/in-race-to-secure-covid-19-vaccines-worlds-poorest-countries-lag-behind-11598998776.

Sherman, E. (2019). Drug companies have big R&D expenses and still make large profits. *Fortune*. http://fortune.com/2019/03/01/drug-companies-rd-profits/.

Social Mobility Commission. (2016). 2016 State of the Nation report on social mobility in Great Britain. https://www.gov.uk/government/news/state-of-the-nation-report-on-social-mobility-in-great-britain#:~:text=the%20social%20mobility%20commission%20is,promote%20social%20mobility%20in%20england.

Stewart A. (2016). *Basic statistics and epidemiology: a practical guide*. CRC Press, Taylor & Francis Group, 218.

Šumilo, D., Nichols, L., Ryan, R. & Marshall, T. (2018). Incidence of indications for tonsillectomy and frequency of evidence-based surgery: a 12-year retrospective cohort study of primary care electronic records. *British Journal of General Practitioners*, 5 November 2018. https://doi.org/10.3399/bjgp18X699833.

Taylor, A. (2020). The beginning of the end of the coronavirus pandemic. *The Washington Post*. https://www.washingtonpost.com/world/2020/12/03/britain-pfizer-vaccine-nationalism/.

The Lancet. (2020). Editorial, 23 May 2020. https://www.thelancet.com/journals/lancet/article/piis0140-6736(20)31200-9/fulltext.

The Lowdown. (2020). £10bn spend on private hospitals to bridge gap in NHS capacity, 24 August 2020. https://lowdownnhs.info/private-providers/10bn-spend-on-private-hospitals-to-bridge-gap-in-nhs-capacity/.

Tobacco-Free Kids. (2020). The global tobacco epidemic. 2020 Campaign for Tobacco-Free Kids. https://www.tobaccofreekids.org/assets/global/pdfs/en/global_tobacco_epidemic_en.pdf.

Victoria, C.G., Bahl, R., Barros, A.J., et al. (2016). Lancet Breastfeeding Series Group. Breastfeeding in the 21st century: epidemiology, mechanisms, and lifelong effect. *The Lancet*, 387(10017):475–490.

Vieira, M. & Moon, S. (eds). (2019). Research synthesis: public funding of pharmaceutical R&D. Knowledge Portal on Innovation and Access to Medicines. https://www.knowledgeportalia.org/public-funding-of-r-d.

WHO. (1995). Global Programme on AIDS, Progress Report. 1992–1993. http://data.unaids.org/publications/irc-pub06/epiupdate98_en.pdf.

WHO. (2017). *Ten Years in Public Health 2007–2017. Chapter 7: Access to Medicines: Making Market Forces Serve the Poor*. WHO: Geneva.

WHO. (2019a). *WHO Report On The Global Tobacco Epidemic 2019: offer help to quit tobacco use. The MPOWER package*. Geneva: WHO. https://www.who.int/teams/health-promotion/tobacco-control/who-report-on-the-global-tobacco-epidemic-2019.

WHO. (2019b). *Delivered by Women, Led by Men: A Gender and Equity Analysis of the Global Health and Social Workforce*. Human Resources for Health Observer Series No. 24. WHO: Geneva.

WHO. (2020). Global nutrition targets 2025—breastfeeding. https://www.who.int/health-topics/breastfeeding#tab=tab_1.

Worstall, T. (2017). Milton Friedman told us the answer decades ago—now it'll probably be IBM's Watson. *Forbes*, 4 June 2017. https://www.forbes.com/sites/timworstall/2017/06/04/milton-friedman-told-us-the-answer-decades-ago-now-itll-probably-be-ibms-watson/?sh=167187b51bce

Yamin, A.E. (2020). A wake-up call in our upside-down world: three starting-points for advancing health rights and social justice in a post-pandemic future. *Journal of Human Rights Practice*, 1–8. Opinion Piece. Oxford University Press: Oxford. https://academic.oup.com/jhrp/advance-article/doi/10.1093/jhuman/huaa033/5920408.

Yearby, R. & Mohapatra, S. (2020). Law, structural racism, and the COVID-19 pandemic, *Journal of Law and the Biosciences*, 1–20. https://academic.oup.com/jlb/article/7/1/lsaa036/5849058.

7

Changing Medicine, Changing Society

I think Marx matters to medicine for three reasons. First, Marx offers a critique of society ... that enables explication of disquieting trends in modern medicine and public health—privatised health economies, the power of conservative professional elites, the growth of techno-optimism, philanthrocapitalism, the importance of political determinants of health, global health's neoimperialist tendencies, product-driven definitions of disease, and the exclusion of stigmatised communities from our societies ... Second, Marxism defends a set of values. The free self-determination of the individual, an equitable society, the end of exploitation, deepening possibilities for public participation in shaping collective choices, refusing to accept the fixity of human nature and believing in our capacity to change, and keeping a sense of the interdependence and indivisibility of our common humanity. Finally, Marxism is a call to engage, an invitation to join the struggle to protect the values we share (Horton, 2017).

So far, this book has focused on the negative aspects of the medical contribution. This has partly been a conscious attempt to correct the prevalent but unbalanced view that medical interventions no matter how small, can only be good and that health workers always make a positive contribution to health.

What then should be the role of those concerned with health? What should be done by those who see the necessity for the promotion of health, as well as the prevention and cure of disease? How, in short, can health workers, both in rich and poor countries, become part of the solution to underdevelopment and ill-health, rather than part of the problem?

Health problems are rooted in social conditions. This is true in all countries, irrespective of their level of development. In former colonies these social conditions are determined by a global economic and political system that ensures underdevelopment.

Historically, the two most important measures to promote health in developed countries were improved nutrition and better environmental hygiene. The same measures are needed to promote health in poor countries today. But the task of ending underdevelopment is not just a repetition of the development that took place in Britain and the other advanced capitalist countries. We have seen how the accumulation of capital for industrial development in those countries came from exploiting the colonial world. The former colonies today have no colonies to exploit—they have no easy source of capital and only small markets for their goods. Since the advent of imperialism, the economies of former colonies have become increasingly controlled by huge foreign-owned enterprises—transnational corporations (TNCs)—in alliance with a local ruling class.

The Struggle for Health. David Sanders with Wim De Ceukelaire and Barbara Hutton, Oxford University Press.
© Oxford University Press 2023. DOI: 10.1093/oso/9780192858450.003.0007

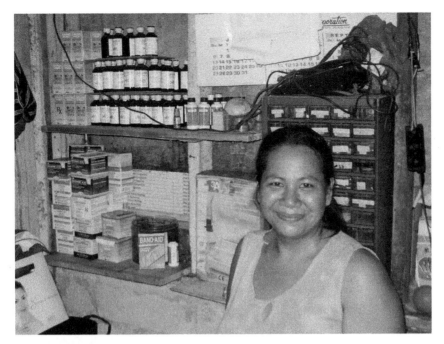

Fig. 7.1 Community pharmacy in one of the slum areas of Manila, the Philippines. A trained community health worker offers a selection of essential medicines to her community members.

Source: Wim De Ceukelaire—Viva Salud.

The possibility of significant independent capitalist development as happened in nineteenth-century Europe no longer exists. There are, however, a few impressive examples of countries where underdevelopment has been successfully tackled and great improvements in people's health achieved. The best known of these examples are China and Cuba, where in the second half of the twentieth century victorious popular struggles resulted in a fundamental change of economic and political systems. Long-stifled human potential was mobilised, foreign-controlled resources reappropriated and the ensuing wealth more fairly distributed, with particular emphasis on health and other social services. That is why we start this chapter by discussing the way in which health promotion grew out of the process that reversed underdevelopment in these countries.

These twentieth-century examples have inspired new and alternative approaches to health care—these will be discussed later in this chapter in the section on 'The community health worker: a possible link', with more recent examples from Ethiopia, India and Iran (see Figure 7.1). Finally, we will describe the global movement for the right to health, the People's Health Movement, which grew out of these alternative approaches.

Health promotion: the Chinese experience

Although the post-colonial world took shape in the decades after World War II, it was not until the 1970s that multinational organisations, like the WHO, began investigating some of the significant inequities in development among former colonies. A landmark collection of case studies, compiled by the WHO in 1975, featured interesting experiences with alternative approaches to tackling health problems in poor, often rural, areas. The largest and most impressive of these case studies was undertaken by Ruth and Victor Sidel, focusing on the early development of health policy and systems, and the implementation of the Primary Health Care (PHC) approach in the People's Republic of China after 1949.

A NOTE ABOUT PRIMARY HEALTH CARE CASE STUDIES

The Alma-Ata Declaration of 1978 drew on a range of influences, including the collection of case studies published by the WHO in 1975, under the title *Health by the People*, edited by Kenneth Newell (see Chapter 4 for more details).

Apart from the Sidels' case studies in the People's Republic of China presented in Newell's collection, Newell also presents two other cases of inspiring PHC, both of which were the product of brilliant medical entrepreneurs—the Aroles in Jamkhed, in India, and the Nugrohos in Solo, in Indonesia. To these we could also add the Karks in Pholela, South Africa (Kark & Kark, 1999); Julian Tudor Hart in Glyncorrwg, South Wales (Warren, 2018); and Jack Geiger in Mound Bayou, Mississippi, USA (Geiger, 2013).

However, none of these other cases achieved scale-up to national programmes (as did that in the People's Republic of China). This is an important lesson which is of particular significance for the NGOs of today, many of which are guided by PHC principles but within the confines of their own domain and funders.

The early years

According to the Sidels, in the 1930s and 1940s, many people in China suffered from the consequence of widespread poverty, unhygienic sanitary conditions, ongoing civil war and rampant disease and ill-health. Available health services were extremely inadequate. At this time, it was estimated that the crude death rate in China was one of the highest in the world—25 deaths per 1000 people. The infant mortality rate was approximately 200 per 1000 live births—in other words, one in every five babies died in their first year of life. Most deaths were due to prevalent infectious diseases, complicated by some form of malnutrition.

Prevalent infectious diseases included bacterial illnesses such as cholera, diphtheria, gonorrhoea, leprosy, meningococcal meningitis, plague, relapsing fever, syphilis, tetanus, tuberculosis, typhoid fever, and typhus; viral illnesses such as Japanese B encephalitis, smallpox, and trachoma; and parasitic illnesses such as ancylostostomiasis (hookworm disease), clonorchiasis, filariasis, kala-azar, malaria, paragonimiasis, and schistosomiasis (Sidel & Sidel, 1975).

Pioneering work was also done from 1932 to 1945 by Dr Chen Zhiqian. He focused on PHC, including area-wide public health and community involvement, in part as a response to the influence of the medical missionaries from the early nineteenth century who practised individualised western scientific sick care (Chen & Bunge, 1989). Further work in education, health, agriculture, poverty alleviation and politics was also undertaken by the Dingxian project—a rural reconstruction project in Dingxian (1926 until the late 1930s), which was run by the Chinese Communist Party (CCP) in liberated areas during the civil war.

The work unit

At the end of the civil war in October 1949 which saw the CCP triumph, sweeping changes were introduced in the People's Republic of China, including in health care. The first National Health Conference, which was held in August 1950, established four guiding principles for health development:

1. Serve the workers, peasants and soldiers (concentrating on rural areas).
2. Put prevention first.
3. Place equal importance on traditional Chinese and western medicine.
4. Mobilise all sectors of the people for health work.

A major structural reform introduced in the early 1950s was the 'work unit'—a coherent social and economic institution which included communes in the country and enterprises in the cities (manufacturing, retail, administration and so on). The work unit resourced enterprise-based health and welfare services, such as clinics, childcare, education and aged care. It also provided the basic organising entity for the National Patriotic Health Campaigns—the platform for promoting the four guiding principles for health development and for implementing major public health initiatives (Horn, 1971).

In the early years, there were few western health care practitioners, and those who were available were largely concentrated in the cities. The initial focus in the rural areas was to build on the health programmes of the Dingxian model. This involved providing basic training to workers and peasants so that they could participate in public health campaigns (environmental hygiene, nutrition, family planning, first aid and so on), as well as providing basic clinical care, largely using traditional Chinese medicine.

CASE STUDY: The Patriotic Health Campaigns

In the first public health campaign, the 'four pests' were attacked—rats, flies, mosquitoes and sparrows (later replaced by bed bugs). People were mobilised to exterminate these pests under the guidance of health personnel. During this assault, more than 74 million tons of garbage were cleared and breeding grounds eliminated (Wylie, 1972). In 1960, it was reported that 1590 million rats, 100 million kilograms of flies and 11 million kilograms of mosquitoes were collected (Christian Medical Commission, 1974).

In later years, the Patriotic Health Campaigns were replaced by 'shock attacks'— short-lived but highly intensive campaigns, often carried out on a regional scale and each dealing with a specific problem. Campaigns then became regular seasonal affairs directed towards eradicating all the major communicable disease as well as the 'four pests' and at improving sanitary conditions. For example, in the 1958 campaign it was reported that 63.27 million public latrines were constructed or repaired—one for every 10 people (Wylie, 1972).

Perhaps the most remarkable achievement was the massive reduction in schistosomiasis (bilharzia).

Mass mobilisation against schistosomiasis (bilharzia)

Schistosomiasis is a chronic disease caused by parasitic worms that live in certain types of freshwater snails. The parasites emerge from the snail into the water and people become infected when their skin comes into contact with the contaminated fresh water. Schistosomiasis is often not highlighted as a public health issue because it mainly affects poor rural communities in low-income countries. In China, however, the public health and socio-economic importance of schistosomiasis was recognised as early as the 1950s. This recognition signalled political will on behalf of the central government and they invested both financial and technical resources in an integrated manner to address the disease (Wang et al., 2008). The approach could be fine-tuned for different eco-epidemiological settings. In the mid-1950s, more than 10 million people were infected with *Schistosoma japonicum* in 12 provinces in southern China. By the 2000s, this number was reduced to less than 1 million. At the same time, transmission of the disease was interrupted in five provinces.

Mass organisation, mobilisation and education were vital to the schistosomiasis reduction. The idea was not only to recruit the people to do the work, but also to mobilise their enthusiasm and initiative so that they would fight the disease. In the 1970s, the Sidels observed that the antischistosomiasis campaign:

> was based on the concept of the 'mass line'—the conviction that the ordinary people possess great strength and wisdom and that when their initiative is given full play they can accomplish miracles.

The population was mobilised in several directions: to move against the snails, to cooperate in case-finding and treatment and to improve environmental sanitation.

The health promotion activities were based on the following: recognition of a problem, important to large numbers of people; analysis of the problem; recommendation of solutions by technical and political leaders; and then—most important—the thorough discussion of the analysis and recommended solutions with the people so that they could fully accept these as their own.

The example below illustrates the various steps in the process.

Antischistosomiasis station in Yukiang County in Kiangsi Province

One million square metres of land in Yukiang County in Kiangsi Province was infested with snails and had been plagued by schistosomiasis for more than a hundred years. After investigating the prevalence of the disease, an antischistosomiasis station was set up in the county in 1953.

- First, the personnel of the station began publicising its purposes, as well as health work in general. They used various media for this, such as broadcasting, wall newspapers, blackboards, exhibits of real and model objects, lantern-slide shows and drama. They also popularised related scientific knowledge.
- To help the peasants raise their political consciousness, break their superstitious beliefs and build their confidence in conquering the disease, personnel organised meetings for recalling sufferings in the old society and to compare with what was happening in the new society.
- Once the population was fully educated in schistosomiasis, a 'people's war' was launched against the snails. From 1955 to 1957, 20 000 peasants, together with voluntary labour from the People's Liberation Army, students, teachers and office workers, filled up old ditches and ponds, dug new ditches and expanded the cultivation area by roughly 36 ha (90 acres).
- After this massive war on schistosomiasis, it was still necessary to check for the recurrence of snails, as well as on water control and waste disposal. So, people were educated in the treatment of human excreta, the provision of safe drinking water and improved personal hygiene. Production teams under the leadership of health workers were responsible for these public health measures.

Using the same techniques of mobilising the general population to participate in the provision of medical care and the prevention of illness, diseases such as smallpox, cholera, typhoid fever and plague were completely eliminated. By the time the Sidels studied China's health situation, venereal disease and kala-azar were practically eliminated and diseases such as malaria and filariasis were being rapidly brought under control.

Assistant doctors: 'barefoot doctors'

The health system received a major shake-up with the **Great Leap Forward** (1957–1958) and the **Cultural Revolution** (1966–1976). Following a famous attack on the Ministry of Health by Mao Zedong in 1964 (he accused it of being 'the ministry of gentlemen's health'—being overfocused on urban problems), there was a dramatic increase in the training of lower-level cadres (assistant or **barefoot doctors**) to scale-up medical skills and numbers in the rural areas. Mao's directive concluded: "*In medical and health work, put the stress on the rural areas!*"

GLOSSARY

Great Leap Forward: an economic and social campaign aimed at transforming private and family-based farming into agricultural people's communes. This period saw positive developments for health, including the introduction of barefoot doctors, but also saw a famine spread through China in the early 1960s.

Cultural Revolution: the Chinese revolutionary movement aimed at reducing inequities between resources in the rural and urban areas and bridging the gap between intellectuals and workers, as well as between government and the people. Despite significant health gains, the period also witnessed human rights abuses sanctioned by the State.

Barefoot doctors: a term for community/village health workers or assistant doctors, who were called 'barefoot doctors' because in many rural areas much agricultural work is done barefoot in the rice paddies.

The introduction of the barefoot doctor scheme was a turning point in the expansion of the health care system and in its reorientation towards the needs of all the Chinese people, and especially those living in poverty. From the early 1960s, there was a rapid expansion in the training of these doctors, with secondary diplomas (two years of senior high-school training) and tertiary diplomas (three years training after finishing high school). Students were usually selected by the people with whom they had worked and whom they were to return to serve. The curriculum was restructured to place greater emphasis on practical work rather than theory, with much more training in Chinese medicine.

Barefoot doctors were employed by the work unit and provided organisational resources for setting up clinics, encouraging environmental health and promoting family planning (see Figure 7.2). They also played a critical role in providing basic health care, drawing on both traditional Chinese and western medicine. They were responsible for environmental sanitation, health education, immunisation and first aid. Perhaps most important, their fellow workers knew them well and trusted them (Sidel & Sidel, 1975).

Although the scheme evolved over the decades, and the term barefoot doctor is no longer used, it was never formally stopped. In the early 1980s, the State Council (the highest executive body) issued a directive that after passing an examination, barefoot doctors could qualify as village doctors. Anyone who did not pass could still work as a health worker but had to practise under the guidance of the village doctors. In the 1980s, village doctors and rural health workers still offered PHC, including prevention, education, maternal and child health care and health data collection.

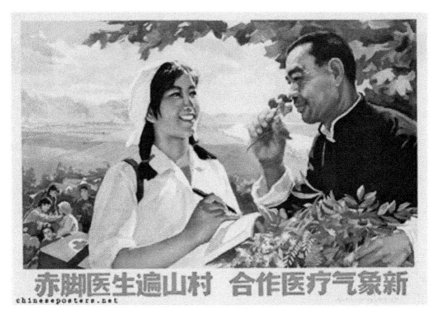

Fig. 7.2 Barefoot doctors are all over the mountain villages; cooperation creates a new atmosphere of medical treatment.
Source: Stefan R. Landsberger Collection.
https://chineseposters.net/posters/e13-659.

Thus, the 1950s and 1960s saw dramatic improvements in population health due to a range of factors, including access to basic health care, improved nutrition and public health programmes. These successes inspired widespread interest well beyond China, mediated in part by visitors such as the Sidels. The perception that formed in the West of the Chinese reforms focused on the barefoot doctors, the National Patriotic Health Campaigns and the integration of western and traditional Chinese medicine under the broad rubric of PHC. The barefoot doctor scheme had a profound influence on the 1978 Declaration of Alma-Ata, and China's experience was also an important part of the inspiration for the WHO to launch the '*Health for All* by 2000' programme.

However, there was less appreciation in the West of the role of the CCP in driving public health campaigns and the role of the work unit as the organisational context for such campaigns. The barefoot doctors were part of the story, but the CCP's policies and strategies were also critical. The National Patriotic Health Campaigns were a product of a partnership between the CCP and the people, and the barefoot doctors were a key instrument of this.

A poorly controlled tiger

PHC in China was not simply a policy for the health sector. It was embedded in a particular political and economic configuration, and while it was critical to the huge improvements in population health that were made, the system of which it was part was not without its drawbacks.

The success of the CCP in sponsoring the PHC movement from the 1950s needs to be balanced against subsequent events, of which the Great Chinese Famine of 1958 and the damage wrought by the Cultural Revolution state-sanctioned murders stand out. A key factor in the genesis of the widespread famine was the culture of setting optimistic (rather than realistic) production targets, being held accountable for them and officials being fearful of being honest about the shortfalls in the harvest.

The system was further convulsed when Deng Xiaoping came to power in 1976 and introduced various reforms. Deng judged that the degree of central planning under Mao had held back economic development and that the economic inefficiency of the work unit was a critical element of this. Central control of capital allocation meant that the work unit was not subject to the disciplines of competition and the need to make a profit. Deng encouraged private enterprise, including with foreign partners, to expose state-owned enterprises to competition as part of forcing them to be more efficient.

From the 1980s onwards, the state-owned enterprises were forced to cut back or shed their enterprise welfare commitments, including their village stations, clinics, small hospitals and their 'health insurance' responsibilities (paying for inpatient care at secondary and tertiary hospitals when needed). As welfare commitments were cut back, barefoot doctors moved into fee-for-service medical practices in the cities and towns. This resulted in a collapse of the cooperative medical system to a payment-based system. According to Zhang and Unschuld (2008), the percentage of rural villages with a cooperative medical system fell from 90% in the 1960s to 5% by 1985 (see Figure 7.3). In the rural areas the return to 'family responsibility' farming and the collapse of the agricultural communes likewise forced the barefoot doctors to return to full-time farming or to try to make a living as fee-for-service village/country doctors (Zhang & Unschuld, 2008). PHC coverage in rural areas declined considerably.

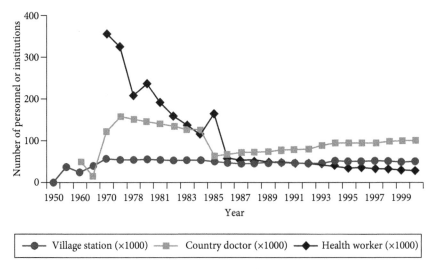

Fig. 7.3 Rural health personnel and institutions in China, 1950–2000.
Source: Zhang & Unschuld. (2008).

The collapse of enterprise-based 'health insurance' had a devastating impact on secondary and tertiary hospital revenues. At a time when public fiscal capacity was limited and policy-makers were convinced of the profit motive as a driver of efficiency, hospitals could charge user fees. This made health care services increasingly unaffordable to the mass of people.

In 2003, the government proposed a new cooperative medical system in which local government pays a fixed amount each year to cover the costs of serious diseases for people under their jurisdiction. Health promotion and prevention were largely ignored.

The achievements of Deng's reforms in terms of economic development made a huge contribution to poverty alleviation and health improvement. However, privatised health care was introduced in the process (a poorly controlled tiger that the central government is still struggling to ride), along with widening inequality.

CASE STUDY: Former barefoot doctors speak out

According to Dr Liu Xingzhu, a former barefoot doctor, health care services in China suffered in the late 1970s and early 1980s when the agricultural sector was privatised. Dr Liu Xingzhu went on to become programme director at the Fogarty International Centre at the National Institutes of Health in the USA. He comments:

> The barefoot doctors, who were paid collectively by the commune, lost their source of income. Many turned to farming or industry. The most direct effect was that few did inoculations or provided primary health care for the peasants. Many diseases that had been eradicated emerged in the countryside again (WHO, 2008a).

Dr Liu Yuzhong, another veteran who started as a barefoot doctor, managed to pass the Ministry of Health exam in 1981 and then practised as a village doctor. When the rural health care system was dismantled in the 1980s because of China's economic liberalisation, he was hired by a local health centre on the outskirts of Beijing. He explained the merits of the barefoot doctor system:

> There are great advantages to having a barefoot doctor in the village. The patients are all my neighbours. I know each family's situation, lifestyle and habits. Since I see my patients very often, even if I cannot diagnose precisely the first time, I can follow up closely and give a better diagnosis the next time (WHO, 2008a).

High-technology, hospital-centric system

The Deng and Jiang Zemin[1] reforms had a particular impact on the hospital sector, partly because of a complex interplay of staff remuneration policies and distorted

---

[1] Jiang Zemin was one of Deng's successors who dominated China's political system in the 1990s.

price controls. The central government had a tight control on wages and salaries but allowed hospitals to supplement medical salaries with large bonus payments, to encourage clinicians to consider 'efficiency' (actually revenues). The central government also kept tight price controls on simple clinical services, such as a consultation, but there were much looser controls over newer technology-intensive services. This led to a perfect storm—outpatient clinics were loss leaders, with huge volumes of patients in low-priced consultations, while senior clinicians had a heavy incentive to overuse high-technology services on those patients who could be admitted to hospital (Likun et al., 2013).

At the same time, the development of the highly technologised, hospital-centric system also reflected a popular demand for modern medicine. Despite repeated attempts to recreate a PHC sector, including boosted training for general practice doctors, urban consumers continued to attend the mega-clinics of the tertiary hospitals because of their perception that they were getting better medicine.

Policy decisions taken in the 1990s committed China to a pluralist health insurance model, which supported the (de facto) privatisation of medical care (Zhao et al., 2005). This reflected a bizarre preoccupation with American health care among many of the senior policy officials under Jiang Zemin.

Under Xi Jinping in 2013 onwards, the central government invested hugely in subsidised health insurance, including for rural dwellers and low-income families in the cities and towns (leading to greatly reduced out-of-pocket costs) and encouraged the development of community health centres. However, PHC practitioners are still marginalised in the highly technologised, hospital-centric and privatised system (in behaviour if not formally). Although the community participation dimension of the earlier PHC regime has virtually disappeared with the rise of privatised health care, the flourishing high-technology hospital sector has contributed to the development of the pharmaceuticals, plastics and electronics industries in China.

Health statistics in China

It was only from about the mid-1970s that some statistics about the health status of China's population were starting to become more available. Scant statistics from Shanghai City in 1975 showed the following per year: six deaths per 1000 of population, with leading causes being cancer, stroke and heart disease; infant mortality rate of nine per 1000 live births; and life expectancy of 70 years (Sidel & Sidel, 1975).

Shanghai City is certainly not representative of the rest of China, or even of its other large cities, but the remarkable changes over the past two decades in Shanghai—the infant mortality rate in 1948 was estimated at 150 per 1000—are probably indicative of rapid changes in health status throughout China (Sidel & Sidel, 1975).

According to Wang et al. (2008), between 1970 and 2007, China experienced a rapid reduction in the yearly incidence of the 18 notifiable infectious diseases, such as malaria and vaccine-preventable diseases like polio, measles, pertussis and diphtheria, as well as gastrointestinal infectious diseases, such as cholera, dysentery, typhoid and

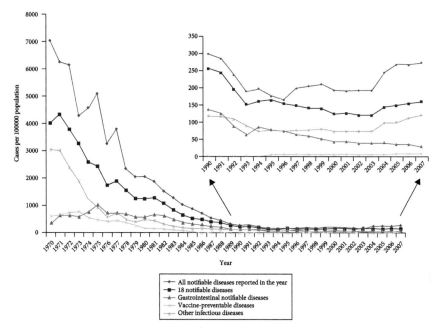

Fig. 7.4 Trends in incidence (cases per 100 000 population per year) of notifiable infectious diseases in China during 1970–2007.

Source: Wang et al. (2008).

paratyphoid. The decrease was between 4000 and 4340 cases per 100 000 population per year in 1970–1971 and between 120 and 250 cases per 100 000 population per year in 1990–2007. As you can see in Figure 7.4, the reported rates in 1990–2007 changed very little.

Reduction in the mortality rate followed a similar pattern for the 18 notifiable infectious diseases. Mortality decreased from eight to nine deaths per 100 000 population per year in 1970–1973 to less than one death per 100 000 population per year in 1991–2007 (Figure 7.5).

In 2006, deaths from infectious diseases accounted for only 1.2% (3.38 per 100 000 population for deaths from infectious diseases, and 530.46 per 100 000 population for overall deaths) of the overall mortality in both urban and rural areas (Wang et al., 2008).

Interestingly, the biggest advances in China's health status predated the rise in living standards. For the first 30 years from the establishment of the People's Republic of China, there was a remarkable increase of life expectancy, from 40 years to nearly 70 years. This increase was all the more remarkable because the nation was relatively poor, and average life expectancy for countries at similar levels of economic development was about 10 years lower than China's. The health success, despite limited economic resources, has been attributed to government commitment and implementation of public delivery systems for food, preventive health care and PHC and other necessities for health (Tang et al., 2008).

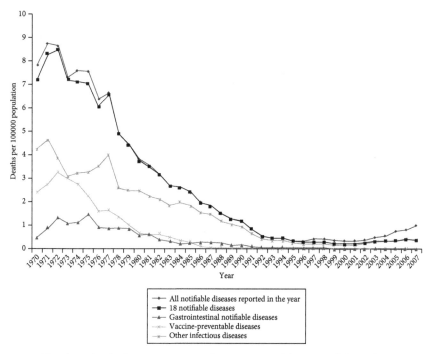

Fig. 7.5 Trends in deaths (per 100 000 population per year) from notifiable infectious diseases in China during 1970–2007.

Source: Wang et al. (2008).

In their study for the WHO, back in 1975, the Sidels concluded:

> *These changes in health status are certainly not the result of changes in health care alone; improvements in nutrition, sanitation, and living standards are at least as important.*

Inequities in health in China

Li et al. (2018) examined differences in health care utilisation in urban and rural China between 1993 and 2011 and revealed that rural areas had a worse health profile compared to urban areas. While the gap was closing, urban Chinese people had better access to health services than rural Chinese people.

According to Tang et al. (2008), there were substantial inequities in child health indicators between rural and urban counties:

- In 2000, infant mortality rates in the poorest rural areas were 123 per 1000 live births, five times higher than in the wealthiest areas, where they were 26 per 1000 live births.
- Between 2000 and 2004, death rates in children under five years ranged from 10 per 1000 in the richest large cities to 64 per 1000 in the poor rural areas.

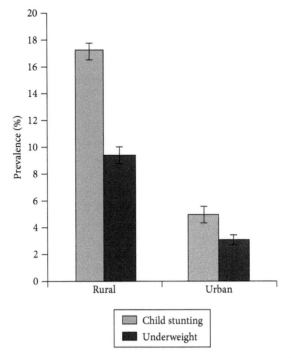

Fig. 7.6 Inequities in child malnutrition between urban and rural areas of China, 2002.
Source: Tang et al. (2008).

- In 2002, the prevalence of child stunting was 17.3% in rural areas compared with 4.9% in urban areas; and 9.3% of children were underweight in rural areas compared with 3.1% in urban areas (see Figure 7.6).

There were also significant differences in health achievements between rich and poor provinces and between population groups. Table 7.1 shows differences in life expectancy gains in the rich urban city of Shanghai (where in the years 1981–2000 there was a 5-year gain) in contrast to Gansu, one of China's poorest provinces (where in years 1981–2000 there was a 1.4-year gain). In 2000, there was a gap of 10.6 years between life expectancy in Shanghai and in Gansu (Tang et al., 2008).

Table 7.1 Life expectancy gains in rich and poor regions in China, 1981–2000

Life expectancy: rich cities	Life expectancy: poor province
Shanghai:	Gansu:
1981: 72.9 years	1981: 66.1 years
2000: 78.1 years	2000: 67.5 years

What can we learn about the evolution of Primary Health Care in China?

The way PHC developed in China reflects the interplay of inspirational individuals (such as Chen Zhiqian), system-wide reform of health systems and enormous changes in wider social, economic and political structures. PHC is not simply a health system model—in China, it arose in revolutionary circumstances where caring for people's health was central to the revolutionary project. It is a vision of how health can be promoted in society, which comes closer to being realised in certain times and places.

Subsequent political and economic reforms altered the organisation of the country's health care system considerably. The Cooperative Medical Scheme was turned into a payment-based system of medical care. Barefoot doctors lost their institutional and financial support and some of them became village doctors. As private practitioners they tended to focus more on treatment of diseases in individuals, and, understandably, the public health of the village became a lower priority.

China has experienced dramatic demographic and epidemiological transitions. With a population that is mainly urbanised and ageing rapidly, China's major health threats are chronic diseases, which now account for more than three-quarters of all deaths. Although China has been successful in the control of infections and maternity-related conditions, these health problems have by no means been eliminated, as exemplified by continuing infectious outbreaks, reproductive health problems and persistent schistosomiasis.

Infectious diseases have substantially increased because of changes and reforms. In the 1970s, for example, sexually transmitted diseases (STDs) were almost eliminated. However, in 1978, with the start of economic reforms, coupled with an increase in internal migrant populations (from rural to urban areas) and in commercial sex, there was once again the proliferation of STDs (Wang et al., 2008).

The example of schistosomiasis control is also instructive. Factors hampering further progress include global warming, increasing population mobility, changes in the snail habitat and distribution due to changes in the ecosystem because of human activity, and privatisation of the health sector. In addition, in 2001 the World Bank terminated its loan for schistosomiasis control. Re-emergence of schistosomiasis, at least in hilly environments of Sichuan province and along the upper Yangtze River, is a growing concern (Wang et al., 2008).

Inequality is on the rise as the fruits of economic reforms have not been distributed evenly among the population. As discussed previously, there is significant and widening inequality in health status between population groups, between poor and wealthy provinces and between and within urban and rural areas. China's national health achievements seem to have shifted from **punching above its weight** in the 1970s to unimpressive health advances by the 1990s (Tang et al., 2008).

GLOSSARY

Punching above its weight: better health than expected from the level of economic development (Baum et al., 2018).

The Chinese government still pledges its commitment to the health of its people and is still mobilising the apparatus of the State to maintain the relatively good health status. It is now increasingly counting on acute health care delivered by conventionally trained formal health care workers. However, China has an acute shortage of health care professionals, with the majority concentrated in provincial urban centres rather than in rural areas.

According to the China Health Statistics Almanac and World Health Statistics, the following were estimates of health care professionals in China (Wu et al., 2016):

- In 2012, 0.43 paediatricians per 1000 children (shortfall of at least 200 000).
- In 2013, 2.05 nurses per 1000 population.
- In 2014, 0.2 psychiatrists per 1000 population (shortfall of at least 40 000).
- In 2015, 0.14 general practitioners per 1000 population (shortfall of at least 161 000).

In 2009, the Chinese government committed to an ambitious health care reform programme, which included universal basic health care coverage for all by 2020. These reforms included: the introduction of a new primary care system as the first encounter with patients, improving the quality of care in all public hospitals; expanding the number of hospitals, clinics, doctors and nurses; and deepening the coverage of the three main health insurance schemes—Urban Employee Basic Medical Scheme, Urban Resident Basic Medical Insurance and New Rural Cooperative Medical Scheme (Jarvis, 2016). The intention was also to resolve public mistrust towards health care providers.

Although much has changed in China, it still has some of the characteristics of the earlier revolutionary period, and the way the whole population was mobilised to combat the disease is still one of them. At the end of February 2020, Dr Bruce Aylward, a senior advisor to the WHO director-general, accompanied an international group of scientists on a mission to learn about the way the outbreak of the Coronavirus disease was handled in Wuhan, China. In their report, the scientists observe that achieving China's exceptional coverage with and adherence to the containment measures had only been possible:

due to the deep commitment of the Chinese people to collective action in the face of this common threat. At a community level this is reflected in the remarkable solidarity of provinces and cities in support of the most vulnerable populations and communities (WHO, 2020).

In an interview, Aylward explained why he was impressed:

> *Nobody was complaining that 'Wuhan got us into this'. Instead, there was this tre-*
> *mendous sense of, 'We've got to help Wuhan'. Other provinces sent 40 000 medical*
> *workers, many of whom volunteered. A lot of civil servants were given new tasks. Road*
> *workers were taking temperatures, distributing food or tracing patients' contacts. I saw*
> *a woman explain how to put on sterile clothing in a hospital. I asked her if she was*
> *the infection control expert. She replied she was the receptionist, but had taken training*
> (McNeil, 2020).

Nonetheless, there are reports of autocratic responses, and some of the outbreak control methods used are hardly imaginable in other countries. However, China's initial response to the COVID-19 pandemic compares well with that of many other countries, including the USA and UK (see Figure 7.7). They managed to control the first outbreak reasonably rapidly and then deal with subsequent outbreaks. The Chinese model has gone through enormous changes and remains a system in transition.

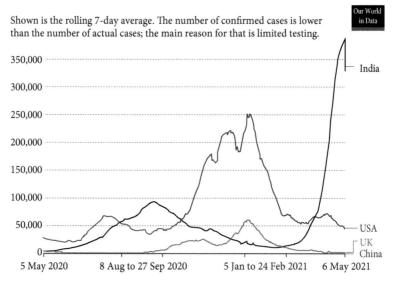

Fig. 7.7 Daily new confirmed COVID-19 cases per million people (USA, UK, India and China), May 5, 2020 to May 6, 2021 (relative to population).
Source: Roser & Ortiz-Ospina. (2021).

Health promotion: the Cuban experience

Cuba has seen a similar evolution to that of China, with spectacular improvements in health in a short span of time. The Cuban Revolution began in 1953 and continued until the end of 1958. When Fidel Castro's revolutionary government was finally installed in power in 1959, health in Cuba was characterised by high rates of infant mortality (138 per 1000 live births) and maternal mortality (70 per 100 000 live births) (Santana Espinosa et al., 2018). This was due to, for example, high illiteracy rates, racial and gender discrimination, limited access to health services and inadequate health infrastructure. Causes of infant death were acute diarrhoeal and respiratory diseases, malnutrition and perinatal conditions; causes of maternal deaths were from lack of attention to complications of childbirth and abortion, and hypertensive disease of pregnancy. Only 10% of the child population received paediatric care and less than 60% of births took place in health institutions (Santana Espinosa et al., 2018).

In the 1960s, the Cuban government enlisted 750 physicians and medical students for a period of their professional lives to work in the mountains and coastal communities. The aim of *el servicio médico rural* or the Rural Medical Service was to provide *"disease prevention and to revitalize health services for those most in need, whether because they are poor, in precarious health or live far from urban centres"* (WHO, 2008b).

An immunisation programme to cover the whole population was established within a few years of liberation. By 1962, 80% of all Cuban children under 15 years of age (over 2 million children) were immunised against poliomyelitis in 11 days. In 1969, a similar task was accomplished in just 72 hours, and in 1970 it was completed in only 1 day (Navarro, 1972).

Figure 7.8 shows how quickly vital health indicators, like infant mortality and child mortality, improved. Infant mortality almost halved by 1970. With further actions implemented over the next five decades, favourable maternal and child health indicators have been achieved, despite economic and resource limitations.

In 2015, the decrease in infant and under-five mortality rates to 4.3 and 5.7 per 1000 live births respectively is noteworthy. These statistics place Cuba, along with Canada, as the countries with the lowest figures in the region of the Americas. In 2015, 99.4% of children survived to age five (and beyond) (Santana Espinosa et al., 2018).

Community-based polyclinic

Cuban health authorities credit the country's impressive health indicators to the preventive, primary-care focus that has been pursued since the 1960s. The backbone of the Cuban health system is the community-based multispeciality polyclinics that were established across Cuba in the 1970s and which gave people local access to primary care specialists.

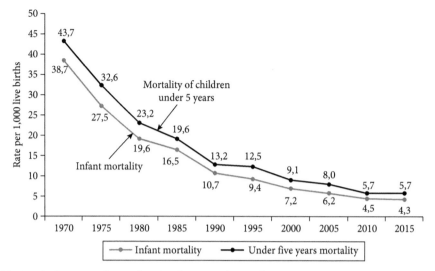

Fig. 7.8 Infant mortality and under-five mortality, Cuba, 1970–2015.
Source: Santana Espinosa et al. (2018).

In the mid-1980s, family doctor-and-nurse programmes were added to the clinics, which enhanced the health system's capacity to provide promotive, preventive and community-health analysis, as well as curative and rehabilitative services. The polyclinics act as an organisational hub for family doctor-and-nurse practices, with the doctor or nurse living in the community. By the 1990s, family doctor-and-nurse practices were servicing more than 95% of the population. According to Yaffe (2020), in 2005 Cuba had:

- One doctor for every 167 people—the highest ratio in the world.
- 449 polyclinics nationwide, serving a catchment area of between 20 000 and 40 000 people.
- Each polyclinic acts as an organisational hub for 15–40 community-based family doctor-and-nurse offices.
- Each polyclinic acts as an accredited research and teaching centre for medical, nursing and allied health sciences students.

The average polyclinic offers 22 services, including rehabilitation, X-ray, ultrasound, optometry, endoscopy, thrombolysis, emergency services, traumatology, clinical laboratory, family planning, emergency dentistry, maternal–child care, immunisation, and diabetic and older people care. Various other specialties—including dermatology, psychiatry and cardiology—are available too, in addition to family and internal medicine, paediatrics, and obstetrics and gynaecology.

CASE STUDY: Cuba—progressive medical education stressing PHC and international and community solidarity

In 1959, Cuba had about 6000 doctors—50% of them left soon after the revolution; there were only 12 Cuban lecturers at the University of Havana's Medical School; and there was one rural hospital (Yaffe, 2020). Medical education in Cuba underwent a radical transformation after the 1959 revolution (Keck & Reed, 2012). Since then, it has emphasised PHC, an interdisciplinary approach, strong community participation, an internationalist focus and a health workforce of sufficient size and skills to meet population needs.

The training of health professionals stresses practical experience so that a lot of the training is in rural polyclinics as part of a primary care team. Moreover, the values of the health workforce include solidarity with poor and disadvantaged communities and a willingness to serve in a variety of challenging settings. Cuban medical education also differs from conventional models by providing graduates with a wider skill set: caregiver; decision-maker; communicator; manager; community leader; and teacher (Sui et al., 2019).

These skills and values mean that Cuban medical graduates are well prepared to practise in poor and under resourced communities and to challenge the nexus between medicine and private fee-for-service practice.

Specialisation in family medicine is a requirement for more than 97% of medical graduates, who spend one internship year and two residency years in training after they receive their degrees. Later, they can apply for a residency in a second specialty. As a result, the ranks in these second specialties are being swelled by physicians who started their careers in family medicine.

Perhaps most importantly, Cuba has achieved impressive improvements in population health, helped by the reforms to medical education (Cooper et al., 2006). Box 7.1 lists the accomplishments in public health achieved by the Cuban health system since the early 1960s until the present (estimates for 2021).

In 1998, Hurricanes George and Mitch caused massive destruction in the region and resulted in 11 000 deaths. In the following year, Cuba established the international medical school, *Escuela Latinoamericana de Medicina* (ELAM)—Latin American School of Medicine (LASM). The aim was to provide medical training to students from the poorest communities who intended returning to practice in those communities. Initially places were offered to students from hurricane-affected countries, but subsequently this was broadened to include students from poor communities in many countries, including from the USA and Africa.

ELAM's mission is to train students to become competent and cooperative doctors who have the same MD (Doctor of Medicine) degree common to medical graduates throughout the Americas. The school is officially recognised by the Educational Commission for Foreign Medical Graduates (ECFMG) and the WHO. It is fully accredited by the Medical Board of California, which has the strictest US

Box 7.1 Indicators of Cuba's accomplishments in public health

First country to eliminate polio—1962

First country to eliminate measles—1996

Life expectancy at birth: 79.41 years—estimate 2021

Death rate: 9.22 deaths per 1000 population—estimate 2021

Infant mortality rate: 4.19 deaths per 1000—estimate 2021

Maternal mortality rate: 36 deaths per 100 000 live births—2017

32 000 people living with HIV/AIDS—2019

Reduction in cardiovascular mortality rate by 45%—2002

Comprehensive health care: 8.42 physicians per 1000 population—2018

Hospital bed density: 5.3 beds per 1000 population—2017

Support of 34 000 health professionals in 52 poor countries

Creation of a national biomedical internet grid (*INFOMED*): network of people and institutions that collaborate to facilitate access to information and knowledge, to improve the health of Cubans and the peoples of the world—established 1992

Source: Adapted from Cooper et al. (2006) and CIA. (2021).

standards. This means that qualified US graduates of LASM are eligible to apply for residency placements in any state of the USA (Keck & Reed, 2012).

The Cuban model is an important example of how models of western medical education can be challenged. A South African study found that graduates from ELAM had stronger intentions than those trained in South Africa to work in rural and underserved communities from which many of them are drawn (Sui et al., 2019).

Cuba developed its own biopharmaceutical and biotechnology sector, which grew out of the need to develop its own vaccine-production capability to circumvent the US embargo which has been in effect since 1959. Public health efforts were coupled with scientific research and the sector is now a source of substantial foreign earnings. For example, Cuba and Brazil cooperated on the production of millions of doses of meningococcal vaccine (A and C) that was prequalified by the WHO for the benefit of those in need (Devi, 2014). And in 2021, Cuba had developed four anti-COVID candidate vaccines which were in different phases of clinical trials (Bergues, 2021) and in April 2021 were looking very promising (Mega, 2021).

Cuba's recommitment to health: 2019

In 2019, the Cuban Constitution was amended to expand people's social, political and economic rights and to extend the right to free, quality, universal public health care for all Cubans. The State recognises its responsibility to protect older people and to realise people's rights to dignified housing, public health, water and food. An important inclusion was the inclusion of amendments to *"promote the conservation of the environment and the fight against climate change, which threatens the survival of the human species"* (*The Lancet*, 2019).

Non-communicable diseases present the biggest health threat to the nation. In 2016, the mortality rate due to chronic non-communicable diseases (NCDs) was 731.4 per 100 000, with heart disease and cancer being the highest (217.7 and 216.3 per 100 000 respectively). These causes together accounted for 49.1% of all deaths in 2016 (Acosta, 2017).

The spectre of communicable diseases also still casts a shadow in Cuba. However, according to the WHO (2021), in 2019:

- 76% of people living with HIV were receiving ART.
- 71% of people living with TB had effective treatment coverage.
- 99% of people had been immunised against measles.
- 99% of one-year-olds had been immunised against Hib (Haemophilus influenza).

In addition, there was 97.8% antenatal care coverage (at least four visits); 92.81% of the population were using at least basic sanitation services; and 44.34% were using safely managed sanitation services (WHO, 2021).

Rapid response to COVID-19
Cuba's rapid response to the spread of COVID-19 received immense praise from the WHO and the Pan American Health Organization (PAHO). A COVID-19 Prevention and Control Plan was primarily led by the primary care network and family-doctor practices and included effective measures to protect the population—quarantines, isolation facilities, dissemination of accurate and clear information to all households through mass organisation, and the increase in production of food for citizens, making food accessible. Treatment for COVID-19 (like all health care) is free. As of March 2021, there have been 55 693 cases of COVID-19 reported and 348 deaths (Burki, 2021). Of significance has been the public's confidence in the government's science-based policies (evident too in its campaigns against HIV, Ebola, dengue fever and the Zika virus), its history of multipronged public service messaging and volunteerism (Hosek, 2021).

Cuba's massive healthcare achievements during the COVID-19 pandemic were not the result of chance, but of a socialist government committed at every level to preventative care and community participation (Wilson, 2021).

Cuba responded to the call from at least 14 countries, including Italy and South Africa, for assistance during the COVID-19 crisis. The arrival of Cuban doctors in northern Italy during the worst days of the first pandemic wave in 2020 was a highly symbolic—and shocking for some—event.

The lessons of China and Cuba

The questions we must ask ourselves after examining the Cuban and Chinese experiences in rapid health improvements are:

- Was the impressive expansion of PHC in both countries responsible for the unparalleled advances in the health of the population?
- Can, for example, the barefoot doctor experience be isolated from the social process in which it evolved and, by implication, be successfully transplanted in societies whose political and economic situations are quite different?

The answer to the first question has already been implied, as the improved health of the Chinese and Cuban population largely predated the widespread increase in PHC facilities. As to the second question, the underlying answer rests in the fundamental change in the organisation of the economy, from one based on individual production for private profit—much of which was appropriated by foreign exploiters—to an economy predominantly based on collective production for social need. Thus, the health care systems were largely financed by the government whose goal was to provide a free service for everyone.

In both Cuba and China, the revolution was the result of long years of struggle involving large numbers of workers and peasants. But in neither case was the seizure of power followed by a people's paradise and certainly not everything that followed in those countries was in the people's interest. Despite any criticisms that can be made, the achievements regarding the people's health status are a fact and make a difference to more than 1 billion people every day.

Both Cuba and China are countries that developed models different to those in the dominant capitalist societies, although they have been criticised for being undemocratic. But undeniably, both countries did and still do display elements of democratic participation, at least at the grassroots level. This participation is important because it was the tool that was used to break the power of the health professionals. It enabled the previously powerless majority to select responsive PHC workers and make them accountable to the community. It also ensured that popular health concerns rather than professional competitiveness influenced the type of training and research carried out in the health sector. While concern has been expressed that the Cuban system may be too reliant on medical knowledge (Werner, 1977), its performance and that of China in the COVID-19 pandemic have been much more impressive than that of countries with populist capitalist government, including the USA, Brazil, India and the Philippines.

Attempts to transplant the barefoot doctor experience into other countries have been largely unsuccessful. The economic resources are not there to sustain such services beyond some relatively small experiments. There is no grassroots democracy, so the barefoot doctor cannot be selected by the community or be answerable to it. A democratised health sector depends on fundamental social change such as that seen in China and Cuba.

Should the concerned health worker therefore abandon health work and become immersed solely in the politics of progressive social change? Clearly this is one possible approach. Indeed, there are several examples of concerned health workers who, after recognising the roots of ill-health, saw their primary roles as agents of social change. Such people include the late presidents of Angola and Chile, Neto and Allende, the Argentinian revolutionary Che Guevara, the Martinican psychiatrist Fanon and President Machel of Mozambique. All were qualified health workers.

In his *Reminiscence of the Cuban Revolutionary War*, Che Guevara recalls the choice facing the socialist health worker. In the first days of the war, the embryonic revolutionary army was ambushed by government troops:

> *This might have been the first time I was faced, literally, with the dilemma of choosing between my devotion to medicine and my duty as a revolutionary soldier. There, at my feet, was a backpack full of medicine and a box of ammunition. They were too heavy to carry both. I picked up the ammunition, leaving the medicine, and started to cross the clearing, heading for the cane field* (Che Guevara, 1969).

But for most of us, partly because of our own class backgrounds and social experience, the understanding and the commitment for such a role is absent. Also, some health workers would reasonably argue that their skills gained from lengthy and expensive training should not be wasted, but should be applied in the most useful way to prevent and cure disease and to ease suffering.

Is there a way of ensuring the more effective performance of useful and necessary medical interventions and *also* assisting in creating the conditions for the promotion of health? In other words, is there a way of both providing effective health care and stimulating within the health sector the growth of popular pressure which could contribute to a movement for progressive social change? This must start with health care workers broadening their focus from a narrow clinical approach to one that understands the social and political determinants of ill-health and the need for community participation and activism.

Changing the medical contribution

The present form of the medical contribution in former colonies and in the countries that dominated them has been determined by the influences of the medical profession, business interests and the State, influences that have been overwhelmingly more dominant than that of the people.

Clearly it is necessary to devise some way of changing this relationship of influences as part of a process of decolonisation. If health promotion is the object, then it is important that such an initiative be part of a wider process aimed at stimulating progressive social change. The essential character of the medical contribution will only be changed when the present economic and political system is transformed. But changes in the balance of power within the health sector—reforms—can help spread popular pressure for thorough-going social transformation. Increasing the power of people (i.e. non-professionals) within the health sector is a necessary part of a struggle for popular control of all areas of society.

Possible general approaches in the health sectors in both rich and poor countries include: weakening the monopoly control of the medical profession over medical knowledge, which allows it to maintain control over health care; fighting for democratic control over health care by representatives of the majority of the people rather than appointees of the State or those sponsored by medical and pharmaceutical transnational operations; and limiting the excesses of medical and pharmaceutical business interests by exposing their operations to the scrutiny of the public.

How can health workers do this, while at the same time contribute to the caring and medically useful functions for which they have been trained?

The community health worker—a possible link?[2]

The high cost of training doctors and the need for improved coverage by official health services was the motivation for the creation of the 'auxiliary worker'. Task shifting became the catch phrase in low-income countries—because of shortage of medical personnel, informally trained health workers perform tasks that are usually performed by formally trained health workers. The problem is that these people often also copy the behaviour of these professionals, become detached from the communities they are supposed to serve and move upwards in the medical hierarchy or just drop out altogether.

Partly as a result of this disappointment and as a response to the success of the barefoot doctor in China and experiences with CHWs in other countries, Lehmann and Sanders (2007), in a publication for the WHO, summed up the characteristics of the CHWs as follows:

- They should be selected by the people from among themselves and should be responsible primarily to them, not to the health professionals.
- They should work part-time so that they can subsist by performing agricultural or other work, possibly receiving a subsidy from either the local community or the national health service.
- They should ideally be people who have been in a health care role, for example as a traditional healer or birth attendant, and should preferably be trained in the community in not only curative but also preventive and promotive functions.

The umbrella term 'community health worker' embraces a variety of community health aides selected, trained and working in the communities from which they come. A widely accepted definition was proposed by a WHO Study Group:

Community health workers should be members of the communities where they work, should be selected by the communities, should be answerable to the communities for their activities, should be supported by the health system but not necessarily a part of its organization, and have shorter training than professional workers (WHO, 2016).

---

[2] Much of this section is drawn from Lehmann, U. & Sanders, D. (2007). *Community Health Workers: What Do We Know About Them?* WHO: Geneva.

Internationally, CHWs have many different titles. Early literature, from before the Alma-Ata Declaration, mentions village health workers (VHWs) who were not only (and possibly not even primarily) health care providers, but also advocates for the community and agents of social change. They functioned as the community mouthpiece to fight against inequities and advocate community rights and needs to government structures.

There is also great variation in the programmes and context within which CHWs work. Some work in large national programmes, such as, most prominently, the Chinese barefoot doctor programme, but also in programmes in India, Indonesia and a number of Latin American and African countries. Tanzania's and Zimbabwe's VHW programmes in their early phase, for example, were set in the political context of wholesale systemic transformation (decolonisation and the Ujamaa movement in Tanzania and the liberation struggle in Zimbabwe), and both focused on self-reliance, rural development and the eradication of poverty and societal inequities (see the case study on Zimbabwe that follows). There are also innumerable smaller programmes run by NGOs, faith-based organisations (FBOs) and community-based organisations (CBOs) within which CHWs work. In the famous words of David Werner, a pioneer of village health care in the Americas, the VHW (or CHW) is a 'liberator' rather than a 'lackey' (Werner, 1977). This view is reflected in the Alma-Ata Declaration, which identified CHWs as one of the cornerstones of Comprehensive Primary Health Care (CPHC).

With the economic recession of the 1980s, together with the spread of neoliberal ideology and policies across the globe, the economies of underdeveloped countries particularly were seriously jeopardised and this brought shifts in their policy environments. The focus on liberation, decolonisation, democratisation, self-reliance and the 'basic needs' approach to development was replaced by World Bank-driven policies of structural adjustment and its successors. CHW programmes were the first to fall victim to new economic stringencies. Most large-scale, national programmes collapsed (although numerous NGOs and FBOs continued to invest in mostly small, community-based health care). (See Chapter 5 for more information on health policies and health care in the context of neoliberal globalisation.)

The collapse was further facilitated by the fact that many large-scale programmes had suffered from conceptual and implementation problems, such as unrealistic expectations, poor initial planning, overloading with too many tasks from different stakeholders, problems of sustainability and the difficulties of maintaining quality. While many policy-makers turned their attention away from CHWs altogether, others, wanting to rescue the concept and practice, suggested subtle shifts.

In 2018, at the occasion of the 40th anniversary of the Alma-Ata Declaration, the WHO developed a *Guideline on Health Policy and System Support to Optimize Community Health Worker Programmes*. This Guideline borrowed the official definition of CHWs from the International Labour Organization's (ILO) International Standard Classification of Occupations (ISCO):

Community health workers provide health education and referrals for a wide range of services, and provide support and assistance to communities, families and individuals with preventive health measures and gaining access to appropriate curative health and social services. They create a bridge between providers of health, social and community services and communities that may have difficulty in accessing these services (ILO, 2012).

Although this concept of CHWs continues to focus on their role in community development and bridging the gap between communities and formal health services, their role as advocates for social change has been replaced by a predominantly technical and community management function. Over the years, and within the prevailing political climate, this pragmatic approach to CHWs has gained currency and undoubtedly today constitutes the dominant approach, although the fundamental tension between their roles as extension workers and change agents remains.

CASE STUDY: Zimbabwe's CPHC Approach of the 1980s[3]

Zimbabwe achieved independence from Britain in 1980, after a protracted liberation war fought by the Black majority against White minority rule. While chronic food problems from historical inequities in land tenure and income distribution had already existed for many years, they worsened dramatically during and after the war due to the destruction of agricultural resources by the old regime and the return of refugees. Extreme income inequality inherited from a century of British colonialism was evident in the wide inequities in people's health. The maldistribution of facilities was matched by a concentration of health personnel, especially professionals, in urban areas. Even the distribution of health care auxiliaries was disproportionately urban.

Zimbabwe's independence saw the ushering in of a PHC approach designed to reduce these inequities, a central feature of this being community participation. The unfolding relationship before and after political independence between the state and the developing institutions of popular organisation is central to understanding the process of community participation in all areas of social development, including health. It is in situations where the old order and power structures are overthrown that CPHC has the best chance of succeeding. It is under such conditions that popular participation in decision-making and collective—rather than individual—self-reliance can grow and flourish. This was the case in Zimbabwe in the 1980s, as it was in revolutionary China and Cuba.

This situation was most evident in the liberated areas where ZANU (PF), the leading party in the national liberation movement, had created popular organisations made up of various tiers of people's councils, set up on village, ward, district and provincial bases. They were initially responsible for supporting the liberation effort, but later structured to perform essential social and economic tasks. Grassroots village committees, for example, dealt with the day-to-day issues of providing basic services to the community, while matters involving larger outlays of money were passed to higher-level committees.

---

[3] This case study has drawn on Sanders (1992), and Werner and Sanders (1997).

Bondolfi VHWs

During a 1980 ceasefire, a health worker at Bondolfi Mission (in Masvingo district) was asked by the District Committee of ZANU (PF) to train popularly elected health workers in nutrition, childcare, hygiene, sanitation and some home treatment. The area was well organised into one political district with 28 branches. Each branch had a committee of 16, who were popularly elected. Of these, two were responsible for community health matters. A six months' training course commenced for 56 branch leaders in May 1980. It included theory and practice—the latter done after planning with their communities. Due to the project's popularity and increasing community demand, the communities decided to have an unpaid VHW for every one to three villages. This resulted in the selection and training of 293 VHWs, 35 of whom were from other districts.

Government VHWs

In late 1981, the government began their own training of VHWs, who were supposed to be selected by their communities in consultation with the District Council. In some areas, real popular involvement in the VHW selection existed at ward level. However, in many areas it was done by the District Council, and in yet others, individual councillors chose the VHWs. District Councils paid the VHWs from a grant received from central government. This meant that VHWs were responsible to the District Councils rather than the villagers they served.

When the government scheme was set up, 10 of the Bondolfi VHWs were taken on and trained. The training was more formal, with more time spent in the clinic or hospital. Because of their lower concentration in the population, government VHWs had to cover a considerably larger area than the Bondolfi VHWs. This meant that most of them were full-time workers. By mid-1984, although still functioning, the Bondolfi VHW scheme was down to about 100 workers. There were several reasons for this, but as one local VHW organiser said, "*When the government scheme started, and some were paid Z$33 a month, others stopped working because they were not paid.*"

Here a general political problem is illustrated. In contrast to the original VHWs, who were directly selected by meetings in the villages and answerable to the local people, the government VHWs were chosen and paid by the District Councils. Although these bodies were democratic this was only in a distant and representative way. If responsibility for the VHW is delegated to a remote state structure, then the crucial element of popular mobilisation is missing. The VHW is no longer directly answerable to the community and cannot be recalled by them. They become just another health service employee—more appropriate perhaps, but still answerable to an outside body.

A comprehensive approach to malnutrition within a PHC framework

To forestall an impending hunger crisis in the 1980–1981 planting season, the Ministry of Health and concerned NGOs developed a nutrition intervention programme. Provincial committees comprised of different levels of health workers, school teachers, community development workers and women's advisors were set up in high-risk areas. The intervention had three important objectives: immediate short-term relief; long-term nutritional education; and collective food production.

Immediate short-term relief: supplementary feeding (curative and rehabilitation)

The community-based administrative infrastructure that had developed during the war permitted a more rapid and better-organised implementation of the nutrition programme than would otherwise have been possible. Mothers were taught to use a Shakir strip to measure and record their children's upper-arm circumferences and evaluate their children's nutritional status. This is a good example of simple and appropriate technology that can be used by a community to assess a major health problem in their midst. Those children with mid-upper arm circumferences less than 13 cm were included in the programme (see Figure 7.9). The reasons for this cut-off point were explained to all parents. The mothers established the locations for the supplementary feeding schemes close to their homes and fields, and they cooked the food and fed the underweight children. The programme emphasised supplements prepared with high-energy, commonly used local foods. It offered a daily meal—based on maize, beans, groundnuts and oil—that provided a portion of the daily energy needs of children; the rest was provided by the parents or community.

The first feeding point was opened in January 1981 and at the peak of the drought helped to feed over 250 000 children. Subsequent droughts severely affected the programme and the nutritional status of all groups.

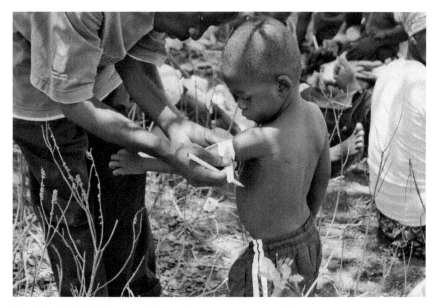

Fig. 7.9 A VHW checks a child's mid-upper arm circumference.
Source: USAID Zimbabwe.

Long-term nutritional education (prevention)

An informative poster in the local languages (and in English) was displayed and discussed at the feeding points and in health facilities. The poster helped to reinforce the message that high-energy foods that could be grown locally would provide a nutritious meal for young children if added to the staple maize and meal porridge (Sadza) (see Figure 7.10). In this way, the relief effort prompted greater self-reliance by affirming the value of locally cultivable foods.

Through community discussions, it was agreed that communal farming plots should be established to move the programme from relief and education to local production. The harvest from these plots would go to the pre-school centres. It was calculated that roughly 0.5 ha of land could yield enough groundnuts to provide seven children with 30 g of groundnuts each day, leaving 10% for seed for the following season. The land was taken from communal grazing lands that had been allocated by the local government authorities. The National Feeding Programme Committee provided the initial seed and fertiliser. Such community decisions were possible because the popular mobilisation during that period of Zimbabwe's history was significant in influencing both national and local development thinking and programmes.

By 1983–1984, there were 292 supplementary food production units in 31 districts. Unfortunately, because of severe and recurrent drought, most of these failed.

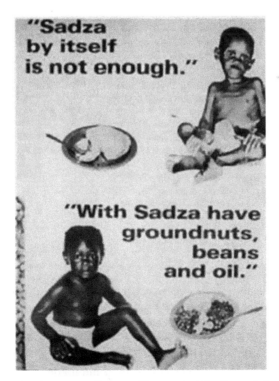

Fig. 7.10 Educational poster to discuss with parents at feeding points.

However, the existing infrastructure facilitated the rapid remounting of relief efforts in 1991 and 1992 when the worst drought once again hit southern Africa.

The expansion and reorganisation of health care in the 1980s also included: greatly improved coverage of immunisation against infectious diseases among children and tetanus among pregnant women; the rollout of a reliable local rehydration solution which VHWs (and hospitals) used and which they taught mothers to use; and the treatment of malaria and pneumonia. The rural–urban differential in antenatal care was significantly reduced; and Zimbabwe also attained the highest rate of contraceptive use in Sub-Saharan Africa.

What can we learn from the Zimbabwe case study?
The democratisation of health care also implies changing the ideology of health care, demystifying the causes of ill-health and giving people a vital role in resolving their own health problems. Initially, the central government of Zimbabwe helped to initiate an empowering, community-based health care programme providing preferential benefits to those with the greatest need. Strong community decisions were possible because the popular mobilisation during this period was successful in significantly influencing both national and local development thinking.

Unfortunately, by late 1981, the beginnings of bureaucratisation and the undermining of popular initiative started to emerge, when the government began its own training of VHWs. By 1988, this scheme was handed over to the Ministry of Community and Cooperative Development and Women's Affairs. VHWs and Home Economics demonstrators were combined into a single group of 'village community workers' who, although notionally part-time, had written conditions of service and were regarded as civil service employees.

The nature of the VHW (and the PHC approach) was qualitatively transformed. The possibility of true grassroots involvement in both defining health problems and tackling them collectively receded. Any possibility for popular democratic control of VHWs becoming a focus for democratisation at all levels of the health sector became remote. Most importantly, the larger question of social inequity and increasing economic hardship persist.

What is the primary role of the CHW?

There is a long and unresolved debate about the main role of CHWs and about how many functions or tasks one CHW can effectively perform, considering the potential scope of activities. Evaluation of some experiences found that while CHWs had been set up to be change agents in communities, they were actually functioning as extensions of formal health services—as auxiliaries rather than independent agents.

This finding highlights a key tension in the conceptualisation of CHWs in the post-Alma-Ata period. While developmental and educational activities are considered important, curative services are demanded by communities that do not have access to these services. There is substantial evidence in several countries that CHW programmes floundered due to disappointment among the community about the range of health services the CHWs could provide.

While in some programmes the lines between generalist and specialist CHWs are blurred, many programmes established since the 2000s make use of CHWs to address specific health issues. This is often, but not only, true for programmes run by NGOs, which frequently have a programme-specific focus. Specialisation may also be a response to the difficulty experienced in finding the optimal mix of CHW functions and tasks and the right balance between breadth and depth of tasks. The role of CHWs in child survival has always been a priority area. A 2007 review article on the potential role of CHWs in child survival in *The Lancet* concluded:

> *Although community health workers are not a panacea for weak health systems, the evidence base, despite limitations, does suggest they can have an important role in increasing coverage of essential interventions for child survival and other health priorities. Nearly 30 years after the Alma-Ata Declaration, the time is right to reassess the potential contribution of community health workers in accelerating coverage of essential interventions, particularly in poor and underserved communities* (Haines et al., 2007).

Community health worker (CHW) programmes

Selection of CHWs

Virtually every document discussing programmes involving CHW emphasises that they should be chosen from the communities they will serve; and that these communities should have a say in the selection of their CHWs. But while the practice of selecting CHWs from local communities is widely accepted and implemented, direct and meaningful participation of communities in the selection process is not. In some experiences it was found that as a rule, local bureaucrats, village chiefs, health professionals or other dignitaries held sway over who was selected. This is a common experience, as selection is often considered a form of patronage.

Whether and how communities are actually involved in selection processes will largely depend on issues of governance, forms and structures of broader community participation and the role of formal health services. The most common approach employed by organisations to initiate CHW selection has been the setting up of village or community health committees, which then are responsible for selecting CHW candidates.

Training of CHWs

Training is in many cases conducted by members of the formal health services, either doctors or nurses, or in the case of NGO-driven programmes, by the NGOs themselves. Approaches to training have changed over the years. While in the past, complaints about inappropriate training—which was too theoretical, classroom-based or complicated—were quite common, today competence-based approaches are usually used. The competencies that are achieved during training are also those that should be assessed during supervisory visits or follow-up, frequently with the checklists used during training.

Some programmes recommend that the training take place in the community rather than in health facilities to provide hands-on experience in the work environment of the CHW. In other contexts, training may take place in the facilities because there are more cases of sick children presenting within the training period, thus providing more opportunities for the trainer to demonstrate skills in a real-life situation and for CHWs to practise newly learned skills.

Because CHWs work within the constraints of the community and usually have limited formal education, programmes often develop or adapt training materials and activities specifically for CHWs, rather than use training packages developed for facility-based workers.

Supervision of CHWs

It is widely acknowledged that the success of CHW programmes hinges on regular and reliable support and supervision. It is equally acknowledged, however, that supervision is often among the weakest links in CHW programmes. Small-scale projects are often successful because they manage to establish effective support and supervisory mechanisms for CHWs, often including a significant amount of supervision and oversight by the community itself. National programmes are rarely able to achieve this consistently. There are several reasons for the lack or poor quality of supervision. Most importantly, however, the greatest need for supervision exists in the most remote areas, where health services are most overstretched and ill-equipped.

Community participation in CHW programmes

At the heart of debates around CHW programmes lie questions about who owns and governs these programmes and to whom CHWs are accountable. The literature is unanimous in its assertion that CHW programmes should be owned and driven by communities, and that CHWs should be accountable to their communities. Yet most articles also acknowledge that the reality of programmes often strays quite far from this ideal.

One would be hard-pressed to find an article that does not emphasise the importance of community participation for the success of CHW programmes. However, there is much less clarity about the exact meaning and purpose of community participation. It carries with it several different underlying philosophies and political agendas. In the early 1980s, a distinction was made between community participation as the mobilisation of community resources (people, money, materials) to carry out health programmes, and community participation as increasing people's control over the social, political, economic and environmental factors determining their health. This distinction reflected the Alma-Ata discourse. Today's debates are unlikely to make use of this discourse, although the tension it reflects undoubtedly still exists.

And while twenty-first-century discourse tends to be much more pragmatic and technical, it is nevertheless widely acknowledged that a considerable gulf exists between the ideal of programmes driven and owned by communities and programme realities. It is further agreed that while there are few success stories of lasting community participation, the sustainability and impact of programmes require the ownership and active participation of communities as a non-negotiable precondition.

This appears to be easier to achieve in small-scale programmes initiated within and by communities. There is also experience that active participation of communities in health and social action, including CHW programmes, is more likely to occur and be sustained in conditions of popular mobilisation, such as in the aftermath of a liberation struggle or after the replacement of military or repressive regimes by popular governments. In most of these cases, substantial and time-consuming investments were made in securing the participation of communities and involving communities in all aspects of the programme, including the identification of priorities and project planning. In other words, community mobilisation precedes and accompanies the establishment of CHW programmes. A policy brief summarises the experiences with a project in western Kenya:

> It seems, from the experience of both Kajulu and Nyakach, that the communities have realised the importance of being organised—or, rather, of organising themselves. Their ability to carry on with promoting awareness-raising activities, with training community health workers, with maintaining water supplies, with securing funds ... all these things depend on having the local committee structures that harness local leadership talents. And so, any community-based health care project should put great emphasis on building the capacities of those who volunteer to assist in the management of the various health care or health education initiatives (AKHS Kenya, Community Health Department, n.d.).

Evidence seems to suggest that problems arise when CHWs are expected to take responsibility for mobilising communities, rather than working with the support of already active communities.

Where community participation is institutionalised, it is usually through community or village health committees, known often by different names, which are charged with managing and guiding the work of CHWs. But these committees also play an ambiguous role within CHW initiatives. The position of the committees within community or village hierarchies is not always clear and is often contested, leading to tensions between committee members and other community leaders, becoming the site of political contestation.

Linkages with formal health services

The attitudes and interactions of health personnel in the formal health services with CHWs have an immediate impact on critical aspects of CHW programme management, such as selection, continuing training and supervision. Many health personnel lack the background and orientation to provide a supportive environment for CHW programmes. They are socialised into the hierarchical framework of disease-oriented medical care systems and have a poorly developed concept of PHC. Such paradigms are ill-suited to providing an environment supportive of partnerships and teamwork between different health workers, particularly if some categories are thought of as less important.

In Australia, Aboriginal Health Workers are an important part of the public health care system. A well-development training programme has provided a career path for these workers who are able to increase the cultural safety of the health services. They act as strong advocates for Aboriginal people within the health system and for a range of issues affecting their health including, for example, housing availability and alcohol licencing laws. They are most empowered when they are employed with an Aboriginal Community Controlled Health Service as these services are directly accountable to their communities (with elected boards of management).

Despite the proven value of CHWs, other health professionals often perceive them as lowly aides who should be deployed as assistants within health facilities, often completely misunderstanding their health promoting and enabling role within communities.

Although improving attitudes involves a complex process of educational and institutional reform, giving medical and health science students specific experience of working collaboratively can assist in developing positive attitudes towards CHWs.

CHWs around the world are making significant contributions to improving the health of their communities, yet often their efforts are undervalued, or they are seen as being in the margin of the health system. In most settings, most CHWs are women. This cadre of workers has been important in shifting a health system to a CPHC approach. They have direct links with local communities and can work in curative, rehabilitative, disease prevention and health promotion programmes. They promote genuine rather than tokenistic community participation. They are playing an important role in responding to the COVID-19 pandemic (Bhaumik et al., 2020).

In the case studies below, we examine the role of CHWs in large-scale state-led programmes in three countries—Ethiopia, India and Iran—to illustrate the ways in which they contribute to clinical care, prevention and addressing the impact of social and environmental determinants of health in daily life. The role of CHWs in each of these three countries is very different. These cases demonstrate how the broader context of the health system determines the extent to which CHWs can be liberators (rather than 'lackeys') who have the ability to organise their local community so that they are empowered to advocate for enough, appropriate, high-quality and accountable health services.

CASE STUDIES: Large-scale state-led CHW programmes

Ethiopia

The Health Extension Program (HEP), with a cadre of CHWs known as Health Extension Workers (HEWs), was launched in 2004 in Ethiopia to develop a community-based accelerated expansion of health facilities. HEWs receive basic health training to deliver a range of services across three main packages: Family Health; Disease Prevention and Control; and Hygiene and Environment (Mangham-Jefferies et al., 2014). They are credited with the dramatic progress Ethiopia has made in improving the health outcomes of its population, including the following:

- It accomplished the UN Millenium Development Goal (MDG)4 by reducing child deaths by 67%—from 204 per 1000 live births in 1990 to 59 per 1000 live births in 2012– three years ahead of schedule (Assefa et al., 2019).

- The maternal mortality ratio plummeted from 871 maternal deaths per 100 000 live births in 2000 to 353 per 100 000 in 2015, translating to about 12 000 maternal deaths a year (Banteyerga, 2011).
- There was also a vast improvement in hygiene and sanitation coverage, as well as a reduction in major communicable diseases (You et al., 2015).
- They might also have contributed to reducing the gender gap in life expectancy (Rieger et al., 2019; Baum et al., 2021).

The HEP is composed of a two-tiered CHW system (Leon et al., 2015). The first tier is made up of the lessor known or 'hidden' community/village level volunteers—known as the Health Development Army. The second tier is made up of formal, paid CHWs.

The Health Development Army usually come from and live in the community and they form the link between the community and health system, participate in village health committee structures, and are appreciated by their communities. They have a strong focus on health promotion and disease prevention, through raising community awareness, mobilising communities, facilitating community dialogue and promoting and demonstrating essential family practices, including long-lasting insecticidal nets, infant and young child feeding practices, proper hygiene and immunisation.

What can we learn from this case study?

- This case study shows that a CHW programme can be established and achieve results very quickly when there is political will to support it (Banteyerga, 2011).
- A systematic review in 2019 found that the HEP enabled Ethiopia to achieve significant improvements in maternal and child health, communicable diseases, hygiene and sanitation, knowledge and health care seeking, but noted that there was scope for more action on the social determinants of health (Assefa et al., 2019).
- With the increased momentum towards child survival goals in Sub-Saharan Africa, including Ethiopia, HEWs have increasingly focused on community treatment of malaria, pneumonia, and diarrhoea and acute malnutrition (collectively known as integrated community case management or ICCM), though evidence of the effectiveness of these programmes at scale remains inconclusive.
- Closser et al. (2019) question whether the volunteer scheme (Health Development Army), while having some benefits for the health system, results in women being taken away from their household tasks without any compensation and without gaining much power. We need a better understanding of the 'hidden' contribution of volunteers, what characterises their interaction with community-based and primary care services and how the volunteer system can be improved with the right type of investments.

India: Chhattisgarh State

The CHW programme of the Chhattisgarh state government in central India—where CHWs are known as *mitanins*—has demonstrated the following successes:

- National surveys show that over a 10-year period Chhattisgarh's rural infant mortality rate declined by 45% (from 95 per 1000 live births in 2000 to 52 per 1000 live births in 2010). This was at a greater rate than the decline nationally (31%) (Nandi & Schneider, 2014).
- Infant breastfeeding and anaemia in women and children showed greater improvements than the rest of India.
- A quasi-experimental evaluation of a nutrition intervention in Chhattisgarh suggests that the *mitanin* programme was responsible for 4.22% and 5.64% annual average reductions in underweight and stunting respectively—higher than the national averages (Vir et al., 2014).
- The programme has also been shown to be effective in addressing the social determinants of health (Nandi & Schneider, 2014).

Upper accountability and/or advocates for the community?

One of the dilemmas associated with CHWs is the question of whether they can act as change agents, enhancing the public accountability of government, despite being state-funded actors themselves. Inevitably there is a tension between their upward accountability through a health service bureaucracy and their role in working with their communities to enforce accountability from the health service.

The *mitanin* programme has developed a learning strategy that encourages *mitanins* to enable sustained action on public accountability, whilst also providing health services and education and linking communities with government health care services.

One example of how the *mitanin* programme has enabled them to function as strong advocates for their communities is their mobilisation of protest action around the felling of forests and logging and the disruptions this caused to local people and livelihoods (Nandi & Garg, 2017) (see Figure 7.11). This struggle meant opposing the state government and demonstrated the value of the importance of people's organisations and their struggles for natural resource justice and how the *mitanins* could support the struggle.

What can we learn from this case study?

The *mitanin* programme shows that a focus on iterative learning that is observant of and committed to managing the essential tensions that are inherent in the role of CHWs is the key for sustainable accountability. The programme enabled actors in state and civil society to design institutions and processes appropriate for accountability to emerge and be sustained.

Iran

Iranian CHWs, called *behvarzes* in Farsi, are local health workers with specialised training in the health needs of the rural population (Javanparast et al., 2011). They have been in existence for 40 years and are central to Iran's PHC strategy. *Behvarzes*

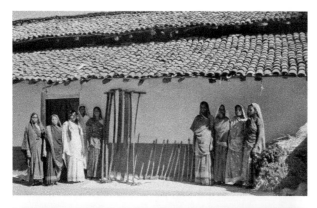

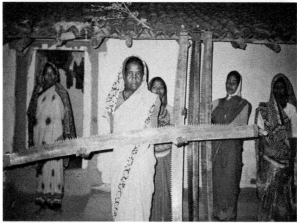

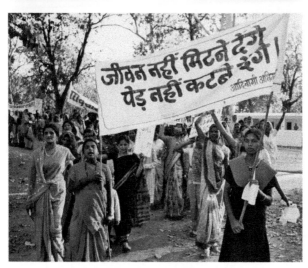

Fig. 7.11 *Mitanins'* forest struggle. On 9 January, about 100 women from three of the surrounding villages stormed the tree-felling site, captured the axes and saws and chased the labourers away. They challenged state action despite threats. The banner says: 'We will not let our lives to be destroyed, we will not let our trees to be felled.'

Source: Adivasi Adhikar Samiti, Chhattisgarh, India (translated as Indigenous Rights Organisation, Chhattisgarh, India).

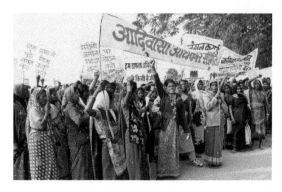

Fig. 7.11 *Mitanins'* forest struggle continued.

are selected from the rural areas where they live and are committed to reside in their area for at least four years after their training. Initially, *behvarzes* were mainly women. More recently, the recruitment of male *behvarzes* has increased and in many rural areas the village health houses from which they work (health delivery facilities) comprise one female and one male *behvarze*.

Behvarzes are permanent employees of and paid by the Iranian health system, which provides a structured and comprehensive two-year training. Their training has been credited with being a central part of improving rural health service provision and health of the rural population.

The tasks of the *behvarzes*

- Their principal role is health education followed by environmental health interventions that address basic determinants of health related to sanitation, potable water, road safety and other physical risks.
- Initially, the *behvarze* programme focused primarily on infectious diseases and maternal and child health; however, changing disease profiles have expanded the range of their responsibilities. An example of the expanded role is their attention to farmers' health and work safety.
- They also contribute to keeping a record of the profile of rural households related to the health house from which they work.
- They attend social events in the rural area and consult with religious leaders and other trusted people.

A study undertaken by Javanparast et al. (2011) showed that *behvarzes* strongly believe that they are crucial in building relationships with members of their rural community and improving programme effectiveness by encouraging people to attend the health house. The study, however, reported that there was room for improving their supervision and recognition of the importance of their role.

What can we learn from this case study?

The *behvarze* programme is firmly embedded in state structures and they do not play a role in ensuring accountability, as the *mitanins* do. This highlights the fact that health systems reflect the broader political context in which they exist. Given the differences in the political context, it is not surprising that *behvarzes* do not have the scope for advocacy on environmental and social issues and for holding the health system accountable to their communities.

What can we learn from all three case studies?
All three case studies demonstrate that CHWs can be liberators in terms of improving the health of their communities, but only the Indian *mitanins* were able to be liberators in addressing broader issues of accountability and fighting for improved environmental and living conditions. To do this type of work CHWs need to be well supported and their work valued by the rest of the health system.

Effectiveness of CHWs in improving health outcomes

Recent interest in CHW programmes focus unilaterally on the effectiveness of CHWs in contributing to improved health outcomes. For example, a research review undertaken by Lu et al. (2020) of 114 low- and middle-income countries that receive aid from various international donors for health purposes showed that:

- CHWs could reduce maternal mortality by 42%–78%.
- Under-five mortality could be reduced by 13%–60% when CHWs prescribe antibiotics for treatment of pneumonia (one of the leading causes of mortality among infants and children younger than five years).
- The long-term impacts of CHWs on social and economic development, including empowering women and increasing jobs, especially in remote poor and rural areas, could result in a positive economic return.
- There is global consensus that CHWs are essential for efforts to achieve the 2030 health-related Sustainable Development Goal (SDG) targets, including the achievement of universal health coverage (WHO, 2020).
- CHWs have played a major role in many countries during the COVID-19 pandemic. In South Africa, for example, they have provided community education, home caring and COVID-19 testing, and have facilitated discussions to address vaccine hesitancy (Peretz, Islam & Matiz, 2020). Unfortunately, they have often been given more tasks with no increase in numbers or remuneration, and there has been insufficient attention in providing them with personal protective equipment (PPE) or enabling them to be in the frontline for vaccination (Mpulo & Mafuma, 2020).

Effectiveness of CHWs as agents of change

Interestingly, since 2000, there has been relatively little interest in the potential of CHWs to empower communities. Equipping CHWs with curative skills does not simply provide health care to more people, more quickly and more cheaply, but also gives CHWs greater credibility in the eyes of the community and enables culturally safe health care. In addition, if through education and the use of appropriate technologies CHWs can equip members of the community with both an understanding of and skills in health care, then the medical profession's monopoly of knowledge and expertise is challenged. The power of the doctor, often based on mystification, can in this way be weakened. And, if certain appropriate health technologies become widely incorporated into health practice, their use can stimulate a critical approach to the expanding range of inappropriately sophisticated, expensive and mystifying technologies. Perhaps the best example is that of pharmaceuticals. Encouragement of the use of a standardised, short list of inexpensive drugs (known by a generic rather than trade name) can reduce inappropriate prescribing practices and begin to undermine the power of the pharmaceutical industry.

Possibly the most important potential of CHWs is their ability to stimulate the growth of a movement for progressive social change. David Werner put it thus:

If the village health worker is taught a respectable range of skills, if he [sic] is encouraged to think, to take initiative and to keep learning … if his judgement is respected, if his limits are determined by what he knows and can do, if his supervision is supportive and educational, chances are he will work with energy and dedication, will make a major contribution to his community and will win his people's confidence and love. His example will serve as a role model to his neighbors, that they too can learn new skills and assume new responsibilities, that self-improvement is possible. Thus the village health worker becomes an internal agent-of-change, not only for health care, but for the awakening of his people to their human potential … and ultimately to their human rights (Werner, 1977).

The special qualifications of CHWs to play the role as an agent of social change derives from two sources, both equally important:

- Through the mechanisms of selection and payment, CHWs are more likely to truly represent the people they serve, rather than the medical profession or the State.
- CHWs can endorse people's ideas that the sources of their ill-health are rooted in their living and working conditions. For, contrary to many misguided assumptions, sociologists have established that villagers do know that disease is caused by food (or its lack), bad sanitation and hygiene, poor water supplies, excessive work and bodily weakness. If CHWs are regarded by the community as their representatives and respected for their responsiveness and health care capabilities, their effect in confirming the community's understanding of the sources of its ill-health has a powerful potential.

Although the assessment of experiences with CHWs has been encouraging and has forced the WHO to keep CHW programmes on the agenda, enthusiasm for CHW programmes is lukewarm at best. Research on aid disbursed to projects that supported CHWs between 2007 and 2017 revealed that development assistance for these projects accounted for less than 3% of total development assistance for health during the 10-year period, with a decrease in the latter half of this period. It accounted for a meagre 1.27% of total development assistance for health in 2017 (WHO, 2020). And even then, the most liberating and empowering potential of CHW programmes has hardly been unleashed. Would that mean that the aid industry is actually afraid of the potential of CHWs to truly empower local communities in low- and middle-income countries?

Engaging CHWs in the COVID-19 response

In 2020, the WHO established the Independent Panel for Pandemic Preparedness and Response, with a mandate to undertake an impartial and independent review of the WHO-coordinated health response to the COVID-19 global pandemic. The aim was to provide evidence-based recommendations to effectively address future health threats, regionally, nationally and globally.

In May 2021, the Independent Panel presented its findings in the report *COVID-19: Make it the Last Pandemic*. A key finding was that those countries that most successfully managed the pandemic established partnerships across governmental departments, NGOs, CHWs, community leaders and the private sector.

> *Community responses and local engagement have been vital resources in the response. Where community structures, such as cadres of community health workers, have been mobilized, they have made a critical difference in establishing trust in government instructions, extending services, and in relaying scientific information* (Independent Panel for Pandemic Preparedness and Response, 2021).

The People's Health Movement

The need for a global People's Health Movement[4]

While the CHW programmes have held promise as a means for organised communities to establish control over their collective and individual health, their relative powerless status against the considerable might of organised medicine and corporate interests in health services means that more is needed. The best hope for extending community and citizen control over health services and the factors that create health is an empowered social movement (see Figure 7.12).

In the decades since the first edition of this book, the power of capital to undermine health has been extended through mechanisms such as trade agreements, widespread privatisation of public services, including health services, deregulation and massive tax evasion which robs public budgets of income. This situation has meant that civil society activism for health must focus more and more on the political and economic structural causes of inequities. This also means that as neoliberalism has intensified, the role of social movements in influencing global policies has been increasingly important, strengthened by the development of global networks and campaigns. Notable successes have included improved mechanisms for debt reduction in low-income

---

[4] Much of this section is taken from Bodini, C. (ed.). (2020). *Building a movement for health*. People's Health Movement (PHM) and Viva Salud. https://issuu.com/m3m-g3w/docs/movement_buildingen.

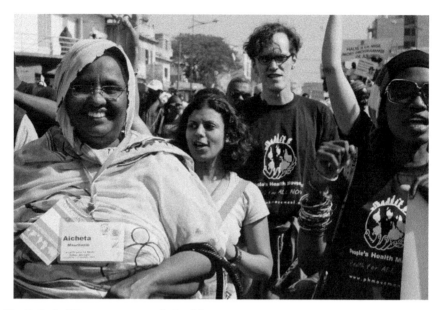

Fig. 7.12 Building a movement for health.
Source: Wim De Ceukelaire—Viva Salud.

countries, blocking the proposed Multilateral Agreement on Investment (MAI), the Doha Ministerial Declaration on Access to Essential Medicines and blocking agreements at WTO Ministerial meetings in Seattle and Cancún. The ongoing international campaign to stop new free trade agreements, such as the Transatlantic Trade and Investment Partnership (TTIP), which can block national measures to improve health, such as tobacco control and access to affordable medicines, has won significant battles, especially to increase transparency in negotiations. (Read more about some of these agreements in Chapter 5.)

However, at best, all these successes have been only able to limit the damage. For example, successes have tried to prevent decisions being taken that would make the situation worse (e.g. MAI, WTO Ministerial meetings and the TTIP); limit the impact of previous adverse decisions (e.g. TRIPS); or in the case of debt, limit the side-effects of the prevailing model of economic structural adjustment, which had already caused devastating health impacts in many underdeveloped countries. Where decisions have successfully been blocked, this has often been temporary. Nonetheless, public interest civil society has a key role to play as a driver of change.

Among the most important priorities for civil society activism is the democratic reform of global economic governance. This includes current reform and better regulation of the global financial system; rejecting austerity measures; implementing a much more progressive taxation system; closing tax havens; supporting a global taxation system; challenging the idea that the current model of growth is indispensable; and reclaiming public space for people's effective participation. Unless and until global governance structures change quite radically, civil society efforts on other issues will inevitably remain limited to damage control, and at best be partially successful.

A global movement to address global economic systems and power structures

The idea of changing our economic system and the underlying power structures that support it can seem like an impossible dream. But the current situation was not given by the laws of nature. Instead, it was created and continues to be shaped by human beings. As such, we can change it! Governance arrangements are both a central cause of why the global economic system fails and the greatest obstacle to overcome.

For centuries there have been individuals, organisations and networks working to address the social determinants of ill-health and to achieve better health care in many different settings and countries. Local, regional and national social movements have played and continue to play a critical role in creating the conditions for better health and for access to affordable decent health care. In the past, these were mostly local struggles addressing local factors, and the 'need' to become part of a global people's health movement was not so pressing. However, in this era of globalisation, the social and political pathways towards better health, decent health care and health equity are increasingly determined globally, nationally and locally. Even the most 'local' issue or struggle has at least some roots in the economic and political dynamics and the global policy-making processes.

Accordingly, the building of a global movement for *Health for All* has been a challenge for civil society activists. The most important movement to emerge in this century has been the People's Health Movement (PHM), which was formed at a People's Health Assembly (PHA) in December 2000 in Bangladesh.

History of the PHM

PHA 2000 was convened by eight global civil society networks concerned that the vision of '*Health for All* by the Year 2000'—promoted by the WHO during the 1980s and 1990s—had not been achieved, and that WHO in particular had progressively moved away from its strategy of comprehensive PHC aimed at achieving *Health for All*. PHA 2000 sought to highlight that the annual World Health Assembly (where ministers of health gather in Geneva as the governing body of the WHO) had become out of touch with people's health needs, hence the convening of a *people's* health assembly.

Prior to PHA 2000, a series of mobilising events were held across the world. The most dramatic of these was in India. For nearly nine months prior to the PHA, local and regional initiatives took place, including people's health enquiries and audits; health songs and popular theatre; sub-district and district level seminars; policy dialogues and translations into regional languages of national consensus documents on health; and campaigns challenging medical professionals and the health system to become more oriented to *Health for All*. Finally, over 2000 delegates travelled to Kolkata, most riding on five converging people's health trains, where they brought forth ideas from 17 state and 250 district conventions. After two days of simultaneous workshops, exhibitions, two public rallies for health and a myriad of cultural programmes, the assembly endorsed the Indian People's Health Charter. About 300 delegates then travelled to Bangladesh, mostly by bus, to attend PHA 2000. Similar preparatory initiatives, though less intense, took place in Bangladesh, Nepal, Sri Lanka, Cambodia, the Philippines, Japan and other parts of the world including Latin America, Europe, Africa and Australia.

Approximately 1500 participants from 92 countries (largely low- and middle-income countries) attended PHA 2000, which lasted five days. It included formal speeches, workshops, cultural programmes, exhibitions, films and testimonies. The programme encompassed the vast experiences of PHC since Alma-Ata; reviewed the impact of structural adjustment and World Bank policies on health; explored a wide range of social determinants of health; and shared the experiences of the wider social movement for health around the world.

The first PHA adopted the People's Charter for Health, which outlined the global health situation, identified the main barriers to *Health for All* and adopted a set of principles, priorities and strategies to guide the people's health social movement globally (People's Health Movement, 2000). The Charter (since translated into more than 40 languages) expressing the commitment of the PHM, has proved to be a powerful leadership document in the decades since December 2000. (See the People's Charter for Health at www.phmovement.org/en/resources/charters/peopleshealth.)

The second People's Health Assembly (PHA 2) followed in July 2005 in Cuenca, Ecuador, with 1492 participants from 80 countries. PHA 2 was organised around nine streams: issues of equity and people's health care; intercultural encounters on health; trade and health; health and the environment; gender, women and health sector reform; training and communicating for health; the right to *Health for All* in an inclusive society; health in people's hands; and PHM affairs.

PHA 3 took place in Cape Town, South Africa, in 2012. It was attended by 800 people from around 90 countries and celebrated the successes of a growing PHM, especially the development of new country circles in Africa. PHA 3 recognised the need to build a more effective and broad-based social movement. To this end, it committed—in a final document called *Cape Town Call to Action*—to building alliances with others who seek progressive and transformative change, including movements of informal and formal health sector workers, the landless, indigenous peoples, women and youth, and those struggling against big dams, nuclear power plants, dangerous mining and hazardous working conditions. Among other things, the *Cape Town Call to Action* also engages the PHM to communicate more broadly its alternative visions, analyses and discourses and to continue providing information and facilitating the sharing of information on the international context and country experiences.

PHA 4 returned to Bangladesh and was held in November 2018 (see Figure 7.13). The Assembly formulated a Declaration entitled *The Struggle for Health is the Struggle for a More Equitable, Just and Caring World* (People's Health Movement, 2018). It noted that the health crisis was a crisis of the capitalism model and called for an alternative organisation of society that would realise Equity, Ecological Sustainability and *Health for All*. It outlined six areas PHM would devote its struggle to health to:

- Gender, Justice and Health
- Environment and Eco-system Health
- Food and Food Sovereignty
- Trade and Health
- Equitable Health Systems
- War, Conflict, Occupation and Forced Migration

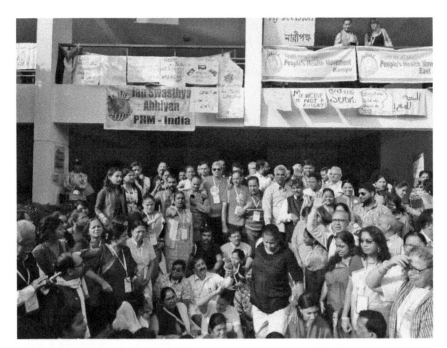

Fig. 7.13 PHA 4 in Bangladesh, 2018.
Source: Wim De Ceukelaire—Viva Salud.

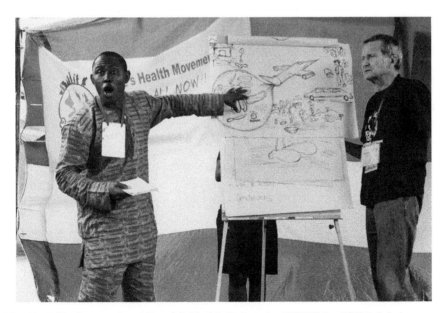

Fig. 7.14 The International People's Health University (IPHU) is a PHM global programme. Activists from different countries meet to exchange information and experiences about strategies in the struggle for health as a right of the people.
Source: Chiara Bodini—Viva Salud.

Details of the action PHM is committed to are detailed under each of these headings. Their scope illustrated the breadth of the PHM vision for health and the huge challenges in reversing the health harms of rampant capitalism. PHM also organises an International People's Health University (see Figure 7.14).

How PHM is organised

PHM as an organisation and the network includes:

- Country circles (core activists plus affiliated organisations).
- Affiliated organisations and networks (globally, regionally and nationally).
- Regional coordinating structures.
- Global structures: the Global Steering Council; Coordinating Commission (CoCo) (executive committee of the Steering Council); and Global Secretariat (the only paid staff of the PHM; its small number varies according to the needs and the available resources) (see Figure 7.15).

PHM Global is not a 'legal person' and does not receive monies or itself enter contracts directly. Since its formation in 2000, PHM has been supported by NGOs which are part of PHM, in most cases in the country where the Global Secretariat is based. These hosting organisations have managed incoming monies, banking, contracting, auditing and reporting. In some cases they have also provided additional administrative support for the Secretariat.

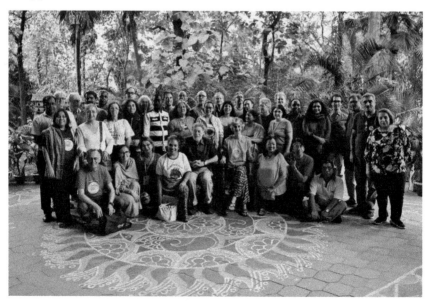

Fig. 7.15 Global Steering Council with representatives of country circles and representatives of the various networks and thematic groups.
Source: Viva Salud.

PHM is part of a much wider people's health movement, not always linked with PHM. This wider people's health movement can be defined as including all of those activists and organisations who are working in various ways to achieve the kinds of outcomes—all of which are essentially integral to health and social equity—that are described in the People's Charter for Health.

What PHM stands for

- **A life with security**: reclaims the security agenda by connecting it to employment, social protection, the environment and our safety and freedom.
- **Opportunities that are fair**: the demand for equal opportunities relates to how a fair taxation regime combined with higher social spending can level gross social inequities.
- **A planet that is habitable**: it is the ecology of the planet that will direct the radical politics of the future.
- **Governance that is just**: the space where states, markets and civil society attempt to manage the crises of capitalist modernity—addresses the issue of social rights and political participation to decide where public investment should be made. People can mobilise in anger for a time, but it takes a larger and more inclusive vision of how we might live to sustain organised movements that can take us forward from there.

Another simple statement of purpose is the vision from the People's Charter for Health, which commits activists to achieving equity, an ecologically sustainable development and peace—a world in which a healthy life for all is made a reality; a world that respects, appreciates and celebrates all life and diversity; a world that enables the flowering of people's talents and abilities to enrich each other; a world in which people's voices guide the decisions that shape our lives. There are more than enough resources to achieve this vision (People's Health Movement, 2000).

There is a further challenge: activists in the progressive health movement need to revalorise the role of the State for its regulatory and redistributive functions—a State that provides the goods and services essential to public health. As activists engage with this task, they need finally to reclaim the public space to fight for this. The world does not have a fiscal crisis. It is a crisis of inadequate taxation of those who are rich and the unaccountable power of corporate capital. We are not living in conditions of scarcity. We are living in conditions of inequality.

Since its formation, the PHM has been building a global social movement, through which global as well as local barriers to *Health for All* can be addressed. The vision of a 'global people's health movement' is not to be seen as aiming to co-opt the huge diversity of individuals, organisations and networks into a monolithic, centrally organised and centrally directed PHM. These individuals and organisations have their own history, commitments and identities, their diverse purposes and ways of working, and identities should not be compromised; indeed, this rich diversity is the strength of the movement.

What makes a movement work?

Important considerations for a global social movement for health are that it is not only 'what' a movement does that brings about change, but also the way we get there, how we get, stay and act together, and the kinds of organisations we build. This determines the nature and quality of what can be achieved. In other words, the process of building the movement through its day-to-day functioning, as well as its actions and ends, should be aimed at promoting health and well-being, starting with the grassroots of people active in the movement. A movement is made by people and can be described as a living system. We need to pay attention to the values, principles and practices that guide the behaviours and actions of the people in the movement, the quality of human relationships, and the way in which the movement responds, learns, grows and changes over time. Being a member of a people's movement means taking part in its coordinated global, regional, national and local actions and sharing the responsibility and ownership of these actions, including their impact on the movement. This implies a need to plan strategically so that the movement helps to build stronger links with existing organisations and networks that also want to strive for health equity. It also implies reaching into constituencies of people who are open to being inspired by a people's movement. Building the movement also involves working to create a shared culture that supports and spreads the values and aspirations of the movement.

Conclusion

In Chapter 6 it was argued that health care systems in high-income countries are dominated by the medical profession and business interests—in opposition to the people. Far from contributing to health, they assist in many ways in maintaining the system that perpetuates underdevelopment and ill-health.

This chapter has shown how the promotion of health is intimately related to the process of ending underdevelopment. This relationship is not confined to the economics—that is, the freeing of resources which are then available for the improvement of social conditions and thus health. It is most importantly a political relationship, for it is the political dimension—specifically popular pressure—that both is responsible for the reclaiming of resources in the first place and can ensure their direction to areas of pressing social and health need.

The COVID-19 pandemic has shown many times over the extent to which national responses reflect the political colour of the governments. Thus, the USA was slow to respond to the pandemic, and this slowness was influenced mostly by the desire to 'protect the economy', unlike the Cuban government which put 'people before profit'. Other governments (e.g. South Korea, New Zealand, Kerala State in India) have been successful at minimising responses to the virus by putting health considerations above those of the economy. This pandemic has also highlighted the importance of popular support for the actions of governments.

To change the nature of the medical contribution means creating a situation in which health care is no longer a commodity owned and purveyed by transnational corporations, doctors and other health workers. This can only be achieved by establishing an economic system that differs from the capitalist one, which is based on the generalised production and exchange of commodities for private profit. Indeed, it is only in those countries where the capitalist system has been overthrown and the economic system is oriented to social need rather than private profit that the medical contribution has changed fundamentally. Changes in the health sector and health outcomes follow rather than precede fundamental social change. While we have capitalism, greed, inequality and imperialism, the struggle for health will always be part of the struggle for a better world.

References

Acosta, L.F. (2017). Chronic non-communicable diseases remain the leading cause of death in Cuba Granma. http://en.granma.cu/cuba/2017-04-20/chronic-non-communicable-diseases-remain-the-leading-cause-of-death-in-cuba.

AKHS Kenya, Community Health Department. (n.d.). *Policy Brief No. 3, Best Practices in Community-Based Health Initiatives—Sustaining Community-Based Health Initiatives.* Community Health Department, Kenya.

Assefa, Y., Gelaw, Y.A., Hill, P.S., Taye, B.W. & Van Damme, W. (2019). Community health extension program of Ethiopia, 2003–2018: successes and challenges toward universal coverage for primary healthcare services. *Globalization and Health*, 15:24.

Banteyerga, H. (2011). Ethiopia's health extension program: improving health through community involvement. *MEDICC Review*, 13:46–49.

Baum, F., Popay, J., Delany-Crowe, T., et al. Punching above their weight: a network to understand broader determinants of increasing life expectancy. *International Journal for Equity in Health*, 17(1):117.

Bergues, L.C. (2021). In the face of attempts to defame Cuba and overshadow our achievements, we will defend the truth. http://en.granma.cu/mundo/2021-02-25/in-the-face-of-attempts-to-defame-cuba-and-overshadow-our-achievements-we-will-defend-the-truth.

Bodini, C. (ed.). (2020). Building a movement for health. People's Health Movement (PHM) and Viva Salud. https://issuu.com/m3m-g3w/docs/movement_building_en.

Burki, B. (2021). Behind Cuba's successful pandemic response. *The Lancet Infectious Diseases*, 21(4):465–466.

Che Guevara, E. (1969). *Reminiscences of the Cuban Revolutionary War*. Pelican: London.

Chen, C.C. & Bunge, F.M. (1989). *Medicine in Rural China: A Personal Account*. University of California Press: Berkeley.

Christian Medical Commission. (1974). *Health Care in China*. Christian Medical Commission: Geneva.

CIA. (2021). The World Factbook, Cuba—Central America. https://www.cia.gov/the-world-factbook/countries/cuba/.

Closser, S., Napier, H., Maes, K., et al. (2019). Does volunteer community health work empower women? Evidence from Ethiopia's Women's Development Army. *Health Policy and Planning*, 34:298–306.

Cooper, R.S., Kennelly, J.F. & Orduñez-Garcia, P. (2006). *Health in Cuba. International Journal of Epidemiology*, 35(4):817–824.

Devi, S. (2014). Cuba's economic reforms prompt debate about health care. *The Lancet*, 383(9914):294–295.

Geiger, H. (2013). Civil Rights History Project Interview completed by the Southern Oral History Program under contract to the Smithsonian Institution's National Museum of African American History & Culture and the Library of Congress. https://www.crmvet.org/nars/geiger_j.pdf.

Haines, A., Sanders, D., Lehmann, U., et al. (2007). Achieving child survival goals: potential contribution of community health workers. *The Lancet*, 369:2121–2131.

Horn, J.S. (1971). *Away with all Pests*. Monthly Review Press: New York, p. 125.

Horton, R. (2017). Medicine and Marx. *The Lancet*, 390(10107):2026.

Hosek, J.R. (2021). How Cuba is getting so much right on COVID-19. *The Conversation*. https://medicalxpress.com/news/2021-03-cuba-covid-.html#google_vignette.

ILO. (2012). *International Standard Classification of Occupations: Structure, group definitions and correspondence tables*. International Labour Office, Geneva.

Independent Panel for Pandemic Preparedness and Response. (2021). *COVID-19: Make it the Last Pandemic*. WHO, Geneva.

Jarvis, E. (2016). The pursuit of healthy China, 2020. *Asia Outlook*, 19. https://www.apacoutlookmag.com/industry-insights/article/538-the-pursuit-of-healthy-china-2020.

Javanparast, S., Baum, F., Labonté, R. & Sanders, D. (2011). Community health workers' perspectives on their contribution to rural health and well-being in Iran. *American Journal of Public Health*, 101:2287–2292.

Kark, S. & Kark, E. (1999). *Promoting Community Health: From Pholela to Jerusalem*. Witwatersrand University Press.

Keck, C.W. & Reed, G.A. (2012). The curious case of Cuba. *American Journal of Public Health*, 102(8): e13–e22.

Lehmann, U. & Sanders, D. (2007). *Community Health Workers: What Do We Know About Them?* WHO: Geneva.

Leon, N., Sanders, D., Van Damme, W., et al. (2015). The role of 'hidden' community volunteers in community-based health service delivery platforms: examples from sub-Saharan Africa. *Global Health Action*, 8:27214.

Li, J., Shi, L., Liang, H., et al. (2018). Urban–rural disparities in health care utilization among Chinese adults from 1993 to 2011. *BMC Health Services Research* 18(102).

Likun, P., Legge, D. & Stanton, P. (2013). The need for hospital management training in China. Wiley Online Library. https://doi.org/10.1177/103841110003800303.

Lu, C., Palazuelos, D., Luan, Y., et al. (2020). Development assistance for community health workers in 114 low- and middle-income countries, 2007–2017. *Bulletin of the World Health Organization*, 98(1):30–39.

Mangham-Jefferies, L., Pitt, C., Cousens, S., Mills, A. & Schellenberg, J. (2014). Cost-effectiveness of strategies to improve the utilization and provision of maternal and newborn health care in low-income and lower-middle-income countries: a systematic review. *BMC Pregnancy and Childbirth*, 14:243.

McNeil Jr., D.G. (2020). Inside China's all-out war on the coronavirus. *The New York Times*, 4 March 2020. https://www.nytimes.com/2020/03/04/health/coronavirus-china-aylward.html.

Mega, E.R. (2021). Can Cuba beat COVID with its homegrown vaccines? *Nature*, 29 April 2021. https://www.nature.com/articles/d41586-021-01126-4.

Mpulo, N. & Mafuma, T. (2020). COVID-19: community healthcare workers vital to SA's response. *Daily Maverick*, 21 April 2020. https://www.dailymaverick.co.za/article/2020-04-21-covid-19-community-healthcare-workers-vital-to-sas-response/.

Nandi, S. & Garg, S. (2017). Indigenous women's struggles to oppose state-sponsored deforestation in Chhattisgarh, India. *Gender & Development*, 25:387–403.

Nandi, S. & Schneider, H. (2014). Addressing the social determinants of health: a case study from the Mitanin (community health worker) programme in India. *Health Policy and Planning*, 29:ii71–ii81.

Navarro, V. (1972). Health, health services and health planning in Cuba. *International Journal of Health Services*, 2:403–404.

People's Health Movement. (2000). The People's Charter for Health. www.phmovement.org/en/resources/charters/peopleshealth.

People's Health Movement. (2012). Cape Town Call to Action. https://phm-na.org/2012/07/pha3-cape-town-call-to-action/.

People's Health Movement. (2018). Declaration of the 4th People's Health Assembly (PHA4). https://phmovement.org/declaration-pha4/.

Peretz, P.J., Islam, N. & Matiz, L.A. (2020). Community health workers and COVID-19—addressing social determinants of health in times of crisis and beyond. *New England Journal of Medicine*, 383:e108.

Rieger, M., Wagner, N., Mebratie, A., Alemu, G. & Bedi, A. (2019). The impact of the Ethiopian health extension program and health development army on maternal mortality: a synthetic control approach. *Social Science & Medicine*, 232:374–381.

Roser, M. & Ortiz-Ospina, E. (2021). Daily new confirmed COVID-19 cases per million people. OurWorldInData.org. https://ourworldindata.org/explorers/coronavirus-data-explorer?ysc ale=log&zoomtoselection=true&time=2020-03-01..latest&pickersort=asc&pickermetric= location&metric=confirmed+cases&interval=7-day+rolling+average&relative+to+populat ion=true&align+outbreaks=false&country=usa~gbr~chn.

Sanders, D. (1992). Health in Zimbabwe since independence: the potential & limits of health sector reform. *Critical Health*, 40:52–62.

Santana Espinosa, M.C., Esquivel Lauzurique, M., Herrera Alcázar, V.R., et al. (2018). Atención a la salud maternoinfantil en Cuba: logros y desafíos. *Revista Panamericana de Salud Publica*, 42:e27. http://iris.paho.org/xmlui/bitstream/handle/123456789/34931/v42supplcuba2018. pdf?sequence=1&isallowed=y.

Sidel, V. & Sidel, R. (1975). The health care delivery system of the People's Republic of China. In: Newell, K.W. (ed.). *Health by the People*. WHO: Geneva.

Sui, X., Reddy, P., Nyembezi, A. et al. (2019). Cuban medical training for South African students: a mixed methods study. *BMC Medical Education*, 19(1):216.

Tang, S., Meng, Q., Chen, L., Bekedam, H., Evans, T. & Whitehead, M. (2008). Health system reform in China 1: tackling the challenges to health equity in China. *The Lancet*, 372(9648):1493–1501.

The Lancet. (2019). Post-Castro Cuba: new constitution expands health rights. *The Lancet Editorial*, 393(10180):1477.

Vir, S., Kalita, A., Mondal, S. & Malik, R. (2014). Impact of community-based mitanin programme on undernutrition in rural Chhattisgarh State, India. *Food and Nutrition Bulletin*, 35:83–91.

Wang, L., Wang, Y., Jin, S., et al. (2008). Health system reform in China. Emergence and control of infectious diseases in China. *The Lancet*, 2(372):1598–605.

Warren, P. (2018). Julian Tudor Hart: visionary general practitioner who introduced the concept of the 'inverse care law'. *BMJ*, 362:k3052.

Werner, D. (1977). The village health worker—lackey or liberator? Politics of Health Knowledge Network. http://www.politicsofhealth.org/index.php?option=com_content&view=arti cle&id=81:lacky-liberator&catid=44:davidwerner&itemid=73.

WHO. (2008a). China's village doctors take great strides. *Bulletin of the World Health Organization*, 86(12):914–915.

WHO. (2008b). Cuba's primary health care revolution: 30 years on. *Bulletin of the World Health Organization*, 86(5):321–416.

WHO. (2016). *Community health workers: a strategy to ensure access to primary health care services*. WHO. Regional Office for the Eastern Mediterranean.

WHO. (2018). *Guideline on Health Policy and System Support to Optimize Community Health Worker Programmes*. http://apps.who.int/iris/bitstream/handle/10665/275474/9789241550 369-eng.pdf.

WHO. (2020). Report of the WHO-China Joint Mission on Coronavirus Disease 2019 (COVID-19). https://www.who.int/docs/default-source/coronaviruse/who-china-joint-mission-on-covid-19-final-report.pdf.

WHO. (2021). The Global Health Observatory. Cuba. https://www.who.int/data/gho/data/countries/country-details/gho/cuba?countryprofileid=acf51fec-7198-4457-b679-34e51 c9c0400.

Wilson, H. (2021). Cuba's COVID-19 containment vs. Pennysylvania's COVID-19 catastrophe. *Militant Journalism*. https://phillyliberationcenter.org/2021/03/09/cubas-covid-19-cont ainment-vs-pennsylvanias-covid-19-catastrophe/.

Wu, Q., Zhao, L. & Ye, X.C. (2016). Shortages of healthcare professionals in China. *BMJ*, 354: i4860.

Wylie, R. (ed.). (1972). *China, the Peasant Revolution*. WSCF: London.

Yaffe, H. (2020). Leading by example: Cuba in the COVID-19 pandemic. *Counterpunch*. https://www.counterpunch.org/2020/06/04/leading-by-example-cuba-in-the-covid-19-pandemic/.

You, D., Hug, L., Ejdemyr, S., et al. (2015). Global, regional, and national levels and trends in under-5 mortality between 1990 and 2015, with scenario-based projections to 2030: a systematic analysis by the UN Inter-agency Group for Child Mortality Estimation. *The Lancet*, 386:2275–2286.

Zhang, D. & Unshuld, P.U. (2008). China's barefoot doctor: past, present, and future. *The Lancet*, 372(9653):1865–1867.

Zhao, J.-S., Manno, D., Beaulieu, C. & Louise, P. (2015). Zhao 2005 IJSEM suppl Table. https://www.researchgate.net/publication/281442571_zhao_2005_ijsem_suppl_table.

Postscript
The Role of the Concerned Health Worker

David Sanders dedicated the first edition of *The Struggle for Health* "*to the children and their mothers living in poverty in Zimbabwe, who made me learn something about the struggle for health*".

For anyone who has finished reading this book, the importance of the knowledge that resides in the people and in communities will be clear. Health equity cannot be achieved without the actions of the people themselves. Concerned health workers can contribute to this struggle for health.

In Chapter 7, we touched briefly upon the example of Che Guevara, who joined the revolutionary struggle in Cuba in order to address the causes of health inequalities and social injustice in the country. Other doctors including Norman Bethune, Frantz Fanon, Lakshmi Sahgal, Nawal El Saadawi and many others have also chosen this path.

This is not the only option for the concerned health worker. Even Che Guevara acknowledged in a speech on 'Revolutionary Medicine' that, "*the doctor, in the function of soldier and revolutionary, should always be a doctor*". He went on to criticise the one-sided radicalism of the young revolutionaries: "*It seemed dishonorable to us to remain at the side of a wounded man or a sick one, and we looked for any way possible of grabbing a rifle and going to prove on the battlefront what we could do.*"

By 1960, circumstances had changed; Cuba had been liberated from the Batista dictatorship and imperialist domination. Che now called on health professionals to practise their craft side-by-side with the people:

We shall see that the doctor has to be a farmer also and plant new foods and sow, by example, the desire to consume new foods, to diversify the Cuban nutritional structure, which is so limited, so poor, in one of the richest countries in the world, agriculturally and potentially. We shall see, then, how we shall have to be, in these circumstances, a bit pedagogical—at times very pedagogical. It will be necessary to be politicians, too, and the first thing we will have to do is not to go to the people to offer them our wisdom. We must go, rather, to demonstrate that we are going to learn with the people, that together we are going to carry out that great and beautiful common experiment: the construction of a new Cuba.

There are many different ways in which doctors, nurses, psychologists, scholars, technicians, engineers, writers and intellectuals can contribute to the struggle for health—working with and learning from the families and communities whose struggle it is.

We can be modern Che Guevaras. Widening inequalities, the erosion of democracy and civil liberties, institutional racism and patriarchy are ingrained in our social and economic systems and are existential threats to health care and population health. They have to be addressed. We might not face the choice between the medicine pack and the ammunition box, but as 'a doctor is still a doctor' we can also contribute to transforming health care.

Community health workers can play a critical role as a link between the people and outside health professionals. Health activists can contribute to strengthening such community health worker programmes. Encouraging community engagement in the governance of Primary Health Care and working with the community to improve health care and population health are critical. In such partnerships, practitioners can learn to reflect on the norms of professionalism (and their links to the wider power structures) and can work towards demystifying medical knowledge and practice.

Even in more institutional settings, such as hospitals and universities, where working with the poorest and most disempowered people is more difficult, the same principles of democratisation and demystification apply. However, institutional hierarchies and culture can prevent individual practitioners from breaking through the norms of professionalism. This points to the importance of working collectively to challenge the prevailing power structures and working to decommodify and decolonise health care.

Climate change and pandemics—two of the most urgent health threats of our times—are threatening people's health on a global scale, as are the global inequities that have persisted beyond the colonial era. It is more necessary than ever to locate the struggle for health at the international as well as the community level.

David Sanders was involved in the struggle for health at all levels. He picked up the basics from the children and their mothers living in poverty in Zimbabwe, applied it to his work with communities in Southern Africa, while organising other intellectuals and health workers and building a global movement.

The Struggle for Health became his life. But the Struggle for Health is not an individual endeavour. It is a collective undertaking.

You can become part of it.

Wim De Ceukelaire

Glossary

Agribusiness: large-scale business that earns most or all of its revenue from agriculture, including from production, processing, manufacturing, packaging and distribution of products.

Autocracy: power concentrated in the hands of one person whose decisions are not subject to legal restraints or other regulations.

Average GDP per person or per capita: calculated by dividing the GDP by the total population. If, for example, two countries have the same GDP but one is twice as populated as the other, it will have a lower GDP per capita than the other country. In other words, the less-populated country is more productive.

Balance of payment (BOP): record of all the financial transactions between countries—for exports, imports, loans and investments.

Barefoot doctors: community health workers or assistant doctors, who were called 'barefoot doctors' because in many rural areas much agricultural work is done barefoot in the rice paddies.

Biomedical approach: assumes that the causes of disease and illness are wholly physical and biological in nature—that they occur when there is a deviation from the norm of measurable biological variables.

Burden of disease: a comprehensive measure of the health status of a nation attained by assessing the morbidity (diseases, injuries and impairments) and mortality (death) rate in a population in a certain period of time.

Cash-crop production: an agricultural crop that is grown for sale to make a profit, rather than used to feed the producer's own family or livestock. It includes, for example, plants grown for animal feed or biofuels, coffee, cocoa, tea, sugarcane, cotton and spices, as well as non-food crops like fresh-cut flowers.

Colonialism: domination of one people or power over other people or areas, usually with the aim of economic and political control. Generally, it involves the transfer of population to the new territory where they become settlers but remain loyal to their country of origin (adapted from *Stanford Encyclopedia of Philosophy*, 2017).

Commercial determinants of health (CDoH): factors that impact people's health that have been developed for financial gain, such as the marketing and promotion of harmful goods including unhealthy foods, tobacco, sugar-sweetened beverages and alcohol.

Commercialisation of health care: provision of health care goods and services to those who can afford it, to make a profit. It includes providing services through market relationships to those who can pay, an investment in those services to make a profit and a payment system based in individual payment or private insurance (Mackintosh, 2003).

Commodities derivatives market: a market that trades in the primary economic sector, e.g. in agricultural products (maize, wheat, soy, coffee, sugar, fruit) and mined commodities like gold and oil.

Compulsory licence: government forces a company that holds the patent to grant other companies a licence to manufacture their product (unlike a voluntary licence in which the patent holder chooses to negotiate with others or not).

Cost-effectiveness analysis: analysis focused only on certain easily measurable interventions and proposed limited 'packages' of mainly personal and preventative and personal curative care—reminiscent of Selective Primary Health Care (SPHC).

Cultural Revolution: revolutionary movement aimed at reducing disparities between resources in rural and urban areas and bridging the gap between intellectuals and workers, as well as between government and the people.

Decolonisation: the deconstruction and dismantling of colonisation.

Deforestation: the destruction of huge forests from an area of land.

Demographic transition: the change from high death rates matched by high birth rates; to low death rates with still high birth rates; then finally to low death rates with low birth rates.

Depression (economic): ongoing, long-term downturn in economic activity characterised by decreasing production and business activity, falling prices and unemployment.

Deregulation: the government reduces or removes restrictions or barriers (especially taxes on imports and exports) that prevent free trade between nations. In a free market economy, prices for goods and services are set freely by the forces of supply and demand, without intervention by government policy.

Derivative: a contract that derives its value from the performance of the underlying asset or commodity (e.g. crops).

Desertification: a process by which land becomes increasingly dry until almost no vegetation grows on it, making it a desert.

Disability-adjusted life years (DALYs): a summary measure that combines the following:

- YLD – years of healthy life lost due to time lived with disease or disability.
- YLL – years of healthy life lost due to premature death.

One DALY is generally thought of as one healthy year of life lost.

Disease mongering: the practice of turning ordinary conditions into medical problems, seeing mild symptoms as serious, treating personal problems as medical and seeing risks as diseases, in order to expand markets for treatment and new products.

Emerging markets: 'newly industrialised' countries which are rapidly developing economically due to growing their manufacturing capabilities and increasing their export trade.

Epidemiology: *"the study of the distribution and determinants of health-related states or events in specified populations, and the application of this study to the control of health problems"* (Last, J.M. (ed.) (2001). *Dictionary of Epidemiology*, 4th edn. Oxford University Press: New York, p. 61).

Equality: equal treatment and access to resources and opportunities, regardless of need or outcomes; based on sameness.

Equity: different treatment and access to resources and opportunities, recognising that disadvantaged groups might need more support or resources to achieve equal outcomes; based on fairness.

Equivalisation: process of accounting for the fact that households with many members are likely to need a higher income to achieve the same standard of living as households with fewer members.

Essential medicines: those medicines that satisfy the health care needs of the majority of the population. They should be available at all times in adequate amounts and in appropriate dosage forms, at an affordable price. The WHO develops and continually updates a 'model' essential medicines list. However, each country is encouraged to prepare their own list, taking local priorities into account.

Excess deaths: the number of deaths from all causes, in excess of what is normal for a country and time period, based on historic averages.

'Foetal origins' or Barker hypothesis: put forward in the early 1990s by epidemiologist David Barker, it shows a link between undernutrition in foetal life and early childhood and the propensity to develop obesity, cardiovascular disease, hypertension and adult-onset diabetes later in life when exposed to a calorie-rich environment (Edwards, 2017).

Food insecurity: people do not have access to sufficient, safe and nutritious food necessary to live a healthy and active life (FAO et al., 2020).

- **Severe food insecurity**: people have run out of food and have gone a day or a few days without eating (FAO et al., 2020).
- **Moderate food insecurity**: people are unsure about their ability to access food and are forced to compromise on the quality and/or quantity of food they consume (FAO et al., 2020).

Food security: food being physically available; people having economic and physical access to the food; using the food in a way that satisfies energy and nutrient intake; and food stability over time (FAO et al., 2020).

Fragile context: fragility is assessed along five dimensions which can affect all countries, not only those traditionally seen as 'fragile' or affected by conflict: violence, access to justice, accountable and inclusive institutions, economic inclusion and stability, and capacities to prevent and adapt to social, economic and environmental shocks and disasters (OECD, 2015).

Free competition: a system in which industries operate without much government regulation or control. Prices are determined by the relationship between the amount of goods for sale and the amount that people want to buy, i.e. supply and demand.

Futures contracts ('futures'): a forward contract or agreement to buy or sell something—a commodity like crops—in the future at a predetermined price agreed today.

Gender: "*socially constructed norms that impose and determine roles, relationships and positional power for all people across their lifetime. Gender interacts with sex, the biological and physical characteristics that define women, men and those with intersex identities*" (2020 Global Health 50/50 Report).

Gender-based violence (GBV)/violence against women and girls: any form of violence—physical, sexual, psychological harm and controlling behaviour—that is perpetrated against an individual because of their gender.

Genetically modified organism (GMO): "*an organism whose genome has been altered by the techniques of genetic engineering so that its DNA contains one or more genes not normally found there*" (dictionary.com).

Geopolitics: how geography, economics and demography influence the politics and foreign policies of states (Labonté & Sanders, Unpublished).

Germ theory of disease: the accepted scientific theory that micro-organisms or 'germs', which are too small to see without magnification, invade humans, other animals and other living hosts and can lead to disease.

Global health governance: "*actions and means adopted by a society to organise itself in the promotion and protection of the health of its population*" (Dodgson et al., 2002). It includes the political collaboration of different actors, across different levels (local, national and global), to develop and institute health policies and to resolve problems. It uses an infrastructure of global agreements and institutions.

Global private-public partnerships (GPPPs): a collaborative relationship between at least three parties, including one in the private for-profit sector and an intergovernmental organisation and perhaps a recipient government—which transcends national boundaries (Buse & Walt, 2000).

Global replacement fertility: "*The total fertility rate at which the population size stays constant. If there were no mortality in the female population until the end of the childbearing years, the replacement fertility would be exactly 2*" (Roser, 2014b).

Global warming: the effect of human activities, particularly the burning of fossil fuels (coal), that release heat-trapping greenhouse gases that profoundly affect our global climate system and cause the average temperature of the Earth to rise.

Great Leap Forward: an economic and social campaign aimed at transforming private and family-based farming into agricultural people's communes.

Gross domestic product (GDP): the total value of all the goods and services produced by all the citizens within a country's borders, usually in one year.

Gross national income (GNI) per capita: a country's final income in a year (before tax), divided by its population, reflected in US dollars. GNI is said to be a good reflection of the general standard of living enjoyed by the average citizen in a country.

Gross national product (GNP): the total value of goods and services produced by all citizens of a country, inside and outside its borders, in a year. Anything produced by foreign residents in the country's borders is excluded.

Health equity: those who have greater need get more services; the absence of systematic differences in health between different social groups in society; allowing all people to access the social, economic and political conditions they need to realise their fundamental human rights, including their right to health. The concept is built on the principles of social justice and fairness.

Health expenditure per capita: amount spent on health care per person per year calculated by dividing the total health expenditure by the number in the population.

Hidden hunger: experienced by a person who does not get enough essential vitamins and minerals (UNICEF et al., 2020).

Imperialism: "*comes from the Latin term* imperium, *meaning to command. Thus, the term imperialism draws attention to the way that one country exercises power over another, whether through settlement, sovereignty, or indirect mechanisms of control*" (*Stanford Encyclopedia of Philosophy*, 2017).

Individual responsibility: this replaces the concept of public goods and services—which are administered by the government and paid for collectively through taxation (WHO, 2015).

Individualism: to place the responsibility (and blame) for problems or conditions with the individual rather than with the structures that may influence or shape behaviour and experience.

Inequalities: unequal treatment or access to resources and opportunities.

Intellectual property rights (IPRs): "*those rights given to persons over the creations of their minds*" (WTO, 2006). This includes ideas and knowledge, products (such as medicines) and processes (such as a method of producing the chemical ingredients of a medicine). IPR includes copyright (the rights of authors of literary and artistic works) and industrial property (distinctive signs, e.g. trademarks, and other types of industrial property protected by patents).

Intersectionality: "*the interconnected nature of social categorization such as race, class and gender, regarded as creating overlapping and interdependent systems of discrimination or disadvantage*" (*Oxford English Dictionary*, 2015).

Intersectoral: collaboration between health and other government sectors to jointly improve the health of populations; there may also be partnerships with government, private and non-profit groups.

Kwashiorkor: a form of malnutrition which typically occurs in children in the one- to five-year age group.

Libertarian: a political philosophy and movement that upholds liberty, i.e. being free from control or oppressive restrictions imposed by authority, as a core principle.

Life expectancy: "*the number of years a person can expect to live*" (Roser et al., 2019).

Low birthweight (LBW): weight that is less than 2500 g in a live birth.

Marasmus: a form of malnutrition that typically occurs in children who are under one year. It leads to dehydration and weight loss, and may include chronic diarrhoea and stomach shrinkage.

Marketisation: introduction of competition into the public sector in areas previously governed through direct public control.

Maternal mortality: death of a woman during pregnancy, at delivery or soon after delivery.

Means of production: everything that is needed and used to produce goods and commodities, e.g. factories, equipment, materials.

Medicalise: treating a natural human condition as if it were a medical condition that needs intervention.

Merit award: a monetary award that can be given to a consultant for outstanding professional services.

Monoculture: a single crop is cultivated at a time over a wide area, again and again. This has an adverse impact on the environment as well as on agriculture.

Monopoly: a single seller controls the market and sets the price of goods because there is no competition.

Monopoly ownership: a group or person has complete ownership of the entire supply of goods or a service.

Morbidity: illness, a diseased state, disability or poor health.

Mortality: death.

Multilateral donors/organisations: wealthy donor nations that give aid to international aid agencies, such as the International Monetary Fund (IMF) and World Bank.

Multilateralism: alliances between multiple countries; intergovernmental platform.

Multinational corporations (MNCs): 'stateless companies' that operate, produce goods, deliver services or have investments in more than one country. Most are the result of mergers of companies based in different countries. They usually have management headquarters in one country (the home country) but operate in a variety of other countries (host countries), either in their own name or through subsidiaries (referred to as transnational corporations [TNCs]).

Neoliberalism: "*new political, economic and social arrangements within society that emphasize market relations, re-tasking the role of the state, and individual responsibility*" (Springer et al. 2016, in Labonté & Sanders, Unpublished).

New International Economic Order (NIEO): after the devastating effects of the global oil crisis in 1973 on underdeveloped countries, there was a call by non-aligned countries for a review of the existing Bretton Woods international economic system and a proposal for a new system that would empower underdeveloped countries to have more control over economic independence and political sovereignty (Gebremariam, 2017).

Non-aligned countries: a group of countries that do not want to be officially aligned with or against any major power bloc.

Non-communicable diseases (NCDs): non-infectious and non-transmissible conditions or diseases, such as heart attacks, stroke, cancer, chronic respiratory diseases, diabetes or a mental health condition (WHO, 2020b). NCDs may be chronic, i.e. of long duration and slow progression, or they may result in more rapid deaths.

Obesity: severe form of overweight (UNICEF et al., 2020).

Organisation for Economic Co-operation and Development (OECD): an intergovernmental economic organisation founded in 1960 to stimulate economic progress and world trade. Its 35 member countries have high-income economies and are regarded as developed countries.

Organization of the Petroleum Exporting Countries (OPEC): established in 1960 to unify and coordinate the petroleum policies of oil-rich nations.

Overweight: a person's weight is too high for their height (UNICEF et al., 2020).

Parallel importing: importing medicines from another country without the permission of the intellectual property (IP) owner.

Patented drugs: those drugs for which pharmaceutical companies have a formal licence which grants them exclusive ownership and IPR to ensure that the drugs cannot be copied by other companies for 20 years.

Plant breeding: the art and science of changing the genes of plants to determine the type of traits they have and to produce desired characteristics.

Population growth rate: the difference between birth rates and death rates.

Population pyramid: the age and gender structure of a country's population. It can be represented as a graph, with the population distributed along the horizontal axis, with males shown on the left and females on the right, represented as horizontal bars along the vertical axis. The youngest age groups are at the bottom and the oldest at the top. The shape of the population pyramid gradually evolves over time based on fertility, mortality and international migration trends.

Privatisation: a reduction in government spending and increase in private ownership.

Promotive health care: addresses the social determinants of ill-health through advocacy and lobbying government and policy-makers, for example to ban smoking in public places; intersectoral interventions directed at households or communities to improve water supply, sanitation, housing, etc.; and interventions that occur at the policy level, e.g. interventions to regulate alcohol or the food system.

Protein-energy malnutrition (PEM) or protein-energy undernutrition (PEU): a form of malnutrition that occurs due to a deficiency of protein and/or calories. It is likely to be due to malnutrition over a long period. It includes:

- **Wasting:** a child is too thin for their height. This is the result of sudden and quick weight loss or failure to gain weight. The child does not get enough calories from food and faces increased risk of death.
- **Stunting:** a child is too short for their age. This is the result of chronic or repeated undernutrition. The physical and cognitive effects can last a lifetime.
- **Underweight:** a child has low-weight-for-age. The child may be wasted, stunted or both.

Punching above its weight: better health than expected from the level of economic development.

Purchasing power parity (PPP): a measure that is used to compare the cost of living and inflation rates in different counties, by converting their currencies to a common currency—US dollars. This makes it possible to determine the quantity of the currency (in US dollars) that is needed in each country to buy the same common basket of goods and services.

Real wages: wages adjusted for inflation; or wages in terms of the amount of goods and services that can be bought.

Social determinants of health: *"The conditions in which people live and die, [which] are in turn shaped by political, social and economic forces"* (Marmot, 2005).

Social exclusion: Not having access to the same rights and privileges as the dominant social group, as a result of belonging to a minority social group.

Social medicine: based on an understanding that human health and disease are affected by social and biological factors; also incorporates preventive medicine.

Speculators: people or institutions whose objective is to make a profit based on the future difference in the prices of assets, rather than to invest in and add value to a commodity or asset.

Sub-prime loan: a type of loan offered at a rate above prime to individuals who do not qualify for prime rate loans—the interest rate that banks charge most credit-worthy customers.

Tariffs: taxes on imports and exports between independent nations.

Total fertility rate (TFR): the number of children born per woman.

Total health service expenditure: total amount of government and private money spent on health care in a given year; shown as a percentage of a country's GDP.

Transformative drugs or drug classes: those that are innovative and have groundbreaking effects on patient care.

Triple burden of malnutrition (TBM): simultaneous occurrence of undernutrition, hidden hunger and overweight and obesity in the same country, community, household or individual.

Under-five mortality rate (U5MR): the chances of a child dying before they reach the age of five years old.

Undernourished (hunger): a chronic condition that occurs when a person does not eat or absorb enough nutrients to grow (UNICEF, 2019).

Important terminology

In the 1950s and 1960s it was common to refer to countries as First World (liberal market economies, generally aligned with the USA), Second World (the Eastern bloc socialist states, aligned with the USSR) and Third World (the non-aligned often neocolonial countries).

From the late 1960s onwards, other terms were introduced, dividing countries as 'developed' (industrialised) and 'underdeveloped' (largely agrarian), the latter soon replaced with 'developing'. This categorisation reflects the idea that all countries should follow the economic model of the wealthier industrialised nations.

More recently, the World Bank developed a classification based on the economic aspect of 'development', where countries are grouped based on GNI per capita (low-income, lower-middle income, upper-middle income, high income).

In addition, the UN has a category for 'least developed countries' based, in part, on the lowest rankings in the UN Development Programme's Human Development Index, which includes health and education measures in addition to income.

(*Source*: Adapted from Ron Labonté and Arne Ruckett, *Health in a Globalising Era: Past Challenges, Future Prospects*, OUP, 2019.)

Index

For the benefit of digital users, indexed terms that span two pages (e.g. 52–53) may, on occasion, appear on only one of those pages.

Notes: Tables, figures, and boxes are indicated by *t*, *f*, and *b* following the page number *vs.* indicates a comparison